T0041612

HOMEMADE

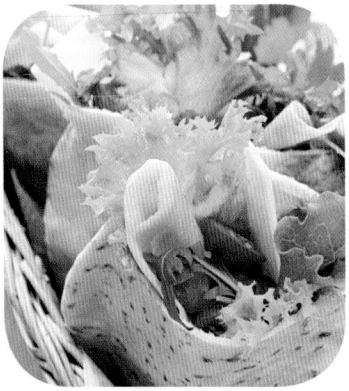
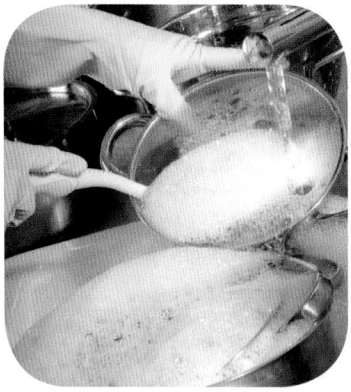
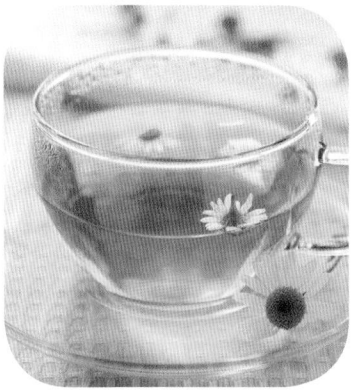
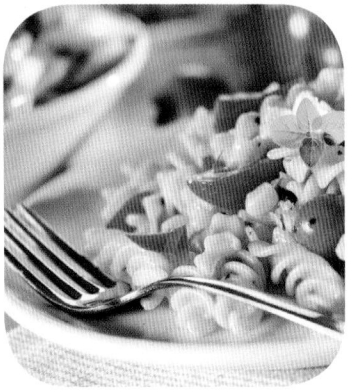
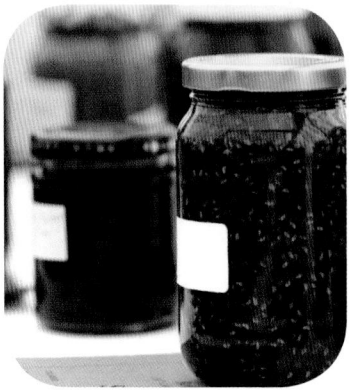
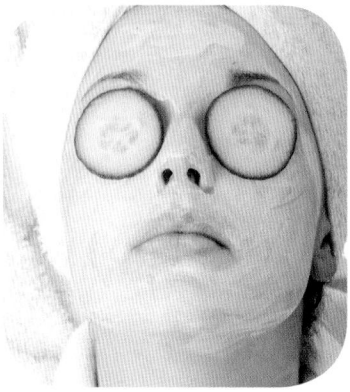
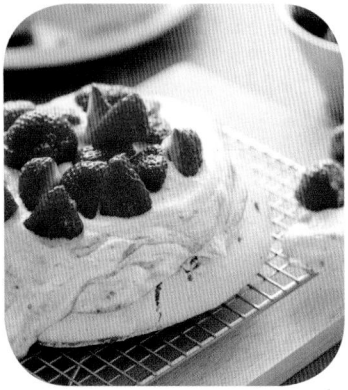
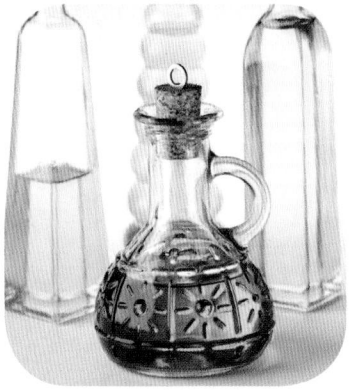
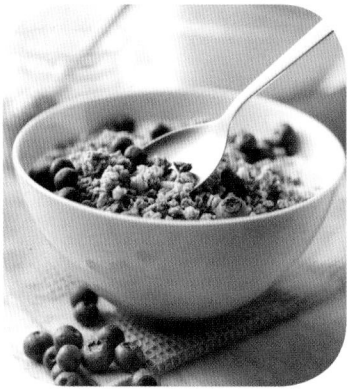
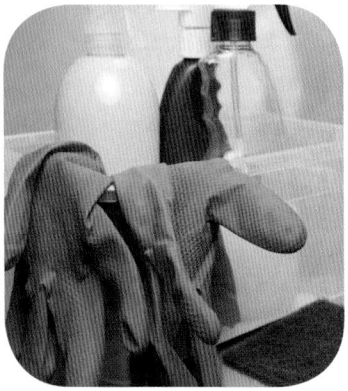
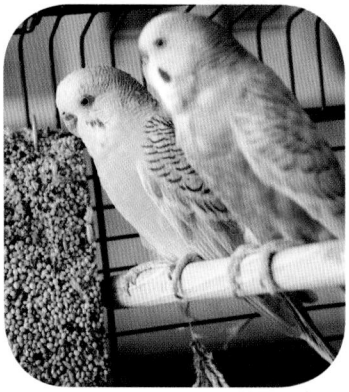
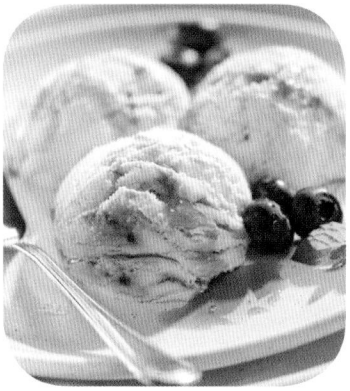

HOMEMADE

707 PRODUCTS TO MAKE YOURSELF TO SAVE MONEY AND THE EARTH!

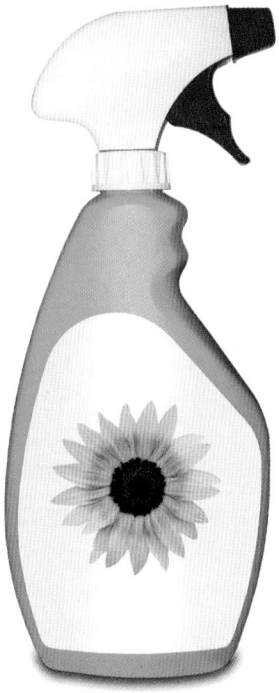

Reader's digest

New York, NY | Montreal

Copyright ©2017 by Trusted Media Brands, Inc.

All rights reserved. Unauthorized reproduction, in any manner, is prohibited.

Reader's Digest is a registered trademark of Trusted Media Brands, Inc.

ISBN 978-1-62145-380-2

Library of Congress catalogued the original edition of this book as follows:
Homemade : a surprisingly easy guide to making hundreds of
everyday products you would otherwise buy. -- 1st ed.
p. cm.
Includes index.
ISBN 0-7621-0753-7 (hardcover)
ISBN 978-0-7621-0904-3 (paperback)
1. Home economics. 2. Recipes. I. Earnest, Don, 1938- II.
Reader's Digest Association.
TX158.H625 2006 640--dc22
2006026506

We are committed to both the quality of our products and the service we provide to our customers. We value your comments, so please feel free to contact us.

Reader's Digest Adult Trade Books
44 South Broadway
White Plains, NY 10601

For more Reader's Digest products and information, visit our website:
www.rd.com (in the United States)
www.readersdigest.ca (in Canada)

Printed in China

10 9 8 7 6 5 4 3 2 1

Note to Readers
The information in this book has been carefully researched, and all efforts have been made to ensure its accuracy and safety. Trusted Media Brands, Inc., and the individual contributing consultant-writers do not assume any responsibility for any injuries suffered or damages or losses incurred as a result of following the instructions in this book. Before taking any action based on information in this book, study the information carefully and make sure that you understand it fully. Observe all warnings. Test any new or unusual repair or cleaning method before applying it broadly, or on a highly visible area or a valuable item. The mention of any brand or product in this book does not imply an endorsement. All prices and product names mentioned are subject to change and should be considered general examples rather than specific recommendations.

The Magic of Homemade

Many of us have a similar shopping ritual. Once a week we go to the supermarket, grab a cart, and load up with a box of this and a bottle or a carton of that. If you also add visits to your local convenience store for extra supplies, it s a whole lot of shopping—and spending—week after week after week.

But what do we get with all these packaged products? We get reliability and convenience, and we get choices—supermarket aisles are packed with mind-boggling variations of the same product. But that's not all we get. Many everyday food items are filled with unwanted chemicals and preservatives, and goods come with wasteful packaging. You also get to see your name-brand products on TV—but it's your money that pays for all those advertisements.

All of this is modern life, but when a window cleaner comes with "citrus orange" or "mountain berry" varieties, or a kitchen bench cleaner is produced in five different "natural fragrances" to try and get our attention, consumerism seems to be getting out of control.

You do, however, have options. You can make your own alternative versions of hundreds of items that you buy at the supermarket, and they will be cheaper, healthier and effective. That is exactly what *Homemade* is all about. In this book, you'll find more than 700 recipes for substitutes for the most common items bought in stores. And they are not just for food items. Beauty products, toiletries, pet supplies, cleaning and garden products and even everyday medicines can be made at home easily, quickly and effectively.

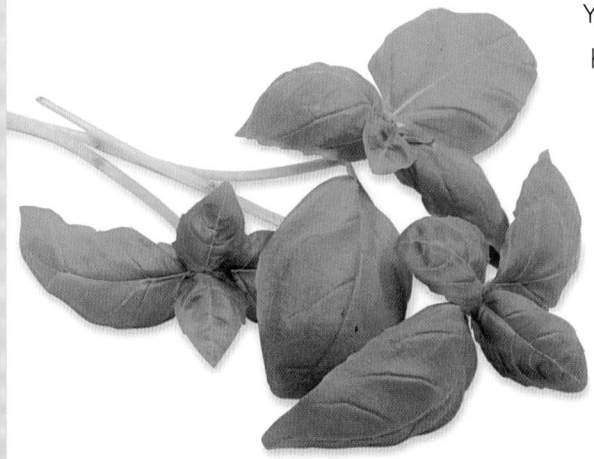

You will not only save a lot of money, but also have great fun and get a real sense of pride from making these easy and clever recipes. You'll love the quality, you'll love the savings and, most of all, you'll love the feeling of accomplishment.

The Editors
Reader's Digest

Contents

Introduction

8 The Joy of Homemade Living
10 The Rewards of Making It Yourself
12 Creating Your Own Food Products
15 Creating Health and Beauty Products
19 Making Products for the House and Garden

Part 1 22 In the Kitchen

24 Pantry Staples
26 Breakfast Cereals
28 Condiments and Spreads
34 Salad Dressings
41 Seasonings
47 Marinades
49 Cooking Stocks
52 Sauces
58 Dessert Sauces
61 Dry Mixes
62 Pasta

64 Pickled, Preserved and Frozen Foods
66 Pickles and Relishes
74 Chutneys
76 Jams, Jellies and Marmalades
85 Frozen Vegetables
88 Frozen Fruit

90 Baked Goods You Can Make
92 Quick Breads
99 Yeast Breads
107 Muffins
110 Rolls
116 Cakes
123 Pies and Meringues
128 Cookies, Slices and Brownies

134 Snacks, Nibbles and Drinks
136 Fast Foods and Snacks
139 Breakfast Treats
143 Appetizing Nibbles
150 Dips
154 Cold Drinks
160 Hot Drinks

164 Take-Out and Prepared Food
166 Deli-Style Dishes
176 Main-Dish Pies
179 Pasta Dishes
187 Soups
195 Salads

202 Easy-to-Make Sweet Treats
204 Candy
211 Custards, Mousses and Puddings
217 Fruit Desserts
220 Ice Cream
228 Frozen Yogurt
230 Ices, Granitas, Sherbets and Sorbets
235 Frozen Pops

Part 2 238 Health and Beauty Care

240 Your Own Beauty Products

242 Face Care
251 Care for Lips and Mouth
254 Shampoos, Conditioners and Rinses
257 Body Care Treatments
263 Bath Products
268 Nail, Hand and Foot Care
272 Just for Men

274 Healthy Home Remedies

276 Digestive Distress
279 Colds, Congestion and Fever
284 Bug Bites, Hives and Itching
288 Skin Outbreaks
291 Cuts, Bruises and Burns
295 Foot Care Products
297 Lips and Mouth
299 Dental Care
301 Joints and Muscles
304 Women's Problems
305 Headaches
307 Anxiety and Fatigue

310 Natural Pet Care Products

312 Dog Food
315 Dog Care Products
319 Cat Food
322 Cat Care Products
324 Treats for Birds
327 Food for Other Pets

Part 3 330 Around the House

332 Clever Solutions Cleaning Products

334 General Housecleaning
337 Air Fresheners
338 Furniture Polishes
339 Mold and Mildew Removers
340 Metal Polishes
342 In the Kitchen
345 In the Laundry
347 In the Bathroom
350 Cleaning the Car

352 Useful House and Garden Products

354 Household Compounds
358 Craft-Making Supplies
364 Household Pest Repellents
368 Garden Helpers
371 Garden Soil Care
374 Garden Pest Deterrents
382 Houseplants

386 Index

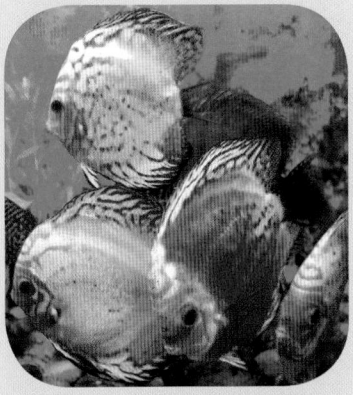

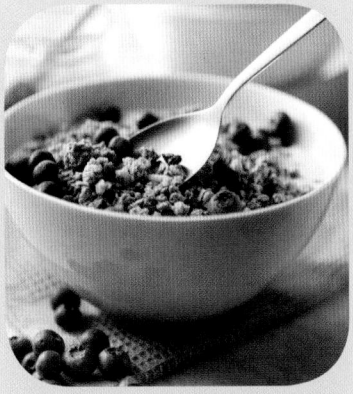

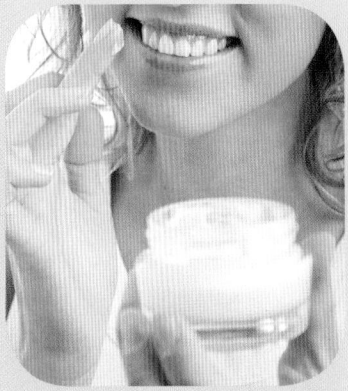

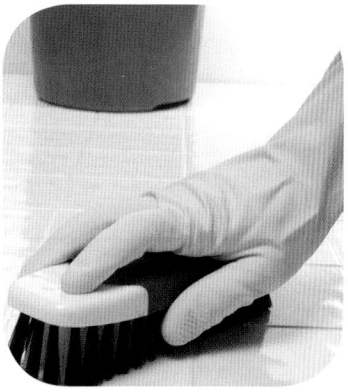
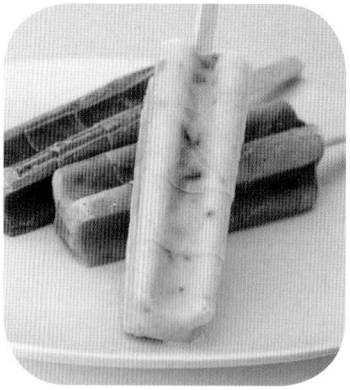
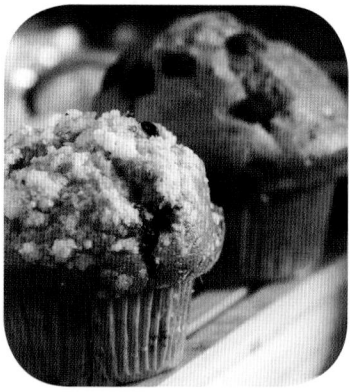
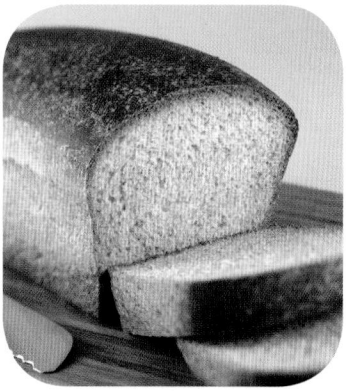
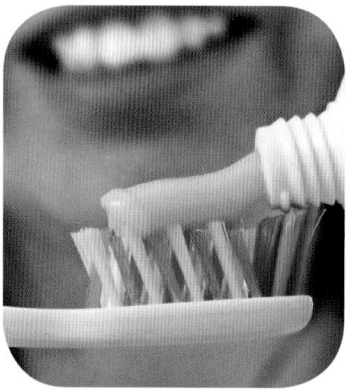
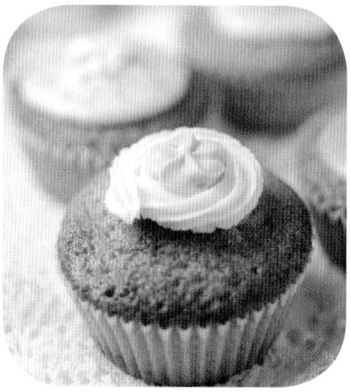
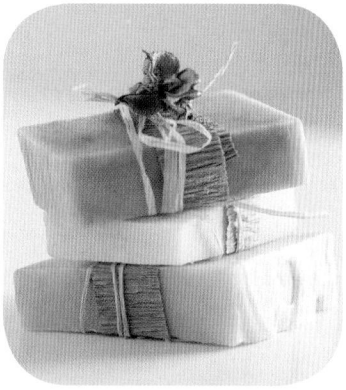
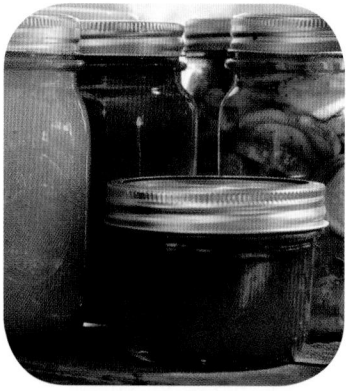
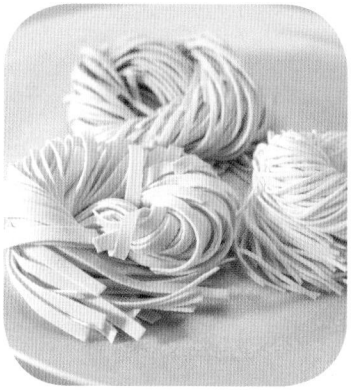
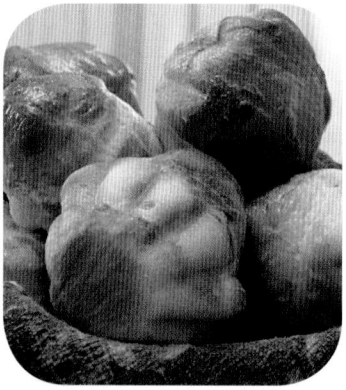
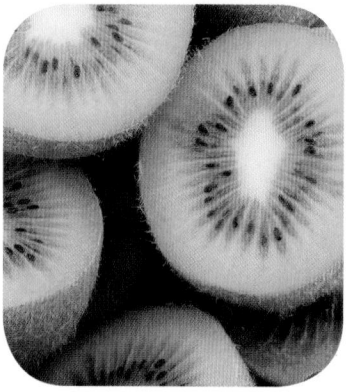
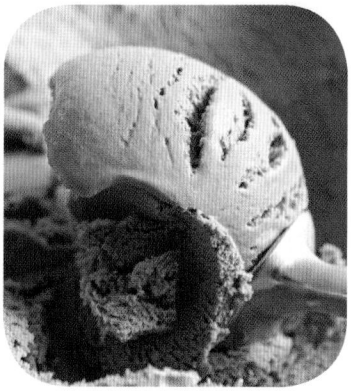

The Joy of Homemade Living

Picking up a bottle of shampoo or jar of mayonnaise at the supermarket is not that much trouble—and in the grand scheme of things neither seems particularly expensive. And if you are buying a name brand, you can feel relatively confident that you are getting products of reliably consistent quality that will do the job—a shampoo that cleans your hair with lots of bubbly lather or a condiment that will add a creamy tang to your sandwiches and salads. Multinational food and home products corporations are adept at putting out innocuous uniform products with a long shelf life and eye-pleasing packaging.

So why bother to make them yourself? There are many reasons that we'll explore on the following pages. The recipes that we provide are not "replication" recipes. We don't claim to have the formula for a famous brand cleanser or a secret herbs-and-spices mix. Our versions of everyday products won't smell or look like many of the name-brand products they are replacing. But rest assured that they work—and work terrifically well.

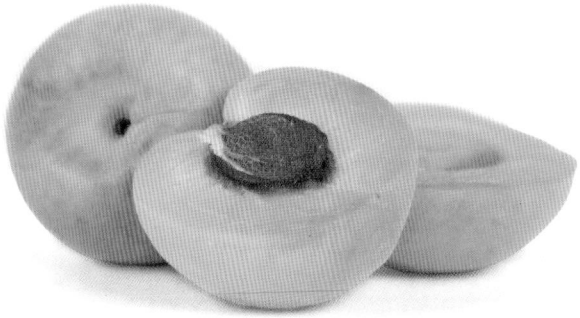

The Rewards of Making It Yourself

There are many good reasons and real, tangible benefits to making common household products yourself. In many cases, you'll find that the quality of the homemade product is superior to the equivalent store-bought item. You'll not only save money, but when you make something yourself, you know exactly what goes into it. You'll know for sure that it contains no questionable extenders, stabilizers or other artificial ingredients, and you can also adjust the recipe to meet your own needs or tastes. Not only that, when you make something yourself, you create a lot less waste, so you can feel good about doing your bit to help the environment. And ultimately, you gain a reward that can't be duplicated by anything that you buy—a great feeling of personal satisfaction that you actually made the product yourself.

Saving Money

Don't overlook the savings when you make something yourself, because the more you make, the more you save! Every time you buy a bottle of tomato sauce, a cream for an itch or liver treats for your dog, only a small percentage of the money goes to cover the cost of making the product. Indeed, if you leave out the cost of manufacturing, the ingredients in most products account for only a tiny fraction of the total. The rest covers the costs of advertising, packaging, shipping, overheads and the retailer's bottom line.

Healthier and More Natural

A commercial product may need to survive weeks or months from the time it is manufactured until it is finally picked up and used. Depending on the product, it could be pumped full of stabilizers, plasticizers, extenders, fillers and other chemicals. Some additives are there to facilitate the manufacturing process, making the product move faster, release from a mold easier or create less interference to the smooth flow of production. Other artificial ingredients are added to help the item withstand heat and cold and to be less likely to clump, precipitate or adhere to packaging.

Still other chemicals are used to cut the cost of using natural ingredients. Why use expensive, perishable, real strawberries when you can add a few pinches of a chemical compound that simulates their smell and taste? Most things that you make yourself are likely to be more natural and healthy for you than manufactured products—whether it's a food, a beauty product or a cleaning compound. And in the case of food, it's going to taste a lot fresher.

Suit Your Own Needs

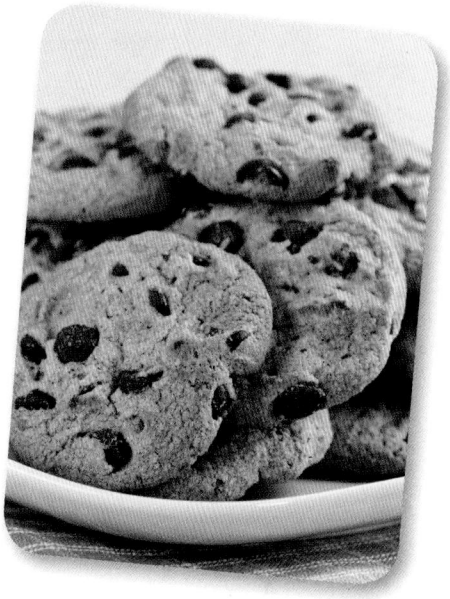

Another great advantage of making products yourself is that you can customize them to be just the way you want them. If you like your moisturizer to be fresh smelling and restorative without being greasy and overwhelmingly perfumy, it can be. If you like your chocolate cookies to be extra chocolatey, they can be. If you want your spaghetti sauce tangier, your soup thicker, your mustard spicier, or if the doctor told you to cut back on the salt or sugar, you can. Nearly all the recipes in this book are flexible and can be adjusted to suit you. Experiment until you get a product just the way you like it.

Make Less Waste

When making your own staples, you'll reduce the amount of waste and rubbish you produce. You won't be throwing away packaging and you'll be reusing jars, bottles and other containers. You'll also cut waste by making things in batches that you use up without throwing anything out if it goes bad. For cleaning, laundering and polishing, you will also be using compounds that are much gentler and less damaging to surfaces and fabrics—and to drains. So when you make it yourself, you'll be doing your bit for the environment.

Creating Your Own Food Products

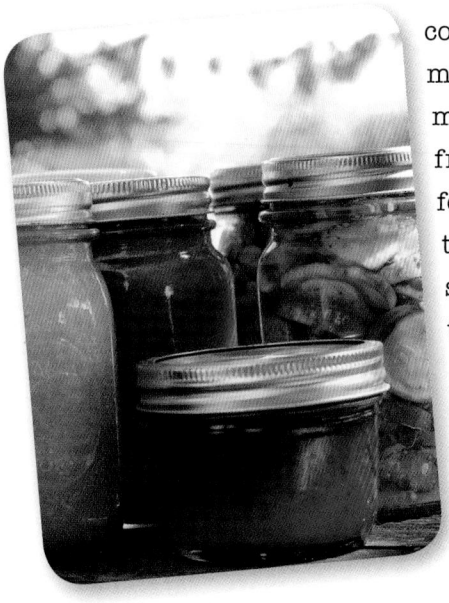

The recipes in Part 1 of this book cover some 350 commonly purchased food products that you can make in your own kitchen. There are recipes for making items to stock your pantry, refrigerator and freezer—or for creating fast on-the-spot replacements for such items. And there are recipes for many foods that you would normally buy already prepared—spending a great deal of money in the process. All told, they cover condiments, seasonings, sauces, pickled and preserved foods, baked goods, snack foods, drinks, take-out foods, candy, ice cream and other sweets. You don't need a large kitchen or a whole battery of equipment, but certain well-designed tools will make your work in the kitchen go faster and more smoothly. See page 14 for a listing of the pots, pans and other gear for food preparation and cooking that make life in the kitchen easier.

Before You Start ...

Take stock of your pots and pans. You want your pots and pans to conduct heat evenly, and you want at least one pan with a nonstick coating for low-fat cooking. Here are your choices:

- Cast-iron cookware heats slowly and evenly, but it is porous, absorbs flavors, and reacts badly to acidic foods.
- Enameled cast iron has all the advantages of cast iron, plus it is nonreactive, but it is heavy to lift.
- Aluminum cookware conducts heat well but reacts badly with acidic food.
- Anodized aluminum is heavier and less prone to warping. Its surface finish makes it less reactive than plain aluminum.
- Stainless steel metal pots are made of several metals fused together to take advantage of each one's properties—copper for even heat and stainless steel for easy cleaning, for example.
- Tin-lined copper pots cook as well as other pans but need to be polished and regularly retinned on the inside.

Check out your large appliances. Use an oven thermometer to check that your oven actually registers the heat it is set for. If it is only 5 to 10 degrees off, you can compensate by setting it higher or lower than the recipe requires. More than 10 degrees off, and it may need recalibrating. Check the temperatures of your freezer and refrigerator with a refrigerator thermometer. The freezer should read 0°F and the refrigerator 40°F.

Evaluate your freezer space. Making your own food is most efficient when you do it in batches large enough to last for a while. When you make a large pot of stock, for example, freeze some of it in ice cube trays and the rest in 1 cup (250 ml) or 2 cup (500 ml) containers. If you put the frozen stock cubes in a freezer bag, you will find it easy to add a little stock to a sauce or gravy to make it more flavorful. Save larger containers for making soups and stews that call for homemade stock. You also need space for containers of Savory Meat Mix (page 166), which gives you a head start on many fast dinners. Use plastic containers or heavy-duty plastic self-sealing bags. Extra pancakes, scones or muffins can also be frozen in freezer bags to make speedy breakfasts or snacks. Freezing the best seasonal produce at its peak will require room, too.

As a Precaution ...

- When bottling, sterilize jars and use only fresh seals.
- If you are worried about salmonella, cook eggs at 160°F for a minute or two to be safe.
- Label and date everything that you freeze or bottle.
- If anything has an "off" color or odor, discard it immediately.

When You Are Finished ...

Store leftover foods in covered containers or plastic bags and put in the refrigerator right away. Never leave cooked meat, poultry or fish at room temperature for more than 2 hours. Foods in a slow cooker are kept at 165°F, just hot enough to kill harmful bacteria.

A well-equipped kitchen

When making the food recipes in this book, you don't need any specialized kitchen equipment beyond what you would ordinarily use for preparing meals. Here is a list of recommended items.

Pots and Pans
10-inch frying pan or skillet with a tight-fitting lid
7-inch frying pan or skillet
3-quart saucepan with a tight-fitting lid
1-quart saucepan with a tight-fitting lid
4- to 5-quart Dutch oven or heavy casserole
4-gallon stockpot/pasta pot
Roasting pan, 13 x 9 x 2 inches with rack
Broiler pan with rack

Baking Equipment
2 baking sheets
1 jelly-roll pan
Loaf pan, 9 x 5 x 3 inches
1-quart microwave-safe casserole
2-quart microwave-safe casserole
3 nesting mixing bowls
2 six-cup muffin pans
8-inch or 9-inch cake pans
8-inch or 9-inch pie pans
2 wire cooling racks

Knives
8- to 10-inch chef's knife
2- to 4-inch paring knife
9- to 10-inch serrated bread knife
6-inch utility knife

Small Appliances
Blender or food processor
Coffee maker
Ice-cream maker (optional)
Microwave oven
Slow cooker
Waffle iron (optional)

Accessories
Bottle opener
Can opener
Candy thermometer
Citrus juicer
Colander
Corkscrew
Cutting board
Egg slicer
Expandable steamer
Flour sifter
Funnels
Grater
Kettle
Knife sharpener
Ladle
Long-handled spoon
Measuring cups
Measuring spoons
Pastry blender
Pepper grinder
Rolling pin
Rubber spatulas
Salad spinner
Scales
Sieves
Slotted spoon
Tongs
Vegetable peeler
Whisks
Wooden spoons

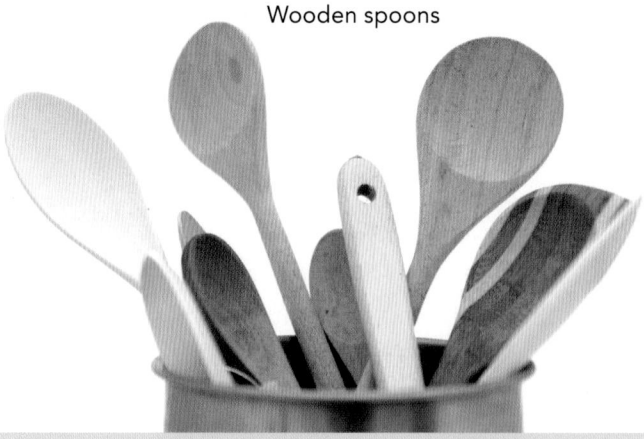

Creating Health and Beauty Products

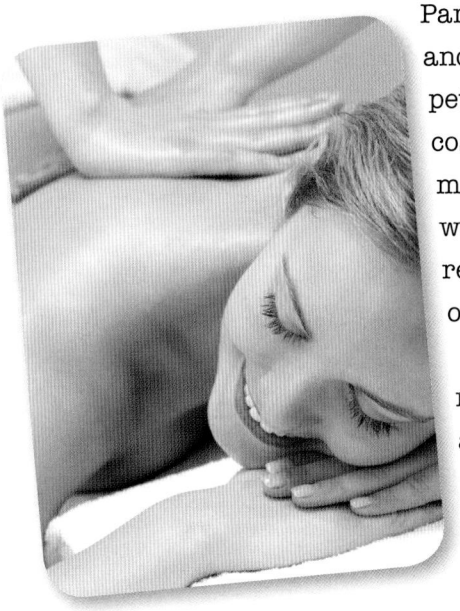

Part 2 of this book covers more than 200 homemade beauty and health products, and food and health products for your pets. You may at first be skeptical about making your own cosmetics or home remedies. Commercial over-the-counter medications and beauty products are expensive (and well advertised) and promise so much that you may feel reluctant to compete—or to compromise your skin, hair or health, or that of your pet.

You should have no such trepidations. Both home remedies and homemade beauty products have a long and honored tradition. In the case of homemade beauty products, it's best to start slowly—with a single moisturizer, for example, and see how it feels and smells on your skin. Try treating your hair after a shampoo with a vinegar hair rinse. Then try one of the facial masks and a toner. Little by little, you will be won over to using these fresh, natural products and want to make more and more of them on a regular basis.

Being able to create your own home remedies instantly is reassuring. You don't have to run to the drugstore or call the doctor every time you or another family member feels a little ill. In this book, you'll find more than 100 remedies for everyday ailments. Remember, however, that home remedies do not take the place of conventional medicine—they complement it. If you don't respond to a home remedy, see a doctor and let the doctor know how you have treated yourself.

Making your own pet supplies gives you control over the quality of the food and care that your animals receive. Making nontoxic flea dips and ear oils, for example, will keep your dogs and cats healthy and make them less dangerous to the people who pet them. Commercial flea collars are poisonous to people, too, remember.

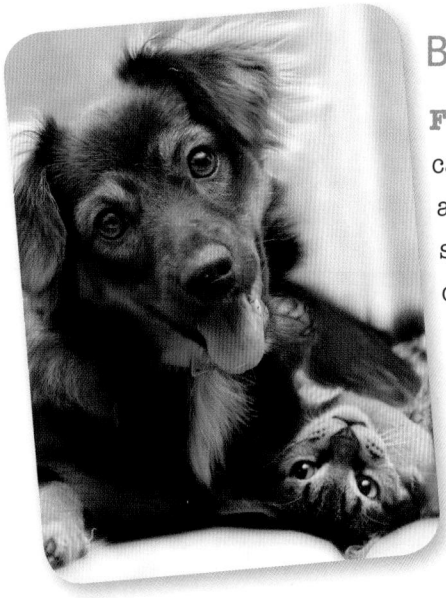

Before You Start ...

Follow the recipe closely. Read the recipes carefully and don't be tempted to use more of any ingredient than what is specified. Make sure you know the difference between regular oils and essential oils. Regular, or "fixed," oils, such as olive or canola oil, are the nonvolatile, mostly seed-derived oils that we use for cooking, while essential oils, such as geranium, lavender or lemon oils, are highly concentrated volatile distillations of leaves and flowers. They are called "essential" because they capture the essence of the plant. Most essential oils must be diluted in a fixed oil before they are applied to the skin. In this case, the fixed oil is known as a carrier oil. You need very little essential oil in each recipe—to conserve your supply, keep them in a cool, dark place but not in the refrigerator.

Source your ingredients. You can buy the ingredients for most home remedies and beauty products in health food stores, the supermarket, drugstores or online. Ideally, grow and dry your own herbs. You can buy seeds or seedlings for many fresh herbs at garden centers and nurseries; plant them in a sunny spot.

The ingredients for pet foods and care products are available in supermarkets, pet shops, health food stores or garden centers. None are particularly exotic or difficult to locate.

Take care with equipment. Although you use ordinary cookware to make home remedies or beauty products, it is best to keep this equipment separate from your regular kitchenware to avoid contaminating foodstuffs. A list of the items you may need is provided in the table opposite. Making pet products doesn't involve any special equipment other than what you probably already have in your kitchen.

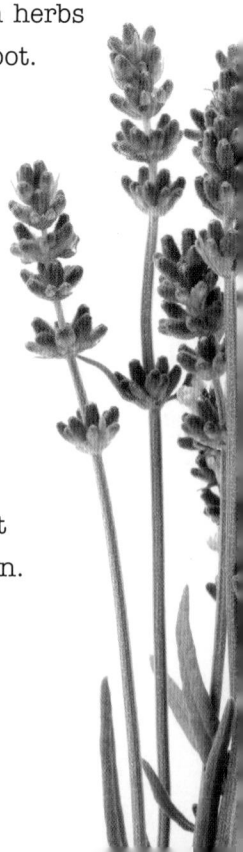

Equipment for home remedies and beauty products

To make either beauty or health products:
You will need nonreactive equipment to protect your health or beauty products from chemical changes in color and odor. That means avoiding uncoated aluminum, iron or copper cookware.

- Glass, stainless steel or enameled double boiler
- Set of nonreactive mixing bowls
- Stainless steel or ceramic funnel
- Stainless steel measuring and stirring spoons
- Wooden stirring and mashing spoons
- Stainless steel or ceramic lemon squeezer
- Kettle
- Ceramic tea bowls and cups
- Tea strainer
- Candy thermometer

Select safe storage jars and dispensers. Look for small opaque jars with wide mouths and tight-fitting lids for storing your beauty creams or skin ointments. Because they have no preservatives, they need to be kept away from light and air. Tinted or colored glass—amber, white or blue—protects creams from light. Keeping a cream in a small container that it fills almost completely protects the cream from air. When you use up half a jar of cream, decant the remaining cream into a smaller jar to protect it further. Tight-fitting lids are important to keep out air and prevent evaporation. Cork lids are too porous to be safe.

You'll also need spray bottles and pint-sized (500 ml) bottles with tight lids. You can reuse many of the jars you need from your regular kitchen and bathroom supplies. Sterilize any storage jars before you use them. Wash plastic spray bottles thoroughly in soap and hot water, rinse thoroughly, and let them air-dry.

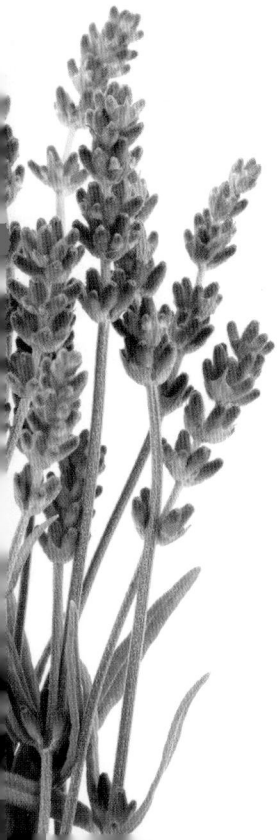

As a Precaution ...

- If you are taking prescription medication, talk to your doctor about possible interactions between it and any herbs or essential oils suggested in this book.
- If you have allergic reactions to any foods or medications, consult your doctor before taking any home remedy that might contain the allergen.

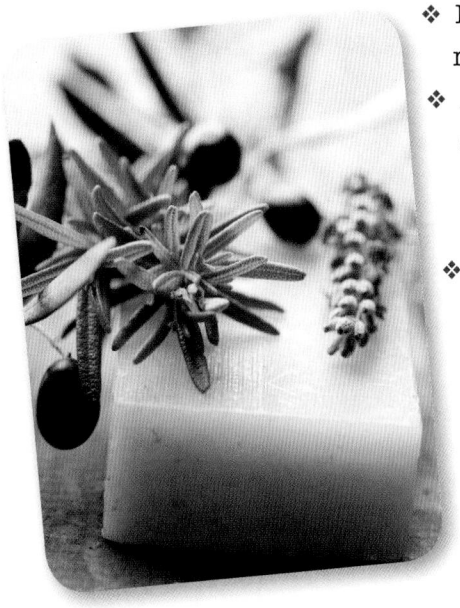

- If you are pregnant, don't take any herbal medications without consulting your doctor.
- Although side effects from using natural cosmetics are uncommon, allergic reactions can occur in susceptible people. If you have a reaction, stop using the product immediately.
- When planning to use an herb or product that is new to you, patch-test it first. Rub the herb against the tender skin on the underside of your arm right above the elbow or in the elbow crease. Wait overnight. If redness or irritation occurs, don't use it.
- Check with a doctor before using products with essential oils if you have a chronic or acute disorder such as heart disease, epilepsy, asthma, diabetes or kidney disease, or if you are pregnant. Keep containers sealed and out of reach of children.
- If an essential oil is accidentally swallowed, do not induce vomiting. Call a poison hotline or get the person to an emergency room immediately.

When You Are Finished ...

Be sure to label each new jar or bottle of a product as you fill it. Write the product's name and the date of preparation. If you give a homemade beauty product as a gift, list its ingredients as well (you don't want to inadvertently cause an allergic reaction).

Store natural products in a cool, dark, dry place, and check them often. Heat, moisture, light and contact with air can all cause deterioration. In summer, the refrigerator is probably the safest place to store homemade beauty products (away from young children). Inspect them regularly to be sure that they have not lost their potency. If a product is discolored or has a funny smell, discard it and make a new batch.

Making Products for the House and Garden

Part 3 of this book covers more than 100 useful household and gardening products—including cleaning and polishing compounds, glue and craft supplies, pest repellents, weed killers, fertilizers and soil conditioners—even houseplant food and whitewash. Having simple, nontoxic aids and remedies for house and garden makes maintenance chores more pleasant and much cheaper.

Whether you are dealing with a cleanser, a polish, a bleach, a weed spray or an insecticide, some commercial products may contain harsh and toxic chemicals that are hard on grime, tarnish, stains and bugs, but that are also hard on furniture, floors, clothes, shrubs—and on your skin, eyes and lungs.

The good news is that there are many inexpensive, time-proven products that will help your garden to flourish and your house to sparkle, smell good and gleam invitingly without such effects. You probably already have most of the ingredients for these homemade products on hand. Try making one of the cleaning recipes and using it. It won't take long or cost much money. Expect to be happily surprised.

Once you discover that there are easy, inexpensive ways to foil the pests that have plagued your woolens in the past, you won't find putting away winter clothes so onerous. Keeping ants and cockroaches out of the cupboards is not a problem either when you get out the borax.

And as you find inexpensive, nontoxic ways to keep pests out of the garden, you may finally be able to grow the herbs and vegetables that you have dreamed about.

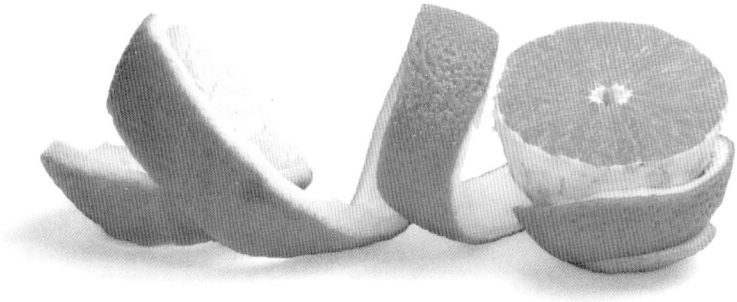

Before You Start ...

Find your ingredients. None of the ingredients required is particularly exotic. If you don't already have them at home, you can buy most of them at your supermarket or hardware store.

- Get the largest, cheapest sizes of baking soda, cider vinegar and white vinegar available. You don't need giant sizes of chlorine bleach or ammonia, however, because the recipes that do use them call for very little of either.
- You'll find borax and washing soda among the detergents in a supermarket.
- Look for castile soap, glycerine and essential oils at health food stores and on many Internet sites.
- Inexpensive house brands of rubbing alcohol are readily available from any supermarket.
- Boiled linseed oil and materials needed for paints and finishes are available at paint, art supply or hardware stores. You can find equipment and wax for candle-making at craft stores.
- Pure soap flakes can be found in the supermarket or you can make your own by lightly grating a bar of pure soap on a coarse grater.

Make garden potting easier. For mixing soil and making compost tea, you can use plastic trash cans or find large buckets at cleaning supply stores. If you have unusually clayey, sandy or other problematic soil, test the soil before adjusting it with homemade nutrients. To get your soil tested, ask at your local garden center or look on the Internet for a service in your area.

Devise a potting table—a place to take care of your container plants, and where you can keep extra pots, homemade fertilizers and pesticides, potting soil and other supplies. The table should be waist high and have shelves above for storing fertilizers and pesticides out of reach of children, and shelves below for large containers of compost, vermiculite or sand. You can make your gardening workstation in the garage or on a covered porch.

As a Precaution ...

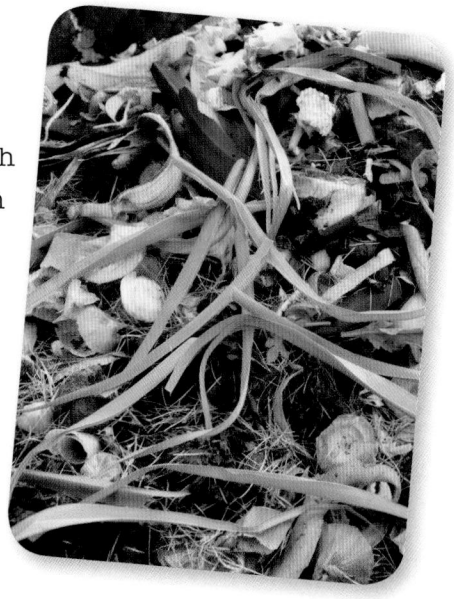

- Never combine chlorine bleach and ammonia. They can form a noxious gas if mixed.
- Label cleaning compounds, pesticides, compost teas and other fertilizers, and keep the containers out of reach of children.
- Wear appropriate vinyl gloves to protect your hands when mixing and using household and gardening products.
- If an essential oil is accidentally swallowed, don't induce vomiting. Call a poison hotline or rush the patient to an emergency room.

When You Are Finished ...

Most of the household and gardening products in this book are best prepared just before you use them so that you get the maximum potency and best results. Most are simple enough to whip up in a few minutes. But as the recipes advise, you can store some products, such as scouring powders and some cleaning and bug-control compounds, for periods ranging from a few days up to a couple of weeks. When you do, be sure to put them in tightly closed labeled and dated jars or spray bottles.

Recycle rags and spray bottles

There are many simple ways to keep down the cost of household supplies:

- One is to recycle worn or outgrown family clothing as rags for cleaning, polishing and crafts. Cloth diapers make famously good rags. Old cotton T-shirts and underpants are also good candidates. Well-worn terrycloth towels absorb water better than anything. Best of all, they can be tossed in the washing machine and reused.
- Also, finish cleaning windows with old newspaper. It's not only cheaper but gives a better result, so you may never buy paper towels again (at least for cleaning) or expensive disposable cloths.
- Wash out old empty spray bottles and reuse them for your homemade household or gardening products. (If you do need to buy some, try a garden center or a cleaning supply store; they are listed in the phone book and online.)

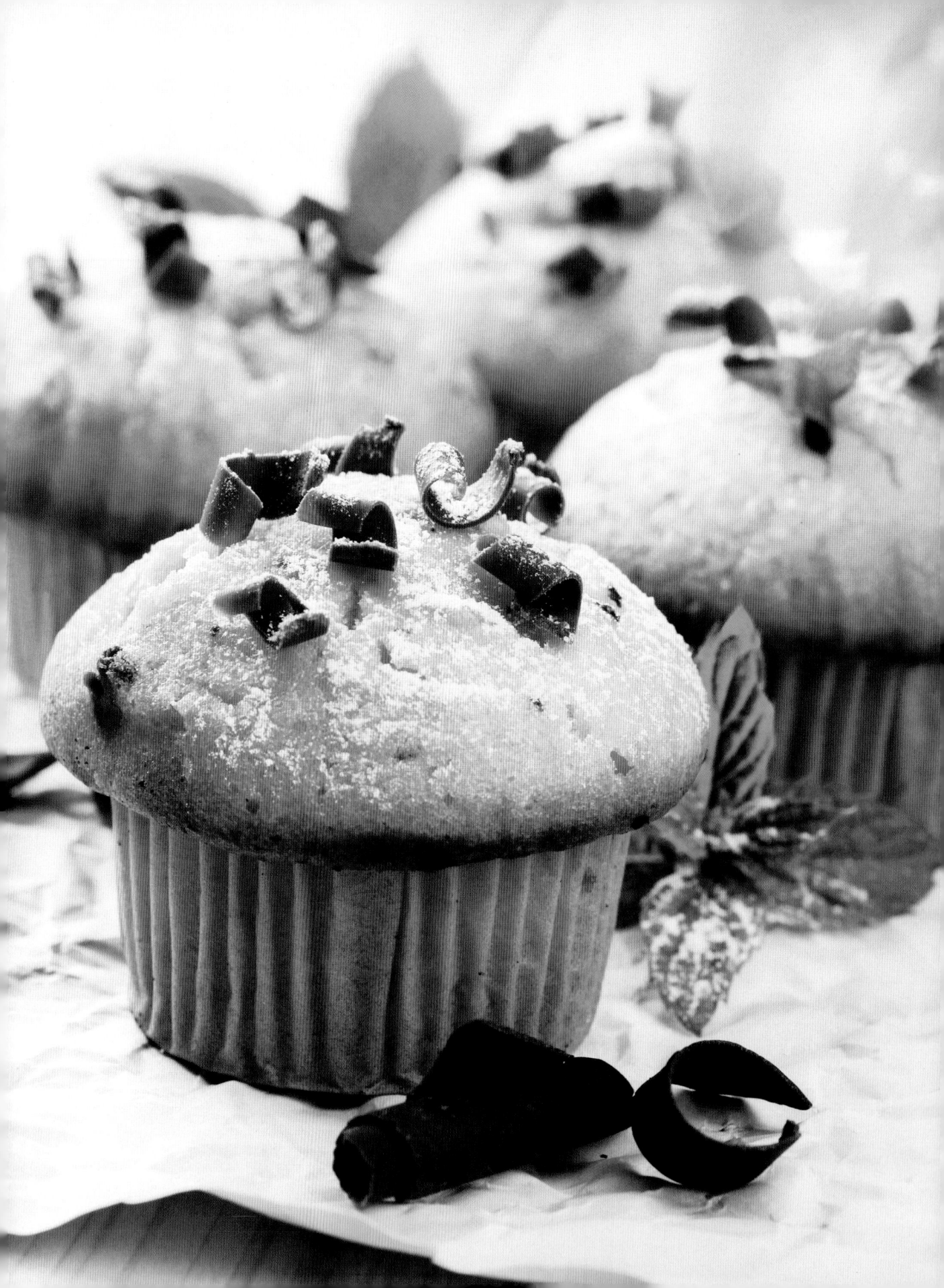

Part 1

In the Kitchen

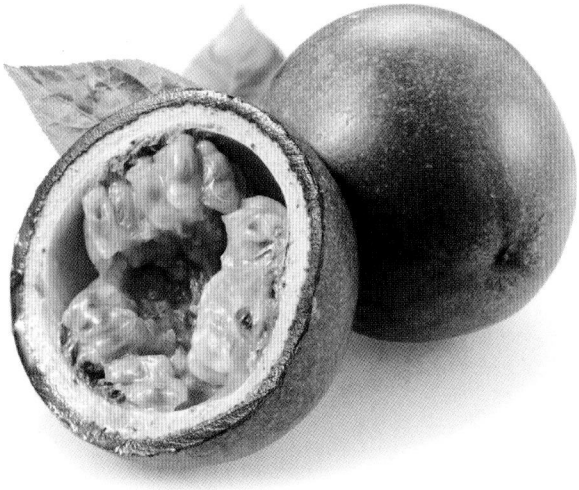

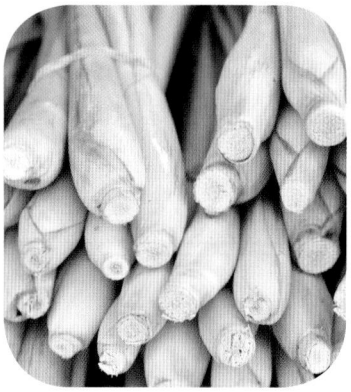

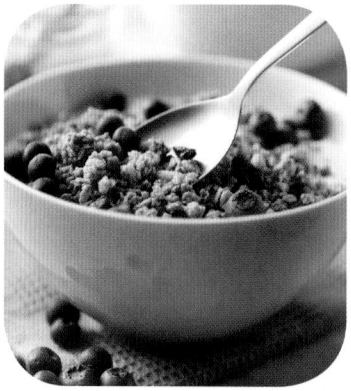

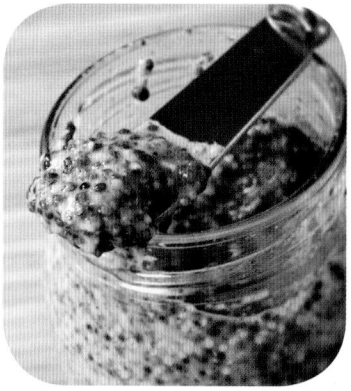

Breakfast Cereals

Muesli ❖ Fruit and Nut Cereal ❖ Granola ❖ Oatmeal Mix

Condiments and Spreads

Ketchup ❖ Seafood Cocktail Sauce ❖ Mustard ❖ Classic Mayonnaise ❖ Aioli (Garlic Mayonnaise) ❖ Tartar Sauce ❖ Spicy Tomato Salsa ❖ Salsa Verde ❖ Sweet Chili Sauce ❖ Peanut Butter

Salad Dressings

Classic Vinaigrette ❖ Herb Vinaigrette ❖ Walnut Vinaigrette ❖ Garlic Vinaigrette ❖ Balsamic Vinaigrette ❖ Raspberry Vinaigrette ❖ Herb Dressing Mix ❖ Herb Dressing ❖ Thai Salad Dressing ❖ Ranch Dressing Mix ❖ Ranch Dressing ❖ Blue Cheese Dressing ❖ Light Blue Cheese Dressing ❖ French Dressing ❖ Italian Dressing ❖ Thousand Island Dressing

Seasonings

Bouquet Garni ❖ Fines Herbes ❖ Herbes de Provence ❖ Italian Herb Blend ❖ Chicken Seasoning Mix ❖ Chili Powder ❖ Cajun Seasoning Mix ❖ Laksa Paste ❖ Chermoula ❖ Caribbean Spicy Meat Rub ❖ Curry Powder ❖ Green Curry Paste ❖ Red Curry Paste

Marinades

Red Wine Marinade ❖ Mustard Marinade ❖ Lemon Herb Marinade ❖ Orange Ginger Marinade ❖ Soy and Sesame Marinade

Cooking Stocks

Beef Stock ❖ Chicken Stock ❖ Fish Stock ❖ Vegetable Stock

Sauces

Barbecue Sauce ❖ Gravy ❖ Plum Sauce ❖ Sweet and Sour Sauce ❖ Mushroom Wine Sauce ❖ Béarnaise Sauce ❖ Tomato Sauce ❖ Satay Sauce ❖ Hollandaise Sauce ❖ Basic White Sauce ❖ Cheese Sauce ❖ Dijon Mustard Sauce ❖ Mushroom Sauce

Dessert Sauces

Blueberry Syrup ❖ Applesauce ❖ Mango and Passion Fruit Sauce ❖ Raspberry Sauce ❖ Custard ❖ Fruit Coulis ❖ Butterscotch Sauce ❖ Chocolate Sauce ❖ Caramel Sauce

Dry Mixes

Pancake and Waffle Mix ❖ Basic Cake Mix

Pasta

Simple Fresh Pasta ❖ Luxury Fresh Pasta ❖ Superfast Fresh Pasta

Pantry Staples

Nowhere do the benefits of making your own pay off more generously than in the kitchen, especially in making replacements for the cereals, condiments, salad dressings, seasonings, sauces and mixes that line your pantry shelves.

To give them an almost indefinite shelf life, these manufactured staples are more likely than any other food products to be packed with fillers, preservatives, stabilizers and other unnatural ingredients. In this chapter, you will not only learn how easy it is to make your own all-natural versions of these staples but also discover how much better a homemade creation tastes.

Homemade stock has real flavor. And there is nothing like freshly ground peanut butter that melts in your mouth or fresh pasta so delectably light that it makes any sauce seem tastier.

None of the staple items here have the extraordinary shelf life of manufactured products. But you will find healthy, nutty breakfast cereals that will keep their fresh taste for weeks, as well as everyday condiments, ranging from peanut butter and mustard that will last for months to fresh salsas that are best eaten in a day or two. Most salad dressings and both savory and sweet sauces are also best if used right away—keep them in the fridge for a couple of days—and there are salad dressing mixes you can prepare ahead of time.

Most herbs, seasonings and dry mixes will keep for weeks or months, as will fresh pasta and stocks if frozen.

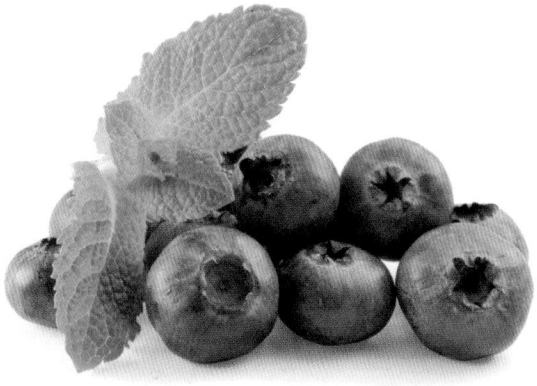

Breakfast Cereals

Muesli

2 cups (200 g) rolled oats
¼ cup (30 g) sunflower seeds
¼ cup (25 g) flaked almonds
¼ cup (25 g) wheat germ
⅓ cup (55 g) finely chopped dates
2 tablespoons oat bran
1 cup (40 g) wheat bran flakes
¼ cup (30 g) raisins
1 tablespoon sugar (optional)

Makes 3½ cups
(about 7 servings)

This traditional cereal is full of healthy grains, seeds, nuts and fruit, plus it's dry-roasted without oil so it will stay fresh for longer. Packaged versions are quite pricey and not nearly as tasty.

1 Preheat the oven to 350°F. In a 15 x 10-inch baking pan, combine the oats, sunflower seeds and almonds. Bake for 10 to 15 minutes, until the almonds are almost golden. Remove the toasted mix to a separate bowl. Add the wheat germ to the baking pan and bake for 5 minutes, making sure it doesn't burn.
2 In a large bowl, combine the dates and oat bran, and stir to coat the dates with the bran. Add the toasted oats mixture and wheat germ, then add the wheat bran flakes, raisins and sugar, if using. Stir to combine all the ingredients.
3 Place the muesli in an airtight container or a self-sealing plastic bag. Label, date and store in a cool, dry place for up to 2 months.

Fruit and Nut Cereal

2 cups (200 g) instant oats
1 cup (50 g) wheat flakes
1 cup (75 g) wheat bran or bran cereal
1 cup (90 g) wheat germ
1 cup (100–150 g) unsalted walnuts, almonds, pecans or cashew nuts
½ cup (80 g) chopped pitted dates
1 cup (175 g) chopped dried prunes, apricots, pears, apples or bananas
1 cup (125 g) raisins
1 cup (100 g) skim powdered milk

Makes about 9 cups
(about 18 servings)

Packed with protein and high in complex carbohydrates, this tasty mix will keep you full until lunchtime.

1 In a large bowl, combine the oats, wheat flakes, wheat bran, wheat germ and nuts. Add the dates and dried fruit, then toss to combine the ingredients and coat the fruit with the oat mixture. Add the raisins and powdered milk, then stir to combine all the ingredients.
2 Place the cereal in an airtight container or self-sealing plastic bag. Label, date and store for up to 2 months in the refrigerator.

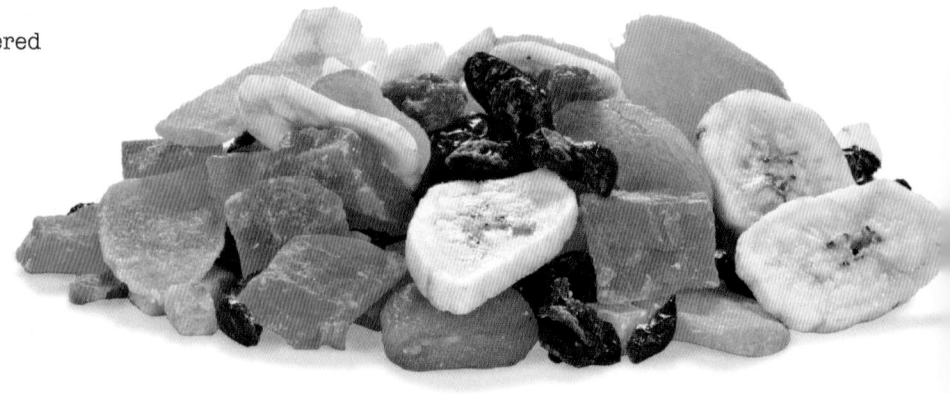

Granola

cooking spray
4 cups (400 g) rolled oats
½ cup (20 g) wheat bran flakes
½ cup (20 g) barley flakes
1 cup (155 g) roughly chopped almonds
½ cup (115 g) firmly packed light brown sugar
1 teaspoon salt
1 teaspoon ground cinnamon
¼ cup (60 ml) apple juice concentrate (available at health food stores)
2 tablespoons butter, melted
2 tablespoons vegetable oil
2 tablespoons honey
1 teaspoon vanilla extract
finely grated zest of 1 orange
1 cup (100 g) dried cranberries
1 cup (125 g) raisins

Makes 7 cups
(about 14 servings)

Packed with nutrition and taste, this granola is the ultimate combination. Eat it with milk for breakfast; sprinkle it on fruit, yogurt or ice cream; incorporate it into crumble toppings for fruit cobblers—or just grab a handful for a healthy, energy-boosting snack. To cut the cost of homemade granola, check out the bulk aisles of health food stores or supermarkets.

1 Preheat the oven to 300°F. Lightly coat a shallow 15 x 10-inch baking pan with the cooking spray and set aside.
2 In a large bowl, combine the rolled oats, wheat bran flakes, barley flakes, almonds, sugar, salt and cinnamon; set aside. In a small bowl, whisk together the apple juice concentrate, butter, oil, honey, vanilla extract, orange zest and ¼ cup (60 ml) water. Pour the juice mixture over the oat mixture and stir to combine the ingredients. Spread the mixture evenly in the prepared pan.
3 Bake, stirring every 15 minutes, for about 1 hour, until golden and slightly crunchy.
4 Remove the pan to a rack to cool completely, about 1 hour. When cooled, stir in the cranberries and raisins. Label, date and store in an airtight container for up to 1 week.

Oatmeal Mix

6 cups (600 g) instant oats
1⅓ cups (135 g) powdered milk
1 cup (175 g) chopped dried apples, apricots, bananas, prunes, raisins or mixed berries
¼ cup (55 g) sugar
¼ cup (45 g) firmly packed soft brown sugar
1 tablespoon ground cinnamon
1 teaspoon salt
¼ teaspoon ground cloves

Makes 8 cups
(about 16 servings)

Ready-to-eat flavored oatmeal mixes are perfect for those busy mornings when you need a healthy breakfast in a hurry. However, the prepackaged mixes aren't cheap, so whip up your own and vary it to suit your family's tastes.

1 In a large bowl, combine all the ingredients and stir until well blended.
2 Store the oatmeal mix in an airtight container or self-sealing plastic bag. Label, date and store in a cool, dry place for up to 6 months.

To use: Shake the mix well before using. In a saucepan, bring ½ cup (125 ml) water to a boil. Slowly stir in ½ cup of oatmeal mix. Reduce the heat and cook, stirring, for 1 minute. Remove the saucepan from the heat, cover, and let stand for 1 minute more or until oatmeal reaches the desired consistency.

Condiments and Spreads

Ketchup

4 quarts tomatoes (3 kg/about 24), peeled, cored and chopped
1 large brown onion, chopped
1 large red bell pepper, cored, seeded and chopped
1½ teaspoons celery seeds
1 teaspoon mustard seeds
1 teaspoon whole allspice
1 cinnamon stick
1¼ cups (285 g) firmly packed brown sugar
1 tablespoon salt
1½ cups (375 ml) cider vinegar
1 tablespoon paprika

Makes 6 cups (1.5 liters)

Forget about buying this staple condiment—homemade sauce is much tastier and an inspired way to use up extra tomatoes at the end of summer.

1 In a very large, nonreactive stockpot or saucepan, combine the tomatoes, onion and bell pepper, then cook over medium heat until soft. Press the vegetables through a food mill or sieve to make a puree. Return puree to saucepan.
2 Over high heat, boil the puree for about 1 hour, until it is thick and has reduced by half.
3 Cut a 4-inch square of cheesecloth. Place the celery seeds, mustard seeds, allspice and cinnamon stick in the center of the cloth, gather up the corners to form a bag, then secure with kitchen string. Add the spice bag, brown sugar and salt to the tomato mixture. Over low heat, cook the mixture gently for 25 minutes, stirring frequently.
4 Stir in the vinegar and paprika. Continue to cook, stirring frequently, until the mixture is thick.
5 Spoon the ketchup into three sterilized pint jars, leaving a ⅛-inch space between the top of the ketchup and the rim of the jar. Wipe the rims, cover and leave for 10 minutes in boiling water (see Safe Bottling and Preserving, page 72). Cool and test for airtight seals. Label, date and store in a cool, dark place for up to a year; the ketchup will be ready to eat in 1 week. Once a jar has been opened, store in the refrigerator.

Seafood Cocktail Sauce

1 cup (250 ml) Ketchup (above)
1 tablespoon horseradish
1 tablespoon lemon juice
½ teaspoon Worcestershire sauce
¼ teaspoon hot red pepper sauce, or more to taste

Makes about 1 cup (250 ml)

This classic sauce adds zest to tasty shrimp. It's cheaper than bottled cocktail sauce, and you can mix the ingredients to suit your taste. To turn up the heat, add more horseradish or hot red pepper sauce.

1 In a small, nonreactive bowl, combine all the ingredients and stir until well blended. Cover the bowl and refrigerate for at least 1 hour before serving.
2 Store in an airtight container in the refrigerator for up to 1 month.

Mustard

⅓ cup (45 g) yellow mustard seeds
3 tablespoons mustard powder
½ cup (125 ml) cider vinegar
½ cup (125 ml) stout or dark beer
2 cloves garlic, crushed
⅓ cup (80 g) firmly packed soft brown sugar
¾ teaspoon salt
½ teaspoon ground ginger
¼ teaspoon ground allspice

Makes about 2 cups (500 ml)

This versatile condiment is easy to make and can be adjusted to your tastes. The basic mix includes 2 to 3 tablespoons of liquid (vinegar, wine, water, flat beer) and about 3 tablespoons mustard powder. You could also add ground turmeric (for a traditional yellow tint), chopped fresh garlic, dried tarragon, sugar or honey, salt and more. Use it to spice up hot dogs, hamburgers or sandwiches, or brush over meats before grilling or roasting.

1 In a small bowl, combine the mustard seeds, mustard powder and cider vinegar. Cover the bowl with plastic wrap and let the mustard mixture stand at room temperature for 3 hours.
2 In a small saucepan, combine the stout, garlic, brown sugar, salt, ginger and allspice. Stir in the mustard mixture. Over medium heat, bring the mixture to a boil; reduce heat to low and simmer for 5 minutes, stirring occasionally.
3 Spoon the mustard into a hot, clean canning jar and seal tightly. Leave the mustard to cool to room temperature before using. Store in a cool, dark place. Once a jar has been opened, store in the refrigerator.

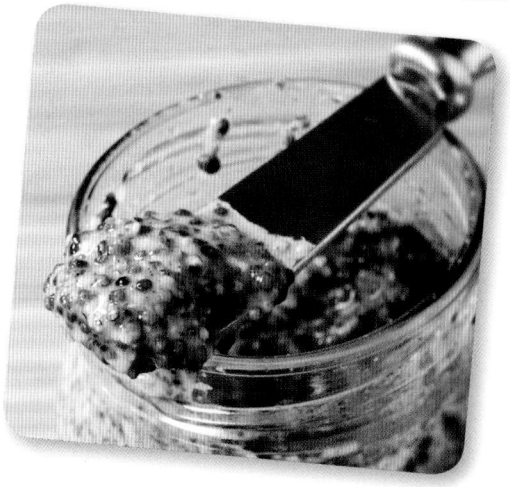

Classic Mayonnaise

4 egg yolks
1 tablespoon white wine vinegar
1½ cups (375 ml) vegetable oil or a combination of vegetable and extra virgin olive oils
1 pinch ground white pepper

Makes about 2 cups (500 g)

Homemade mayonnaise is a tasty addition to most salads and sandwiches. You can experiment with the flavor by using different oils and lemon juice instead of the vinegar. You could also try cayenne pepper in place of the white pepper.

1 In a food processor or blender, process the egg yolks, vinegar and 2 tablespoons water until just combined. With the motor running, drizzle in the oil very slowly so that the mixture emulsifies; if the oil is added too quickly, it will remain a thin, liquid dressing.
2 Stir in the white pepper. Cool quickly and store in the refrigerator for up to 5 days.

Aioli (Garlic Mayonnaise)

4 egg yolks
1 tablespoon white wine vinegar
1 clove garlic, crushed
½ cup (40 g) fresh white bread crumbs
1½ cups (375 ml) extra virgin olive oil
1 pinch ground cayenne pepper

Makes 3 cups (750 g)

Traditionally served with poached fish, aioli can also be used as a dip for fresh vegetables or seafood, or as a salad dressing. Homemade aioli is delicious and much better value than the prepackaged variety.

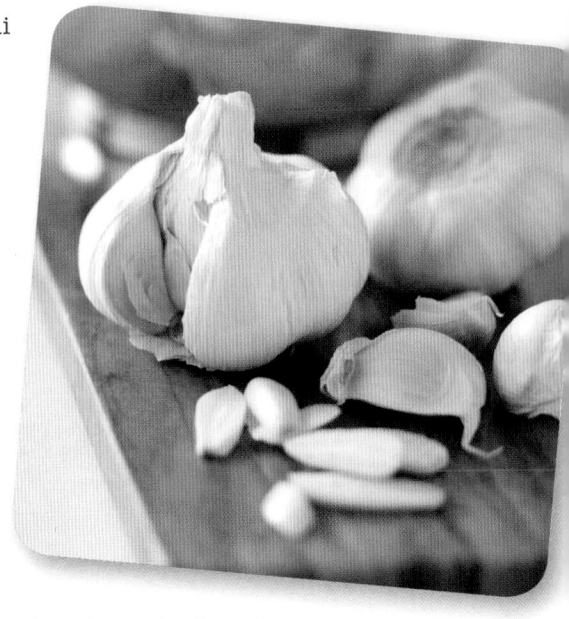

1 In a food processor or blender, process the egg yolks, vinegar, garlic, bread crumbs and 2 tablespoons water until ingredients are just combined. With the motor running, drizzle in the oil very slowly so the mixture emulsifies; if the oil is added too quickly, it will remain a thin, liquid dressing.
2 Stir in the cayenne pepper. Cool quickly and store in the refrigerator for up to 5 days.

A safer way to make mayonnaise

Raw eggs may contain the bacterium salmonella, which can cause illness and is particularly dangerous for pregnant women, very young children, the elderly and anyone who has a serious illness. To reduce the risk of contamination from salmonella, you should boil the mayonnaise. Transfer the blended dressing to the top of a double boiler and cook until a thermometer placed in the mayonnaise registers 167°F. Cool the sauce quickly and store in the refrigerator for up to 5 days.

Tartar Sauce

½ cup (125 g) Classic Mayonnaise (page 29)
½ cup (125 ml) reduced-fat sour cream
6 spring onions, finely chopped
¼ cup (60 g) chopped Sweet Pickles (page 66)
2 tablespoons lemon juice
1 tablespoon capers, rinsed and squeezed dry
1 tablespoon finely chopped fresh parsley
1 tablespoon Dijon mustard

Makes 1¼ cups (310 g)

When you have tasted a homemade version of this classic fish accompaniment, you won't waste your money on prepackaged tartar sauce.

1 In a bowl, combine all the ingredients and stir until they are well blended.
2 Cover the bowl and refrigerate for 2 hours or overnight before using. Store in the refrigerator for up to 5 days.

Spicy Tomato Salsa

3 tomatoes, cored, seeded and chopped
3 small spring onions, trimmed and roughly chopped
1 jalapeño pepper, cored, seeded and finely chopped (wear gloves when handling; they burn)
1 clove garlic, crushed
¾ teaspoon salt
⅓ cup (10 g) roughly chopped fresh coriander leaves

Makes 3½ cups (875 g)

A staple of Mexican cuisine, salsa is now popular everywhere. The spiciness can vary from very mild to tongue-burning hot, depending on the variety and quantity of peppers used. The zesty mix in this basic recipe is not just for tortilla dipping; you can also dollop it on grilled chicken breasts, firm fish, in beef fajitas or omelettes.

1 In a large, nonreactive bowl, combine the tomatoes, spring onions, jalapeño pepper, garlic and salt, then stir until well blended. Let the salsa stand for 1 hour to allow the flavors to mellow.
2 Just before serving, add the chopped coriander and stir. Serve immediately or store in the refrigerator for up to 2 days.

Salsa Verde

⅔ cup (12 g) flat-leaf parsley
⅔ cup (20 g) fresh basil leaves
1 clove garlic, halved
3 tablespoons capers, rinsed and squeezed dry
2 tablespoons chopped anchovies
¼ cup (60 ml) red wine vinegar
⅓ cup (80 ml) extra virgin olive oil
½ teaspoon Dijon mustard
freshly ground black pepper, to taste

Makes about 1 cup (250 ml)

This homemade green salsa—a mixture of fresh herbs, garlic, capers and salty anchovies—is sensational with seafood.

1. In a food processor or blender, process the parsley, basil, garlic, capers and anchovies until smooth.
2. Stir in the vinegar, olive oil and mustard. Add the pepper. Serve immediately or store in the refrigerator for up to 2 days.

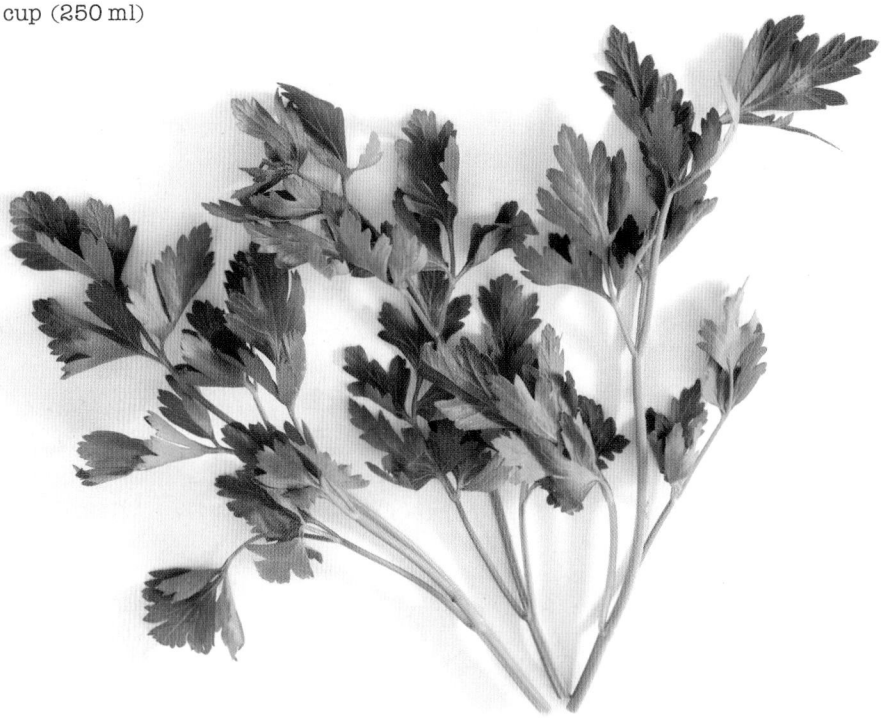

Sweet Chili Sauce

1 red chile pepper, thinly sliced
2 teaspoons arrowroot
⅓ cup (80 ml) lime juice
2 tablespoons rice vinegar
1 tablespoon soft brown sugar
2 teaspoons fish sauce

Makes about ½ cup (125 ml)

It doesn't take long to make a small batch of this sauce fresh for your next meal. If you don't need the whole quantity, try freezing it; using arrowroot as a thickener will ensure it thaws well.

In a small saucepan, combine the chile pepper and arrowroot. Slowly stir in the lime juice, vinegar, brown sugar and fish sauce, until well combined. Over medium–high heat, bring the mixture to a boil, until thickened. Remove from the heat and leave to cool to room temperature. Use immediately, or freeze in an airtight container for up to 1 month.

Peanut Butter

4 cups (650 g) salted, dry-roasted peanuts
1 tablespoon plus 1 teaspoon safflower or other mild-flavored vegetable oil

Makes 1 cup (250 g)

This family favorite can really eat up your budget. Surprisingly, making your own peanut butter in bulk is cheaper, not to mention healthier.

For smooth style: Using a food processor or blender, and working in batches, process the peanuts and the oil until the desired consistency is reached. Stop and scrape down the sides of the bowl as needed.

For chunky style: Using a food processor or blender, roughly chop about one-third of the peanuts; set aside. Working in batches, process the remaining peanuts with the oil until the desired consistency is reached. Scrape down the sides of the container as needed. Stir in the chopped peanuts.

To store: Scrape the peanut butter into a clean container with an airtight lid. Store in the refrigerator for up to 1 month but no longer—without preservatives, the oil can turn rancid.

VARIATION
Replace the peanuts with salted, dry-roasted almonds, hazelnuts or cashew nuts for luxurious nut butters.

About peanut butter

Peanut butter is an excellent source of protein, fiber and B vitamins. These days, peanut butter is a staple of most average households, but in its early years it was mostly only eaten by the wealthy people who frequented health spas. Peanut butter was initially marketed as a protein source for vegetarians.

Salad Dressings

Classic Vinaigrette

¼ cup (60 ml) extra virgin or virgin olive oil
1 tablespoon vinegar (such as white wine, red wine or tarragon) or fresh lemon juice
½ teaspoon salt
freshly ground black pepper, to taste

Makes ¼ cup (60 ml)

This classic salad dressing can be whipped up just before serving, then used over fresh salad greens. All the ingredients are pantry staples, so it's a quick and easy gourmet touch that's not costly.

In a small, nonreactive bowl, whisk together all the ingredients until well blended. Use immediately.

Herb Vinaigrette

¼ cup (60 ml) extra virgin or virgin olive oil
1 tablespoon vinegar (such as white wine, red wine or tarragon) or fresh lemon juice
1 tablespoon finely chopped fresh herbs, such as tarragon, basil, chives or parsley
½ teaspoon salt
freshly ground black pepper, to taste

Makes about ¼ cup (60 ml)

The fresh herbs in this vinaigrette add zest that you will never find in a bottled version.

In a small, nonreactive bowl, whisk together all the ingredients until well blended. Use immediately.

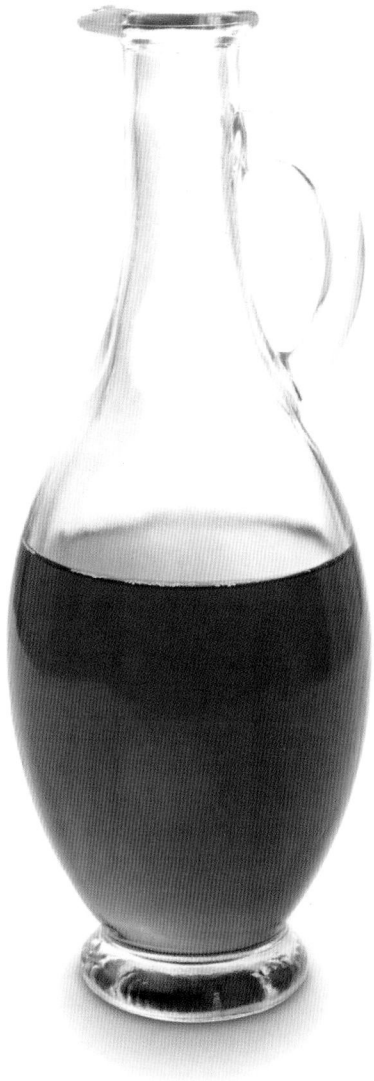

Walnut Vinaigrette

¼ cup (60 ml) walnut oil
2–3 tablespoons red wine vinegar
freshly ground black pepper

Makes about ¼ cup (60 ml)

Make a special bottle of walnut oil go further by using it in this tasty vinaigrette.

In a small, nonreactive bowl, whisk together all the ingredients until well blended. Use immediately.

Garlic Vinaigrette

¼ cup (60 ml) extra virgin or virgin olive oil
1 tablespoon vinegar (such as white wine, red wine or tarragon) or fresh lemon juice
1 clove garlic, crushed
½ teaspoon salt
freshly ground black pepper, to taste

Makes about ¼ cup (60 ml)

Try experimenting with different vinegars and/or lemon juice to vary the taste of this dressing.

In a small, nonreactive bowl, whisk together all the ingredients until well blended. Use immediately.

Balsamic Vinaigrette

¼ cup (60 ml) extra virgin or virgin olive oil
1 tablespoon balsamic vinegar
1 tablespoon finely chopped fresh basil
½ teaspoon salt
freshly ground black pepper, to taste

Makes about ¼ cup (60 ml)

Use the best balsamic vinegar and olive oil that you can afford for this dressing.

In a small, nonreactive bowl, whisk together all the ingredients until well blended. Use immediately.

Flavoring oils with herbs

Surprisingly easy to make, flavored oils pack a powerful flavor punch in salads. They make fabulous gifts, too, but make them in small quantities because they are perishable. The best choices for flavorings are lower-moisture herbs, such as rosemary, thyme or sage, or spices such as coriander seeds or chiles.

❖ **To make a flavored oil**, all you need are several sprigs of fresh herbs or whole spices and enough olive oil to fill the bottles.

1 Spread the herbs or spices on a clean work surface. Using a rolling pin, gently press down on the herbs or spices to lightly bruise them.
2 In a small saucepan over low heat, warm the olive oil. Add the herbs or spices and let them steep for several minutes. Using a slotted spoon, transfer the herbs or spices to sterilized bottles, distributing them equally. Pour the warm oil on top of the herbs or spices, leaving a ¼-inch space between the top of the oil and the rim of the bottle. Wipe the rims, cover tightly and refrigerate for at least 2 days to allow the herbs or spices to infuse the oil.
3 Strain the oil into a new set of sterilized bottles, adding a fresh herb sprig or whole spice to each bottle. Wipe the rims, cover, label and date. Store the flavored oil in the refrigerator for up to 1 month. Keep refrigerated after the oil is opened.

Make your own croutons

A wonderful way to use up stale bread, croutons are so easy to prepare that it makes no sense to spend money on ready-made ones that have been sitting on the shelf.

Cut slices of day-old bread into ½-inch cubes. In a large frying pan or skillet over medium heat, heat some extra virgin olive oil. Add the bread cubes and sauté, stirring constantly, until the cubes are well coated, golden in color and crisp. Transfer the cubes to paper towels and let drain. Add to salads or float on soups. Store the croutons in airtight containers.

To add more flavor to your croutons, first sauté some garlic slices, sprigs of fresh herbs or even whole chile peppers in the olive oil. Remove and discard the flavorings before adding the bread cubes to the flavored oil, and sautéing as above.

Raspberry Vinaigrette

2 jars (12 oz/340 g) raspberry preserves, seedless if available
1¼ cups (275 g) sugar
⅓ cup (50 g) chopped red onion
¼ cup (60 ml) balsamic vinegar
1 tablespoon dried tarragon
1 tablespoon curry powder
1 teaspoon ground white pepper
1 teaspoon freshly ground black pepper
1 cup (250 ml) extra virgin or virgin olive oil

Makes about 4 cups (1 liter)

Sweet, tart and tangy, this dressing will quickly become a family favorite. Homemade not only tastes better, but it's a fraction of the price of the bottled version.

1 In a large, nonreactive saucepan over high heat, combine the raspberry preserves and ¾ cup (165 g) of the sugar and bring to a boil. Remove the saucepan from the heat and let cool slightly. Pour the raspberry mixture into a food processor or blender. Add the onion, vinegar, tarragon, curry powder, white pepper, black pepper, the remaining sugar and ¼ cup (60 ml) water.
2 Cover and process, adding the olive oil in a slow, steady stream, until the ingredients are well blended. Use immediately, or store in an airtight container in the refrigerator for up to 1 week. Bring to room temperature and whisk vigorously before using.

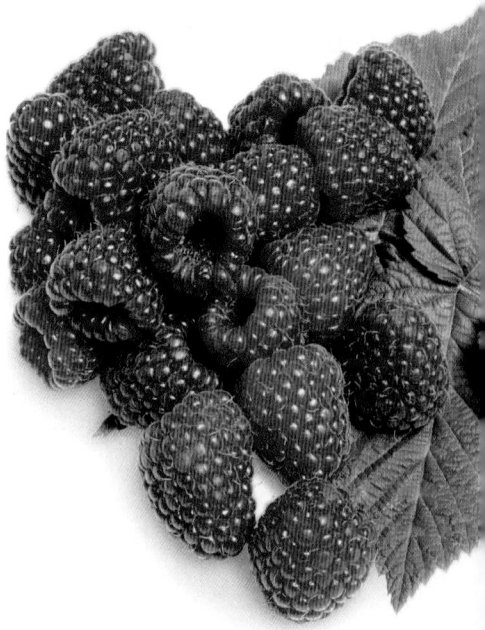

Flavoring vinegars with herbs

It's easy to make your own herb-flavored vinegars—they add a subtle taste to salads, especially those simply dressed with oil and vinegar. But remember, the higher quality vinegar you use, the better the result.

To make flavored vinegar, you only need:

- Several sprigs of fresh herbs
- Sterilized bottles with screw top lids
- Good-quality vinegar to fill the desired number of bottles.

Here's how to proceed:

1. Spread the herbs on a clean work surface. Using a rolling pin, gently press down on the herbs to bruise them lightly. Place 1 sprig in each bottle.
2. In a large, nonreactive saucepan over high heat, bring the vinegar to a boil. Using a funnel, pour the hot vinegar over the herb sprigs in each bottle. Cover the bottles and place them on a sunny windowsill for at least 2 weeks to allow the herbs to infuse. Turn each bottle daily.
3. Place a fresh herb sprig into each of a new set of sterilized bottles. Strain the vinegar, discarding the old herbs. Pour the flavored vinegar into the bottles over the fresh herb sprigs. Cover, label and date. Store the flavored vinegar in a cool, dark place for up to 1 year; it will be ready to use in 2 weeks. Store the flavored vinegar in the refrigerator after opening. The plain vinegar does not need refrigeration.

Herb Dressing Mix

4 tablespoons dried parsley
3 tablespoons dried oregano
3 tablespoons dried basil
3 tablespoons dried marjoram
¼ cup (55 g) sugar
2 tablespoons fennel seeds, crushed
2 tablespoons mustard powder
1 tablespoon freshly ground black pepper

Makes 2 cups (150 g)

All the taste and no preservatives required! Keep this mix on hand to make an Herb Dressing (page 38) that's suited to your taste.

1. In a large jar, combine all the ingredients. Seal the jar and shake until all the herbs are well mixed.
2. Store in a cool, dry, dark place for up to 6 weeks.

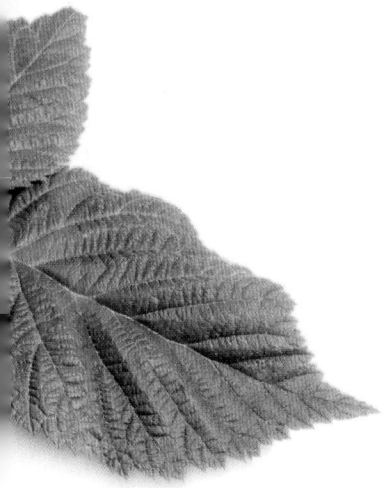

Herb Dressing

2 tablespoons Herb Dressing Mix (page 37)
1½ cups (375 ml) warm water
2 tablespoons olive oil
5 tablespoons (100 ml) white or tarragon vinegar
2 cloves garlic, crushed

Makes 2 cups (500 ml)

You can adjust the strength of this mouth-watering dressing by increasing or decreasing the amount of Herb Dressing Mix you use.

1 In a small, nonreactive bowl, whisk together all the ingredients until well blended. Let the dressing stand at room temperature for 30 minutes; whisk vigorously again and use.
2 Store the dressing in an airtight jar or bottle in the refrigerator for up to 1 week.

Thai Salad Dressing

1 tablespoon peanut or sunflower oil
2 red chile peppers, finely chopped (wear gloves when handling; they burn)
1 tablespoon grated fresh ginger
1 lemongrass stem, white part only, finely chopped
2 cloves garlic, finely chopped
¼ cup (60 ml) lime juice
1 tablespoon fish sauce
1 teaspoon soft brown sugar

Makes about ⅓ cup (80 ml)

This zesty sauce is the one to dress a traditional Thai beef salad, or more contemporary salad combinations, such as seafood, salad leaves and fresh herbs.

1 Heat the oil in a large, nonstick frying pan or skillet over medium heat, then add the chile peppers, ginger, lemongrass and garlic. Cook for 1 minute, stirring.
2 Remove from the heat and allow to cool slightly. In a small bowl, combine the lime juice, fish sauce and sugar. Add the chili mixture and stir until well combined. Use immediately.

Ranch Dressing Mix

2½ tablespoons onion flakes
1 tablespoon dried parsley
2 teaspoons paprika
2 teaspoons sugar
2 teaspoons salt
2 teaspoons freshly ground black pepper
1½ teaspoons garlic powder

Makes about ¼ cup (20 g)

This mix makes it easy to whip up Ranch Dressing on demand, for tossing through salads, dipping with crudités or soothing the heat of spicy chicken wings.

1 In a small, airtight container, combine all the ingredients. Cover and shake vigorously until well blended.
2 Store in a cool, dry, dark place for up to 1 year.

Ranch Dressing

1 quantity Ranch Dressing Mix (page 38)
1 cup (250 g) mayonnaise
1 cup (250 ml) buttermilk or low-fat natural yogurt

Makes about 2 cups (500 g)

To make a lower-fat version of this dressing, substitute low-fat mayonnaise for the regular mayonnaise. Buttermilk is made from skim milk, so it is already low in fat and calories. Instead of buttermilk, use runny, low-fat natural yogurt. If you'd like a thicker consistency for dipping, use sour cream.

In a small, nonreactive bowl, whisk together all the ingredients until the dressing is smooth and creamy.

Blue Cheese Dressing

1½ cups (375 g) mayonnaise
½ cup (125 ml) sour cream
¼ cup (60 ml) cider vinegar
4 teaspoons sugar
½ teaspoon mustard powder
1 teaspoon crushed garlic
2 teaspoons finely chopped onion
1 cup (125 g) crumbled blue cheese

Makes about 2 cups (500 g)

You can make this tangy treat or any of the following prepared salad dressings from scratch and keep them on hand in the refrigerator. They are all easy to make and cost a lot less than their commercial counterparts.

In a small, nonreactive bowl, combine all the ingredients except the blue cheese. Whisk to blend until the dressing is smooth and creamy. Gently stir in the blue cheese. Cover the bowl and refrigerate for at least 2 hours before serving. Store, covered, in the refrigerator.

Light Blue Cheese Dressing

½ cup (125 g) low-fat mayonnaise
2 tablespoons skim milk
1 tablespoon lemon juice
½ teaspoon sugar
1 teaspoon crushed garlic
¼ teaspoon mustard powder
½ cup (60 g) crumbled blue cheese

Makes about 1 cup (250 g)

Rich, creamy and loaded with flavor—you'd never guess this is a low-fat dressing.

In a small, nonreactive bowl, combine all the ingredients except the blue cheese. Whisk to blend until the dressing is smooth and creamy. Gently stir in the blue cheese. Cover the bowl and refrigerate for at least 2 hours before serving. Store, covered, in the refrigerator.

French Dressing

1 cup (250 ml) Ketchup (page 28)
½ cup (125 g) low-fat mayonnaise
3 tablespoons cider vinegar
3 tablespoons honey
2 tablespoons water
1 tablespoon olive oil
1 teaspoon lemon juice
½ teaspoon mustard powder
¼ teaspoon salt

Makes 2½ cups (625 ml)

You probably have all the ingredients for this creamy dressing in your pantry. It takes just a few minutes to prepare and is more delicious than the bottled variety.

In a food processor or blender, process all the ingredients until the dressing is well blended, smooth and creamy. Store in an airtight container in the refrigerator.

Italian Dressing

¼ cup (60 ml) extra virgin or virgin olive oil
¼ cup (60 ml) red wine vinegar
1 clove garlic, crushed
1 teaspoon finely chopped onion
½ teaspoon mustard powder
½ teaspoon celery seeds
½ teaspoon paprika
¼ teaspoon Italian Herb Blend (page 42)
2–4 tablespoons sugar

Makes about ⅔ cup (170 ml)

Nothing tastes better—or is more pleasing to the wallet—than homemade Italian dressing.

In a small, airtight container, combine all the ingredients. Cover and shake vigorously until all the ingredients are well blended. Use immediately or store in the refrigerator overnight.

Thousand Island Dressing

2 cups (500 g) Classic Mayonnaise (page 29)
¼ cup (60 ml) chili sauce
¼ cup (60 g) chopped Sweet Pickles (page 66) or similar pickle relish

Makes 2½ cups (625 ml)

For a lighter version of this dressing, substitute low-fat mayonnaise or low-fat natural yogurt for the regular mayonnaise. Using homemade mayonnaise will please both your palate and your budget.

1 In a small, nonreactive bowl, whisk together all the ingredients until the dressing is well blended and creamy.
2 Store in an airtight container in the refrigerator.

Seasonings

Bouquet Garni

1 bay leaf
2 sprigs parsley
1 sprig thyme

This famous combination uses either fresh herb sprigs or dried leaves. Use it for soups, stews and casseroles.

1 Cut a piece of cheesecloth about 4 inches square. Lay the herbs in the center of the cheesecloth, then bring the corners of the cloth together to form a bundle around the herbs. Tie the top of the bundle with kitchen string.
2 Add the herb bundle to a soup or stew. Once the cooking has finished, remove the bundle and discard.

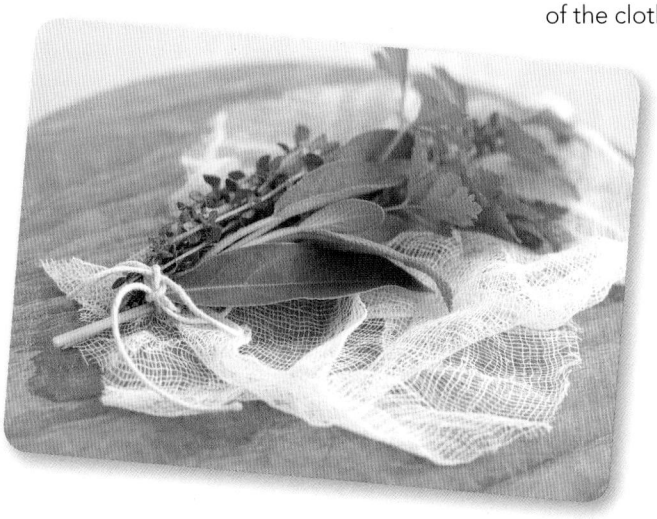

Fines Herbes

4 tablespoons dried parsley
1 tablespoon dried tarragon
1 tablespoon dried chervil
1 tablespoon dried chives

This classic blend of four herbs enhances the flavor of fish, poultry, egg dishes or cooked vegetables.

1 In a self-sealing plastic bag or airtight container, combine all the herbs. Shake until the herbs are well blended.
2 Label, date and store in a dry place at room temperature. Use within 3 months.

How to dry herbs

Drying fresh herbs that you have grown yourself will really save you money. For best flavor, try to use dried herbs within 4 to 6 months after preserving them. Once dried, crumble the leaves with your hands so they are ready to be used in recipes.

❖ **Air-drying** Pick fresh herbs. Gather the herbs in bunches and tie each bunch of stems with string, leaving a long end. Using the long end, hang the herb bunches upside down in a cool, dry place until they are completely dried.

❖ **Drying in an oven** Preheat an electric oven to 100°F. Preheat a gas oven to 200°F, then turn off the oven. Spread the herbs in a single layer over a baking sheet with a rim, then place in the oven until the herbs are completely dried, about 50 minutes.

Herbes de Provence

1½ tablespoons dried oregano
3 teaspoons dried basil
3 teaspoons dried marjoram
3 teaspoons dried thyme
1½ teaspoons dried mint
1½ teaspoons dried rosemary
1½ teaspoons dried sage
1 teaspoon fennel seeds

This popular French herb mixture can be sprinkled over meats, fish or poultry before grilling; stirred into rice or couscous; added to omelettes or scrambled eggs; or whisked together with oil and vinegar for an herbed salad dressing.

1 In a mortar, blender or food processor, crush or pulse all the herbs together until they reach the desired consistency.
2 Place the herb mixture in a self-sealing plastic bag or airtight container, label and date. Keep in a dry place at room temperature. Use within 3 months.

Italian Herb Blend

6 tablespoons dried basil
3 tablespoons dried oregano
2 tablespoons dried parsley
2 tablespoons dried thyme
1 teaspoon dried garlic

This well-loved herb mix is almost essential in pasta dishes and sprinkled on pizza. It is also delicious with chicken or firm fish.

1 In a self-sealing plastic bag or airtight container, combine all the ingredients. Shake until all the herbs are well blended.
2 Label, date and store in a dry place at room temperature. Use within 3 months.

Chicken Seasoning Mix

2 cups (300 g) plain flour, sifted
1 tablespoon paprika
2 teaspoons dried marjoram
2 teaspoons dried thyme
2 teaspoons onion powder
2 teaspoons garlic powder
1 teaspoon dried rosemary
½ teaspoon salt
¼ teaspoon freshly ground black pepper

Makes enough to coat 20 pork chops or four whole chickens

This is a fabulous addition to fried or baked chicken and pork recipes.

1 In a self-sealing plastic bag or airtight container, combine all the ingredients. Shake until all the ingredients are well blended.
2 Label, date and store in a cool, dry place for up to 6 months.

Make it a gift

Jars of herb mixtures are always welcome in a cook's home. You can make herb or spice bags with cheesecloth tied with string, then place the bags in a glass jar—all the cook needs to do is pull out a bag and pop it into whatever's cooking to add extra flavor.

Freezing herbs

Freezing herbs protects their flavor even more than drying them, in the opinion of many knowledgeable cooks. You can freeze herbs as whole sprigs or as chopped leaves frozen in an ice cube.

❖ **Whole sprigs** Wash and spin-dry sprigs of bushy herbs using a salad spinner. Pack in self-sealing freezer bags, label, date and freeze. Remove leaves as needed, returning the sprigs to the bags, then resealing and refreezing them.

❖ **Chopped leaves in ice cubes** Chop leaves of fresh herbs, such as chives, parsley or basil. Place 1 tablespoon of the chopped herb into each container of an ice-cube tray. Pour just enough water into each container to cover the herbs. Place in the freezer until well frozen. Pop out the frozen herb cubes, place in self-sealing freezer bags, label, date and freeze. When using those herbs in a recipe, just add the cube and let it melt.

Chili Powder

3 tablespoons ground chile peppers or paprika
1 tablespoon ground cumin
1 teaspoon ground turmeric
1 teaspoon dried oregano
1 teaspoon garlic powder
¼–1 teaspoon ground cayenne pepper
¼ teaspoon salt
¼ teaspoon freshly ground black pepper

Makes about ¼ cup (30 g)

You don't have to pay fancy prices for fancy spice mixes. Make your own, then slowly start adding a little more of one ingredient or a little less of another until you have your own favorite blend. You can adapt this recipe to your own taste: Make it hotter by adding more cayenne pepper, then add more or less of each spice.

1. In an airtight container, combine all the ingredients. Shake until all the spices are well blended.
2. Label, date and store in a cool, dark place for up to 6 months.

Cajun Seasoning Mix

⅔ cup (65 g) ground cayenne pepper
½ cup (156 g) salt
¼ cup (20 g) garlic powder
¼ cup (20 g) onion powder
¼ cup (20 g) chili powder
2 tablespoons freshly ground black pepper

Makes about 2 cups (350 g)

Sprinkle this spice sensation over popcorn, French fries or chicken pieces, or use it in Cajun dishes.

1. Combine all the ingredients in an airtight container. Shake until all the spices are well blended.
2. Label, date and store in a cool, dark place for up to 6 months.

Laksa Paste

1 onion, roughly chopped
4 cloves garlic
2 tablespoons finely chopped fresh ginger
2 stems lemongrass, white part only, roughly chopped
3 red bird's eye chilies (or serrano or jalapeño peppers), roughly chopped
6 macadamia nuts or toasted candlenuts
2 teaspoons shrimp paste
1 teaspoon ground turmeric
1 teaspoon ground cumin
2 teaspoons ground coriander
10–12 Vietnamese mint leaves
1 cup (50 g) roughly chopped fresh coriander (leaves, stems and roots)
4 kaffir lime leaves, finely chopped
¼ cup (60 ml) vegetable oil, plus extra for storage

Makes about 1 cup (250 g)

Keep this spicy paste in the fridge so you can whip up your favorite laksa recipe in less time than it takes to get to your local takeout.

1. Process all the ingredients in a food processor or blender until a paste forms.
2. Put the paste into a sterilized jar and drizzle over a little extra oil until the surface of the paste is covered, then seal with a tight-fitting lid. Keep the paste in the refrigerator for up to 1 month or divide the paste into ¼ cup portions (the amount required in most laksa recipes to serve 4) and freeze for up to 6 months.

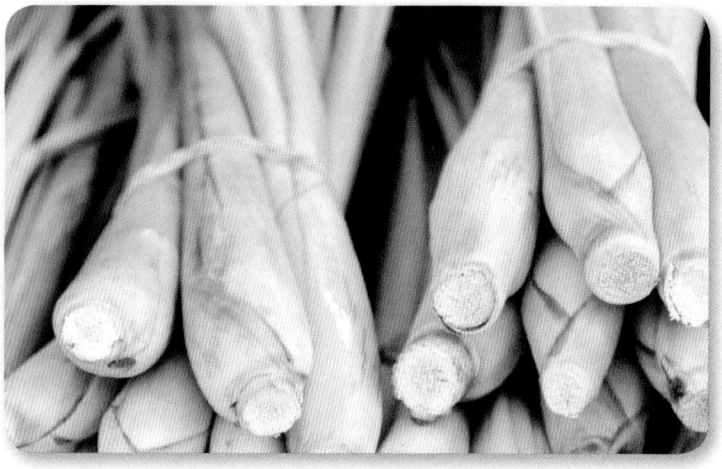

Chermoula

½ cup (15 g) fresh coriander leaves, finely chopped
½ cup (10 g) fresh parsley, finely chopped
1 small red onion, finely chopped
2 cloves garlic, crushed
1 teaspoon ground cumin
1 teaspoon ground paprika
1 teaspoon ground turmeric
1 teaspoon chili powder
½ cup (125 ml) olive oil
2 tablespoons lemon juice

Makes about 1 cup (250 g)

This Moroccan herb and spice mixture can be used as a marinade for meat, poultry and fish. It can also be applied to meat as a paste, which will form a crust during cooking.

In a bowl, combine the coriander, parsley, onion, garlic, cumin, paprika, turmeric and chili powder. Add the olive oil and lemon juice, then stir until well combined.

Caribbean Spicy Meat Rub

3 tablespoons brown sugar
2 tablespoons paprika
2 teaspoons mustard powder
2 teaspoons garlic salt
1½ teaspoons dried basil
1 teaspoon ground coriander
1 teaspoon dried savory
1 teaspoon dried thyme
1 teaspoon freshly ground black pepper
1 teaspoon ground cumin
1 bay leaf, crushed

Makes about ½ cup (85 g)

A pungent, sweet, spicy blend to rub onto just about any kind of meat before grilling, this mix can also be added to sauces and stews. Alternatively, stir 4 tablespoons of the rub into 2 tablespoons vegetable oil and heat just until the aromas are released, then add to any marinade for tougher cuts of meat.

1 Combine all the ingredients in an airtight container. Shake until all the ingredients are well blended.
2 Label, date and store in a cool, dark place for up to 6 months.

Curry Powder

3 tablespoons ground coriander
2 tablespoons ground turmeric
2 teaspoons ground cumin
2 teaspoons ground ginger
2 teaspoons ground allspice
1 teaspoon ground cinnamon
1 teaspoon ground celery seed
1 teaspoon ground black pepper
¼ teaspoon ground cayenne pepper

Makes about ½ cup (60 g)

Try making this basic recipe, then experiment each time you make it to find a blend that's perfect for you by adding or subtracting one of the following: cumin seeds, ground turmeric, black peppercorns, fennel seeds, cayenne pepper, ground coriander, ground cinnamon, nutmeg or mace, ground cloves, tamarind paste or cardamom seeds.

1 Combine all the ingredients in an airtight container. Shake until all the spices are well blended.
2 Label, date and store in a cool, dark place for up to 6 months.

Green Curry Paste

4 shallots, chopped
1 teaspoon shrimp or anchovy paste
3 cloves garlic, quartered
2 dried kaffir lime leaves, crushed, or 1 teaspoon lime zest
4 inch-long piece (10 cm) lemongrass stem, inner stalk chopped
1 tablespoon coriander seeds
1 tablespoon thinly sliced fresh ginger
1 teaspoon freshly grated nutmeg
1 teaspoon cumin seeds
1 teaspoon white peppercorns
6 green chile peppers, seeded and quartered
3–4 tablespoons coconut cream

Makes about ¾ cup (290 g)

This recipe and the one that follows are two staples of Thai cooking. You'll be surprised how often you'll reach for these pastes to add a little exotic flavor to your meals. You can find many of the ingredients at specialty Asian food stores. Stir this paste into poultry or vegetable dishes, or add it to more delicately flavored meat dishes. To release the flavors, sauté the paste in a little vegetable oil before using.

1 In a food processor or blender, process all the ingredients until well blended and smooth.
2 Use the paste at once or place in an airtight container, cover with vegetable oil and store in the refrigerator for up to 4 days. Alternatively, pack the paste into an ice-cube tray, freeze, pop out the paste cubes and store in a self-sealing, freezer-safe plastic bag in the freezer. Use the cubes as needed in recipes.

Red Curry Paste

1 tablespoon coriander seeds
3–6 red chiles, stems removed but not seeded
4 shallots, quartered
1 red onion, cut into eighths
4 cloves garlic, quartered
4 inch-long piece (10 cm) lemongrass stem, inner stalk chopped
¼ cup (7 g) fresh coriander leaves
2 kaffir lime leaves, finely chopped
zest of 2 limes
1 teaspoon freshly grated nutmeg
1 teaspoon cumin seeds
1 teaspoon white peppercorns
2 teaspoons shrimp or anchovy paste

Makes about 1 cup (290 g)

You can adjust the heat of this spicy Thai delight by adding or subtracting the fresh red chiles. As with the Green Curry Paste (above), sautéing the paste in a little oil before using it will fully release the flavors.

1 In a frying pan or skillet over medium-high heat, toast the coriander seeds for about 30 seconds. In a food processor or blender, process the toasted coriander seeds, red chiles, shallots, onion, garlic, lemongrass, coriander leaves, kaffir lime leaves, zest, nutmeg, cumin seeds and white peppercorns until all the ingredients are well blended.
2 In a frying pan or skillet over medium-low heat, dry-roast the shrimp or anchovy paste for 2 to 3 minutes, stirring constantly. Add to the chile mixture and process until smooth. Use the paste at once, or place in an airtight container, cover with vegetable oil and store in the refrigerator for up to 2 weeks.

Marinades

Red Wine Marinade

¼ cup (60 ml) dry red wine
2 shallots, chopped
2 tablespoons balsamic vinegar
½ teaspoon dried rosemary
2 tablespoons olive oil
2 cloves garlic, crushed
½ teaspoon salt
½ teaspoon freshly ground black pepper

There's no need to buy an expensive packaged marinade when you can easily make one. The purpose of any marinade is twofold: An acid, such as lemon juice or vinegar, breaks down the fibers in tough pieces of meat, while the seasonings infuse the meat with piquant flavor. Try marinating chunks of beef or lamb in this rich-tasting marinade before grilling them on skewers.

In a small, nonreactive bowl, stir together all the ingredients until well blended. Pour the marinade into a large, self-sealing bag and add the lamb or beef to be marinated. Place the bag in the refrigerator for at least 4 hours or overnight.

Mustard Marinade

⅓ cup (80 ml) lemon juice
2 shallots, chopped
2 tablespoons soy sauce
2 tablespoons Dijon mustard
2 tablespoons olive oil
¼ teaspoon hot red pepper sauce

Use this tasty mixture to marinate boneless, skinless chicken breasts, either for grilling or cutting into cubes to thread on skewers.

In a small, nonreactive bowl, stir together all the ingredients until well blended. Pour the marinade into a large, self-sealing bag and add the poultry to be marinated. Place the bag in the refrigerator and store for at least 4 hours or overnight.

Make your own tenderizing meat marinades

These marinades not only add flavor but will also tenderize the meat.

❖ **Beer** Place the meat in a nonmetallic dish, pour a bottle of beer over it and place it in the refrigerator for 1 hour or overnight, turning it once or twice. If you're slow-cooking the meat (the best method for tough cuts), use beer as part of the cooking liquid.

❖ **Natural yogurt** Yogurt is great when used as a marinade, especially for lamb and chicken.

❖ **Lemon juice** If you grow your own lemons, you have a terrific tenderizer for nothing! Lemon juice breaks down tough fibers quickly and easily—and adds a bright citrus taste.

❖ **Vinegar** Soak a tough piece of meat in 1 or 2 cups of vinegar overnight in the refrigerator to tenderize it. Try different vinegars with different meats to find out which combinations you prefer.

Lemon Herb Marinade

¼ cup (60 ml) vegetable oil
1 teaspoon grated lemon zest
¼ cup (60 ml) lemon juice
2 cloves garlic, crushed
1 teaspoon dried rosemary
½ teaspoon dried thyme
½ teaspoon salt
¼ teaspoon freshly ground black pepper

Makes about ½ cup (125 ml)

This Greek-style marinade is lovely with lamb chops and great with chicken. It's easy, inexpensive and delicious.

In a small, nonreactive bowl, stir together all the ingredients until well blended. Pour the marinade into a large, self-sealing bag and add the lamb or poultry to be marinated. Place the bag in the refrigerator for at least 4 hours.

Orange Ginger Marinade

¼ cup (60 ml) soy sauce
2 shallots, chopped
⅓ cup (90 ml) orange juice
2 teaspoons grated fresh ginger
2 tablespoons olive oil
2 tablespoons grated orange zest
1 clove garlic, crushed

Makes about ¾ cup (200 ml)

Lend a sweet, tangy flavor to scallops, shrimp or fish with this easy-to-make mixture, which rivals any prepared marinade.

In a small, nonreactive bowl, stir together all the ingredients until well blended. Pour the marinade into a large, self-sealing bag and add the seafood to be marinated. Place the bag in the refrigerator for 30 minutes to 1 hour.

Soy and Sesame Marinade

¼ cup (60 ml) lemon juice
½ teaspoon salt
2 tablespoons sesame oil
1 large clove garlic, crushed
1 tablespoon soy sauce

Makes about ½ cup (125 ml)

Sensational with shrimp, this marinade is also good with chicken or rump steak. Compare your own version with the ingredients in the bottled ones and you'll be glad you saved the money. If salt is an issue, use low-sodium soy sauce.

In a small, nonreactive bowl, stir together all the ingredients until well blended. Pour the marinade into a self-sealing bag and add the seafood, meat or poultry to be marinated. Place the bag in the refrigerator for at least 1 hour.

VARIATIONS

Teriyaki Marinade: In a small, nonreactive bowl, stir together ¼ cup (60 ml) soy sauce, 2 tablespoons mirin or rice vinegar, 2 tablespoons honey, 1 small finely chopped garlic clove and ¾ teaspoon ground ginger until well blended. Use as above.

Cooking Stocks

Beef Stock

4 lb (1.8 kg) meaty beef bones, including marrow and shinbones or knucklebones
2 onions, thickly sliced
2 carrots, thickly sliced
2 celery stalks with leaves, sliced
6 sprigs fresh parsley
2 small bay leaves
1 sprig fresh thyme, or ½ teaspoon dried thyme
10 black peppercorns
1 tablespoon salt

Makes 12 cups (3 liters)

At the heart of every great soup is a great stock. Although prepackaged stocks are convenient, they never have as much flavor as those you make yourself. Plus, when you make your own, you know exactly what goes into it—and what doesn't. When you buy the beef for this rich-tasting stock, ask the butcher to break up the bones into pieces small enough to fit into your stockpot or largest saucepan.

1 Preheat the oven to 400°F. Place the bones, onions and carrots in a roasting pan, then roast for 30 to 45 minutes, until the bones turn a rich brown.
2 Transfer the mixture to a stockpot or very large saucepan. Add the celery, parsley, bay leaves, thyme, peppercorns and salt. Add enough water (about 5 quarts) to cover the mixture.
3 Add a little water to the roasting pan and stir to loosen any browned bits. Pour the liquid and bits into the stockpot.
4 Place the stockpot over medium-high heat, then slowly bring the mixture to a boil, using a slotted spoon to skim off any fat or scum that rises to the surface. Reduce the heat, partly cover the pot and simmer gently for 3 to 4 hours.
5 Line a fine sieve with cheesecloth and set it over a large bowl. Slowly pour the stock through the sieve; discard the solids. Let the stock cool to room temperature. Pour the stock into serving-sized, airtight containers; cover, label and date. Store in the refrigerator for 1 week, or freeze for up to 6 months. If fat congeals on top of the stock while refrigerated or frozen, remove and discard before using the stock.

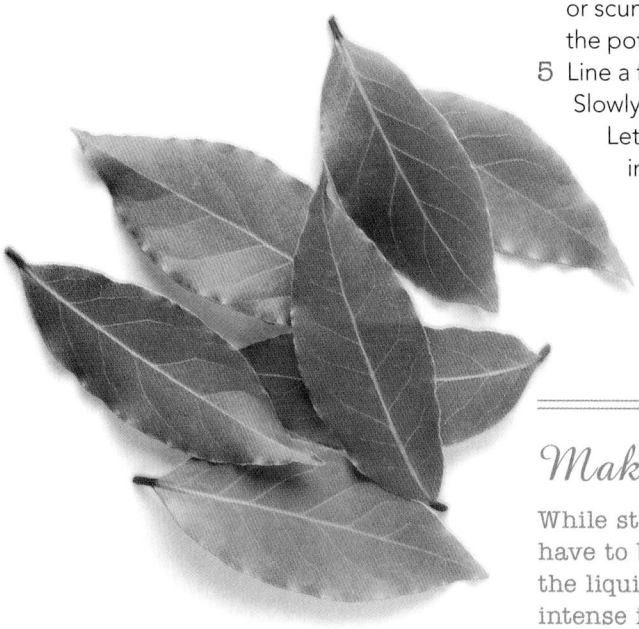

Make your own stock cubes

While stock (bouillon) cubes are convenient, you don't have to buy them. When cooking a pot of stock, cook the liquid down to 2 cups (500 ml)—it will be thick and intense in both flavor and color. Let the reduced stock cool completely, then pour it into ice-cube trays and place the trays in the freezer. When the stock cubes are solid, remove them from the trays, wrap each in foil and store them in a labeled, dated, self-sealing freezer bag. Each cube, diluted, will make 1 cup (250 ml) of stock.

Chicken Stock

5½ lb (2.5 kg) whole stewing hen, or 2 lb (900 g) chicken wing tips, necks and backs
3 celery stalks, sliced
1 large carrot, sliced
1 large onion, quartered
1 leek, white part only, halved lengthwise, cleaned and sliced
6 sprigs fresh parsley
½ teaspoon dried thyme
1 bay leaf
1 teaspoon salt
½ teaspoon black peppercorns

Makes 8 cups (2 liters)

As an alternative to chicken, use the same technique to make turkey stock with Christmas leftovers.

1 In a stockpot or very large saucepan, combine all the ingredients. Add enough water to cover the mixture. Bring slowly to a boil over medium-low heat, using a slotted spoon to skim off any fat or scum that rises to the surface.
2 Reduce the heat, partly cover the pot and gently simmer the stock for about 3 hours, until the stock is well flavored. The longer you simmer the stock, the richer the flavor.
3 Line a fine sieve with cheesecloth and set it over a large bowl. Slowly pour the stock through the sieve; discard the solids. Let the stock cool to room temperature. Pour the stock into serving-sized, airtight containers; cover, label and date. Store in the refrigerator for 1 week, or freeze for up to 6 months. If fat congeals on top of the stock while refrigerated or frozen, remove and discard before using the stock.

Fish Stock

1½ lb (700 g) whole white-fleshed fish, such as cod, snapper or haddock, cleaned and scaled
1–2 celery stalks, sliced
1 small onion, sliced
1 cup (250 ml) white wine, or the juice of 1 lemon
3 sprigs fresh parsley
1 sprig fresh thyme or ½ teaspoon dried thyme
1 small bay leaf
½ teaspoon salt
½ teaspoon black peppercorns

Makes 6 cups (1.5 liters)

An elegant base for seafood soups and stews, this delicately flavored stock can also be used as a poaching liquid for whole fish. Be careful not to overcook fish stock; too much cooking destroys the complex flavor and can give it a bitter edge. After making the stock, use the cooked fish in salads or spreads.

1 Cut off the fish head, slit open the fish and remove the bones. In a large saucepan, combine the fish fillets, head and bones. Add the remaining ingredients and 6 to 8 cups (1.5 to 2 liters) water. Bring the mixture to a boil over medium-high heat, using a slotted spoon to skim off any fat or scum that rises to the surface.
2 Reduce the heat to very low and barely simmer the stock, uncovered, for about 5 minutes, until the fish fillets are just cooked. Using a slotted spoon, lift out the fish fillets and set aside to drain.
3 Simmer the stock for a further 15 minutes.
4 Line a fine sieve with cheesecloth and set it over a large bowl. Slowly pour the stock through the sieve; discard the solids. Let the stock cool to room temperature. Pour the stock into serving-sized, airtight containers; cover, label and date. Store in the refrigerator for 1 week, or freeze for up to 6 months.

Clarifying stock

The best-quality stock is beautifully clear. This is achieved by clarifying the liquid after cooking. There are two methods for clarifying stock: The first will yield fairly clear results; the second method, very clear.

❖ **Straining** Line a fine sieve with cheesecloth and pour the stock through; this will remove any small solids floating in the stock.

❖ **Egg-white method** Separate 2 eggs and whisk together the whites. Crush the eggshells and add to the stock with the egg whites. Leaving the lid off, slowly bring to a simmer. When the egg whites begin to set, remove the stock from the heat. Pour the stock through a sieve or colander lined with cheesecloth into a large bowl; any floating solids or particles will be trapped in the cooked egg whites. Discard the whites and shells.

Vegetable Stock

¼ cup (60 g) unsalted butter
5 onions, chopped
2 leeks, white part only, halved lengthwise and sliced
2 cloves garlic
4 carrots, chopped
4 celery stalks with leaves, chopped
6–8 dried mushrooms, such as porcini
1 small bunch fresh parsley
1 sprig fresh thyme, or ½ teaspoon dried thyme
1 tablespoon salt
½ teaspoon ground allspice
pinch of mace or nutmeg
1 tablespoon red wine vinegar (optional)
1 fresh red chile, halved and seeded (optional); wear gloves when handling—they burn

Makes about 12 cups (3 liters)

Homemade vegetable stock is very economical and a creative way to use up vegetable peelings, leftover vegetables or the parts that are full of nutrition yet not generally served, such as mushroom stems, celery tops, and broccoli and cauliflower stalks.

1. In a stockpot or very large saucepan, melt the butter over medium heat. Add the onions, leeks and garlic and sauté for 5 to 8 minutes, until the onions are golden. Add the carrots, celery, mushrooms, parsley, thyme, salt, allspice, mace or nutmeg and 16 cups (4 liters) cold water.
2. Bring the mixture slowly to a boil, using a slotted spoon to skim off any fat or scum that rises to the surface. Reduce the heat, partly cover the pot, then simmer gently for 2 hours, adding more water as needed to maintain the level at about 12 cups (3 liters). Add the vinegar and red chile, if using, then simmer for 30 minutes longer.
3. Line a fine sieve with cheesecloth and set it over a large bowl. Slowly pour the stock through the sieve, gently pressing with a wooden spoon to squeeze all the liquid from the solids; discard the solids and the red chile. If desired, clarify the stock (see Clarifying Stock, above). If a thicker stock is desired, do not discard the solids after straining; puree about ½ cup of the cooked vegetables and stir the puree back into the stock. Let the stock cool to room temperature. Pour the stock into serving-sized, airtight containers; cover, label and date. Store in the refrigerator for 1 week, or freeze for up to 6 months.

Sauces

Barbecue Sauce

1 onion, chopped
¼ cup (60 ml) vegetable oil
1 cup (250 ml) Ketchup (page 28) or Tomato Sauce (page 55)
2 tablespoons Worcestershire sauce
2 tablespoons sugar
¼ cup (60 ml) cider vinegar
2 tablespoons mustard
1 teaspoon salt
½ teaspoon freshly ground black pepper

Makes about 2½ cups (625 ml)

Great with beef, chicken or pork, this homemade sauce is not only cheaper than bottled ones, but can also be customized to suit your family's taste.

1. In a nonreactive saucepan over low heat, combine all the ingredients and ¾ cup (185 ml) water. Simmer, uncovered, for 20 minutes, then remove from the heat and allow to cool.
2. Store in an airtight container in the refrigerator for up to 1 week, or freeze for up to 6 months.

Gravy

¼ cup (60 ml) pan drippings from roast meat or poultry
melted butter, as needed
2 cups (500 ml) Beef Stock (page 49) or Chicken Stock (page 50)
¼ cup (35 g) plain flour
salt and freshly ground black pepper, to taste

Makes 2 cups (500 ml)

Real gravy, made using the drippings from roasted meat or poultry, is the finishing touch for any roast, especially when you use homemade stock. You can also use prepackaged stock, but the flavor will be less intense.

1. Pour the drippings into a large frying pan or skillet and set aside; if needed, add some melted butter to make up the full amount.
2. Place the roasting pan with the remaining drippings over medium heat. Stir in the stock and simmer, stirring to loosen any browned bits on the bottom of the pan, about 1 minute.
3. Place the frying pan over medium heat and heat the drippings for 1 minute. Blend in the flour and cook, whisking, until the flour is a nutty brown, 1 to 2 minutes. Gradually add the stock, whisking constantly, then cook until the mixture boils and thickens.
4. Reduce the heat to medium-low and simmer, stirring occasionally, for a further 2 to 3 minutes. Add salt and pepper. If the gravy is lumpier than desired, strain it through a sieve. Transfer to a heated gravy boat and serve immediately.

Note: For extra flavor, add chopped fresh or dried herbs to the stock; try rosemary for lamb and tarragon for chicken.

Plum Sauce

3 lb (1.5 kg) plums, washed, stalks removed
2 cups (500 ml) white wine vinegar
1½ cups (345 g) firmly packed soft brown sugar
½ teaspoon salt
½ teaspoon freshly ground black pepper
½ teaspoon ground cayenne pepper
2 cinnamon sticks
2 star-anise
2 teaspoons ground cloves
2 inch (5 cm) piece fresh ginger, grated

Makes about 3 cups (750 ml)

You'll never purchase plum sauce again once you've tasted this spicy homemade alternative. It will keep for months in a cool, dark place.

1 In a large, heavy saucepan, combine all the ingredients and stir over a medium heat, without boiling, until the sugar is completely dissolved.
2 Bring to a boil and simmer, uncovered and stirring occasionally, for about 20 minutes, until the fruit is soft and pulpy and the pits have loosened.
3 Push the mixture through a food mill or coarse sieve, then discard the pits and other spices. Return the sauce to the saucepan and simmer again, until it thickens to the desired consistency.
4 Spoon the sauce into three warm, sterilized, widemouthed, ½ pint jars, leaving a ¼-inch space between the top of the sauce and the rim of the jar. Wipe the rims, cover and leave for 10 minutes in boiling water (see Safe Bottling and Preserving, page 72). Label, date and store the jars of sauce in a cool, dark place; the sauce will be ready to eat in 2 weeks.

Sweet and Sour Sauce

1 oz (30 g) glacé ginger, drained (reserve the syrup) and finely grated
3 teaspoons syrup from the ginger
2 small canned pineapple rings, drained and finely chopped
2 tablespoons soft brown sugar
pinch of ground cayenne pepper
3 teaspoons rice vinegar, white wine vinegar or cider vinegar
salt and freshly ground black pepper, to taste
1½ teaspoons arrowroot

Makes about 1 cup (250 ml)

Try this sauce poured over cooked beef, fish, chicken or pork, or use it for dipping.

1 In a saucepan, combine all the ingredients except the arrowroot. Add ⅔ cup (170 ml) water. Bring the mixture to a boil over medium heat, stirring often. Reduce the heat to low and simmer for 5 minutes.
2 Blend the arrowroot with 2 teaspoons cold water, then stir into the sauce. Return the sauce to a boil, stirring continuously, until it thickens and becomes clear.

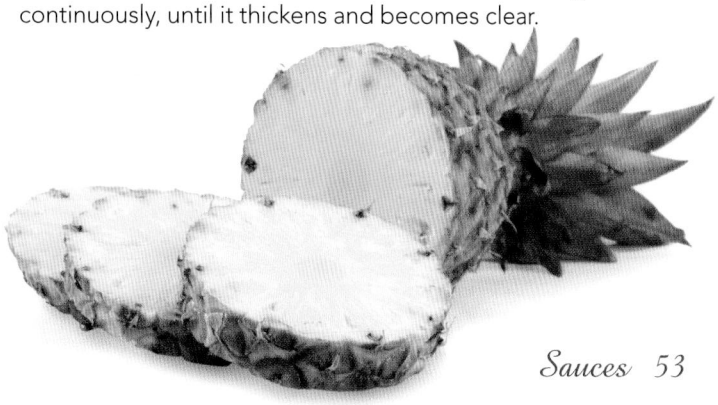

Mushroom Wine Sauce

¼ cup (60 g) unsalted butter
2 oz (50 g) dry-cured ham, such as Virginia, chopped
1 onion, chopped
1 carrot, thinly sliced
¼ cup (35 g) plain flour
3 cups (750 ml) Beef Stock (page 49)
1½ cups (375 ml) Chicken Stock (page 50)
2 tablespoons tomato paste
½ teaspoon salt
¼ teaspoon dried thyme
¼ teaspoon freshly ground black pepper
3 tablespoons butter, extra
2 shallots, finely chopped
8 oz (225 g) button, shiitake or portobello mushrooms, thinly sliced
⅔ cup (170 ml) dry red wine

Makes 3½ cups (875 ml)

Many a steak lover considers this sauce the perfect accompaniment, but it is equally good with veal or chicken. Prepackaged mushroom gravy just doesn't come close, either in taste or economy.

1. In a large, heavy saucepan, melt the butter over medium heat. Add the ham and cook, stirring frequently, until lightly golden, about 8 minutes. Add the onion and sauté for 5 minutes, until soft. Add the carrot and cook for another 5 minutes, until tender.
2. Sprinkle the flour over the mixture and stir until blended. Gradually add the beef and chicken stocks, stirring constantly. Add the tomato paste, salt, thyme and pepper. Cook, stirring frequently and skimming off any scum that rises to the surface, for about 30 minutes, until the sauce thickens and thickly coats the back of a spoon. Strain the sauce through a sieve and discard the solids.
3. In a large frying pan or skillet over medium heat, melt the extra butter. Add the shallots and cook until soft. Add the mushrooms and cook until tender. Pour in the wine, increase the heat and boil, uncovered, until the liquid is reduced by half.
4. Add the mushroom mixture to the sauce, stirring until the ingredients are well blended.

Béarnaise Sauce

⅓ cup (10 g) chopped fresh tarragon
2 tablespoons white wine vinegar
1 tablespoon finely chopped shallot
2 egg yolks
¼ teaspoon salt
½ cup (125 ml) clarified unsalted butter (see How to Clarify Butter, page 57), liquid but not hot
pinch of ground white pepper

Makes 1 cup (250 ml)

Egg-based sauces add immediate elegance to almost any meal. This Béarnaise sauce and the Hollandaise that follows are among the most refined. Once made with raw eggs (or eggs only lightly cooked in a double boiler), these recipes cook the eggs enough to remove any fear of salmonella contamination. Slow and steady is the rule when cooking egg sauces—or you may scramble your culinary plans. Béarnaise is the sauce served with fillet mignon in fine restaurants for sky-high prices, and jars sold in specialty food stores just don't measure up.

1. In a small saucepan, combine the tarragon, vinegar and shallot. Cook over medium-high heat for 1 to 2 minutes, then remove from the heat and leave to cool.
2. In a 4 cup (1 liter) saucepan, combine the egg yolks, salt, tarragon mixture and 2 tablespoons water. Bring to a boil over medium-high heat, whisking constantly.
3. Remove the saucepan from the heat. The mixture will begin to curdle, but continue whisking until the mixture becomes smooth. Stir in the clarified butter, 1 tablespoon at a time. Add the pepper and stir until smooth.

Tomato Sauce

2 lb tomatoes (1 kg/about 10), halved
2 tablespoons olive oil
1 onion, finely chopped
salt and freshly ground black pepper

Makes 2½ cups (625 g)

Try this rich sauce over freshly cooked pasta, as a base for chili con carne or veal parmigiana, or smear it over a pizza base before adding the topping.

1 In a very large, nonreactive stockpot or saucepan, cook the tomatoes, covered, over medium heat for 10 minutes. Press the tomatoes through a food mill or sieve to make a puree. Discard the skins and seeds.
2 In a large saucepan, heat the oil. Add the onion and cook over medium heat, stirring, until the onion is translucent but not brown. Add the tomato puree and simmer for about 30 minutes, until the sauce thickens. Season to taste. Store in an airtight container in the refrigerator for up to 1 week, or freeze for up to 3 months.

Satay Sauce

⅓ cup (90 g) crunchy Peanut Butter (page 33)
1 teaspoon low-sodium soy sauce
1 teaspoon honey
1 teaspoon rice vinegar or cider vinegar
1 large clove garlic, peeled
1 spring onion, chopped
⅓ cup (80 ml) reduced-fat coconut milk
1 tablespoon Sweet Chili Sauce (page 33)

Makes about 1 cup (250 ml)

Full of flavor, this rich, creamy sauce is robust enough to take on meat, tofu and vegetable skewers.

In a food processor or blender, process all the ingredients until almost smooth.

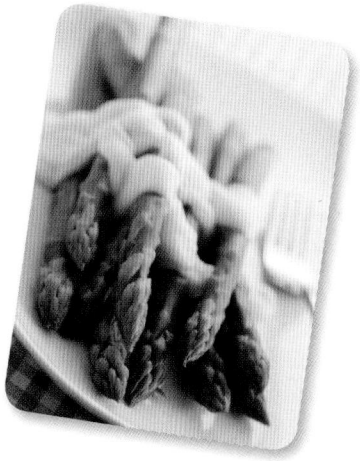

Hollandaise Sauce

2 egg yolks
¼ teaspoon salt
1 tablespoon lemon juice
½ cup (125 ml) clarified unsalted butter (see How to Clarify Butter, page 57), liquid but not hot
pinch of ground white pepper

Makes 1 cup (250 ml)

There is simply no comparison to homemade hollandaise. It's essential for dishes such as eggs Benedict and eggs Florentine, and superb drizzled over fresh steamed asparagus, broccoli, cauliflower or poached fish.

1 In a 4 cup (1 liter) saucepan, combine the egg yolks, salt, lemon juice and 2 tablespoons water. Bring to a boil over medium-high heat, whisking constantly.
2 Remove the saucepan from the heat. The mixture will begin to curdle, but continue whisking until the mixture becomes smooth. Stir in the clarified butter, 1 tablespoon at a time. Add the pepper and stir until smooth.

Basic White Sauce

1 tablespoon butter
1 tablespoon plain flour
1 cup (250 ml) hot milk
¼ teaspoon salt
pinch of ground white or freshly ground black pepper

Makes 1 cup (250 ml)

Thin, medium or thick, white sauce is the most versatile of all sauces and can be adapted to suit many dishes. Thin white sauce serves as a base for creamy soups or stews; medium white sauce is added to casseroles and creamed vegetable mixtures or used as a base for other sauces; thick white sauce works as a binder or a base for dishes such as soufflés or croquettes. Making your own white sauce, starting with this basic version, allows you to make all kinds of other recipes, such as the three that follow.

1. In a small heavy saucepan, melt the butter over low heat. Add the flour and cook, whisking constantly, for 2 to 3 minutes, until the mixture is smooth; do not let the flour brown. Gradually stir in the milk.
2. Increase the heat to medium and cook, stirring constantly, for 3 to 5 minutes, until the sauce is thickened and smooth, and no raw flour taste remains. Remove the saucepan from the heat and stir in the salt and pepper.
3. To store, lay plastic wrap directly on the surface of the sauce to prevent a skin forming. Allow the sauce to cool to room temperature, then refrigerate until needed. Reheat the sauce in the top of a double boiler.

Cheese Sauce

1 tablespoon butter or margarine
1 tablespoon plain flour
½ teaspoon mustard powder
1 cup (250 ml) hot milk
½–¾ cup (60–90 g) grated cheddar
¼ teaspoon salt
pinch of ground white or freshly ground black pepper

Makes 1¼ cups (310 ml)

Remember that you can choose the kind of cheese to use in this sauce. Cheddar is the classic variety, but there are many other possibilities. Pour the sauce over potatoes or steamed vegetables for a simple starter dish.

1. In a small heavy saucepan, melt the butter over low heat. Add the flour and mustard powder and cook, whisking constantly, for 2 to 3 minutes, until the mixture is smooth; do not let the flour brown. Gradually stir in the milk.
2. Increase the heat to medium and cook, stirring constantly, for 3 to 5 minutes, until the sauce is thickened and smooth, and no raw flour taste remains. Remove the saucepan from the heat and stir in the cheese, salt and pepper.
3. To store, lay plastic wrap directly on the surface of the sauce to prevent a skin forming. Allow the sauce to cool to room temperature, then refrigerate until needed. Reheat the sauce in the top of a double boiler.

Dijon Mustard Sauce

1 tablespoon butter or margarine
1 tablespoon plain flour
1 cup (250 ml) hot milk
2 tablespoons Dijon mustard
1 teaspoon white wine vinegar
¼ teaspoon salt
pinch of ground white or freshly ground black pepper

Makes 1 cup (250 ml)

This tangy condiment is wonderful with ham or poached or grilled fish.

1. In a small heavy saucepan, melt the butter over low heat. Add the flour and cook, whisking constantly, for 2 to 3 minutes, until the mixture is smooth; do not let the flour brown. Gradually stir in the milk.
2. Increase the heat to medium and cook, stirring constantly, for 3 to 5 minutes, until the sauce is thickened and smooth, and no raw flour taste remains. Remove the saucepan from the heat and stir in the mustard, vinegar, salt and pepper.
3. To store, lay plastic wrap directly on the surface of the sauce to prevent a skin forming. Allow the sauce to cool to room temperature, then refrigerate until needed. Reheat the sauce in the top of a double boiler.

How to clarify butter

Clarified butter is essential for making certain sauces, such as hollandaise, and for dipping artichoke leaves or steamed lobster into. By clarifying butter, you are removing the milk solids, leaving a clear, golden, rich oil. In a small saucepan over very low heat, melt ½ cup (125 g) butter. When the butter has completely liquefied but not yet begun to cook, remove the saucepan from the heat and let the butter stand until the white milk solids sink to the bottom. Place a piece of cheesecloth over a small glass bowl. Carefully pour the golden-yellow liquid butter into the bowl through the cheesecloth; be careful to stop pouring when the white solids begin to move. Remove the cheesecloth. Cover the clarified butter and store in the refrigerator until required.

Mushroom Sauce

3 tablespoons butter or margarine
½ cup (45 g) chopped mushrooms
1 tablespoon plain flour
1 cup hot milk (250 ml) or Beef Stock (page 49)
¼ teaspoon salt
pinch of ground white or freshly ground black pepper

Makes 1 cup (250 ml)

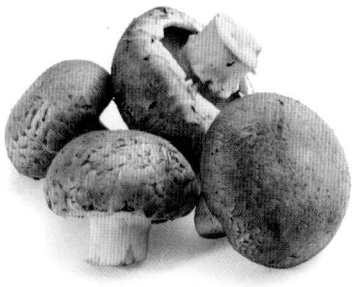

Serve this creamy mushroom sauce with roast meat or poultry, or use it in casseroles. It's a far cry from canned mushroom soup or sauces!

1. In a small frying pan or skillet, melt 2 tablespoons of the butter over medium heat. Add the mushrooms and sauté for 3 minutes, then remove from the heat and set aside.
2. In a small heavy saucepan, melt the remaining 1 tablespoon butter over low heat. Add the flour and cook, whisking constantly, for 2 to 3 minutes, until smooth; do not let the flour brown. Gradually stir in the milk or, if a darker sauce is desired, the stock. Increase the heat to medium and cook, stirring constantly, for 3 to 5 minutes, until the sauce is thickened and smooth, and no raw flour taste remains.
3. Remove the saucepan from the heat and stir in the mushrooms, salt and pepper.
4. To store, lay plastic wrap directly on the surface of the sauce to prevent a skin forming. Allow the sauce to cool to room temperature, then refrigerate until needed. Reheat the sauce in the top of a double boiler.

Dessert Sauces

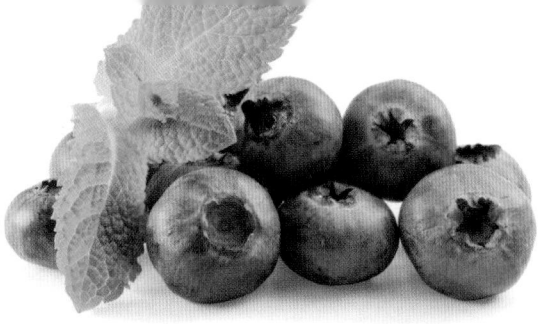

Blueberry Syrup

4 cups (600 g) blueberries, fresh or frozen
2 thin strips lemon zest
3 cups (660 g) sugar
1 tablespoon lemon juice

Makes 3½ cups (875 ml)

This fresh syrup is a perfect match for bread pudding, ice cream or pancakes.

1 In a large saucepan, crush the berries using a wooden spoon. Add the lemon zest and 1 cup (250 ml) water. Over medium heat, bring the mixture to a simmer. Reduce the heat to low and cook, uncovered, for 5 minutes without simmering.
2 Line a colander or large sieve with cheesecloth and set it over a large bowl. Pour the berry mixture into the colander, squeezing the cheesecloth to extract all the juice; there should be about 2 cups (500 ml) blueberry juice. Discard the solids.
3 In a saucepan over medium-high heat, combine the sugar and another 2 cups (500 ml) water. Bring to a boil, stirring until the sugar has dissolved. Continue boiling, without stirring, until a candy thermometer reads 260°F.
4 Add the blueberry mixture and boil, uncovered, for 1 minute. Remove from the heat and let cool, then stir in the lemon juice. Store in an airtight container in the refrigerator for up to 1 month.

Applesauce

3 small cooking apples, peeled, cored and sliced
¼ teaspoon ground allspice
2 teaspoons soft brown sugar
2 tablespoons lemon juice

Makes about 1 cup (250 ml)

Keep this versatile sauce on hand to serve with ice cream or yogurt for dessert—but remember it's also a great match with pork for a main meal.

1 In a small saucepan, combine the apples, allspice, sugar, lemon juice and 1 tablespoon water. Cover and cook over low heat for about 30 minutes, until soft and pulpy.
2 Remove from the heat and mash with a fork. For a finer texture, cool the sauce, then puree it in a food processor or blender.

Mango and Passion Fruit Sauce

1 large mango, pitted, peeled and roughly chopped
½ cup (125 ml) passion fruit pulp (from 6–8 fruit)

Makes 1 cup (250 ml)

The only ingredients in this delicious sauce are fresh fruit. No canned sauce can come close for pure taste.

1 In a food processor or blender, puree the mango and passion fruit pulp until smooth.
2 Chill before serving. Store in an airtight container in the refrigerator for up to 2 days.

Raspberry Sauce

½ cup (110 g) sugar
2 tablespoons orange-flavored liqueur
2 cups (250 g) raspberries, fresh or frozen

Makes about ¾ cup (185 ml)

Simple and sensational, this sauce is quick to make and inexpensive when raspberries are in season. It will quickly become a family favorite, served over fruit salad or ice cream.

1 In a small saucepan, bring the sugar and ½ cup (125 ml) water to a boil. Remove from the heat and let the syrup cool.
2 Add the liqueur and raspberries, then stir gently; let stand for 2 minutes. Pour through a sieve into a bowl, pressing to remove the seeds; discard the solids.
3 Chill before serving. Store in an airtight container in the refrigerator for up to 2 days.

Custard

1½ cups (375 ml) milk
¼ cup (55 g) sugar
pinch of salt
3 egg yolks, lightly beaten
¾ teaspoon vanilla extract

Makes about 1½ cups (375 ml)

Forget thick, prepackaged custard—enjoy this classic creamy sauce with its hint of vanilla, also known as crème anglaise.

1 In a saucepan over low heat, combine the milk, sugar and salt, and heat just until small bubbles appear on the surface. In a bowl, whisk ¼ cup (60 ml) of the milk mixture into the egg yolks, then stir the mixture back into the saucepan. Cook over low heat, whisking constantly, for about 10 minutes, until the mixture coats the back of a spoon.
2 Remove the saucepan from the heat and strain the mixture through a sieve into a bowl. Stir in the vanilla. Let the sauce cool to room temperature, then cover and refrigerate until ready to serve.

Fruit Coulis

2 cups (250 g) berries, fresh or frozen
sugar, to taste

Makes about 1 cup (250 ml)

Here is a versatile sauce that you can whip up to take advantage of berries in season—or less costly frozen ones the rest of the year. You can use raspberries, blueberries, blackberries or strawberries. You can also use fresh peaches or apricots—just lightly poach them before pureeing.

1 Rinse and drain the berries thoroughly (frozen berries do not require rinsing). In a food processor or blender, puree the berries until smooth. If desired, add a little sugar while pureeing.
2 Press the mixture through a sieve into a bowl; discard any solids or seeds. Taste and add more sugar if desired.
3 Chill before serving. Store in an airtight container in the refrigerator for up to 2 days.

Butterscotch Sauce

1½ cups (375 g) unsalted butter
1½ cups (345 g) firmly packed brown sugar
pinch of salt
1 cup (250 ml) heavy cream
1 teaspoon vanilla extract

Makes about 2½ cups (625 ml)

Once you've tried this delicious sauce warm over ice cream in summer or sticky date pudding in winter, you'll never buy the commercial variety again.

1 In a small saucepan over low heat, melt the butter. Add the sugar, salt and cream, and stir until the sugar has dissolved. Simmer for 8 to 10 minutes, stirring continuously so that the sugar doesn't crystallize. Remove the saucepan from the heat and stir in the vanilla.
2 Serve warm or cold. Can be refrigerated in a covered container for up to 1 week.

Chocolate Sauce

2 tablespoons good-quality cocoa powder, such as Dutch processed
½ cup (125 g) unsalted butter
1½ cups (225 g) chopped dark chocolate (85 percent cocoa)
⅔ cup (100 g) chopped dark chocolate (70 percent cocoa)
1 cup (230 g) firmly packed light brown sugar
¾ cup (165 g) sugar
½ cup (125 ml) light corn syrup or glucose syrup
¼ teaspoon salt
1 teaspoon vanilla extract

Makes about 2½ cups (625 ml)

Quality cocoa powder and dark chocolate make for a decadent sauce that can't be matched at any price.

1 In a glass cup, combine the cocoa powder and 3 tablespoons cold water and stir until completely dissolved. In the top of a double boiler, melt the butter over low heat. Add the cocoa mixture and all the chocolate, then stir in 1 cup (250 ml) boiling water, both types of sugar, the corn syrup and salt.
2 Remove the top of the double boiler, place over medium heat and bring the mixture to a boil; boil, uncovered, for 5 minutes (or for 7 minutes for a thicker sauce that will harden when it comes into contact with ice cream).
3 Remove the saucepan from the heat and let the sauce cool to room temperature, then stir in the vanilla.

Caramel Sauce

2 tablespoons unsalted butter
⅓ cup (60 g) soft brown sugar
3 tablespoons cream

Makes about ⅔ cup (170 ml)

This recipe is great for last-minute guests; in less than 10 minutes you can transform just three ingredients into a real crowd-pleaser.

In a small saucepan, slowly melt the butter over medium heat. Add the sugar and stir for about 2 minutes, until it has dissolved. Add the cream and simmer the mixture gently for about 3 minutes, stirring frequently, until it turns a caramel color. Remove from the heat and serve.

Dry Mixes

Pancake and Waffle Mix

6 cups (900 g) plain flour (or half plain flour and half whole wheat flour)
3½ tablespoons baking powder
1 cup (100 g) skim powdered milk
1 tablespoon salt
1 cup (200 g) solid vegetable shortening

Makes about 8 cups (1.2 kg)

This mix will quickly make these favorite treats—see Pancakes and Waffles (page 142).

1. In a large bowl, sift together the flour, baking powder, powdered milk and salt, then stir until well blended.
2. Add the vegetable shortening and, using a pastry blender tool or two knives, "cut" the shortening into the flour mixture, until it resembles coarse crumbs.
3. Put the mix in a self-sealing bag. Label, date and refrigerate for up to 6 weeks.

Basic Cake Mix

8 cups (1.2 kg) plain flour
6 cups (1.3 kg) sugar
¼ cup (50 g) baking powder
1½ teaspoons salt
2¼ cups (450 g) solid vegetable shortening

Makes about 16 cups (3 kg)

Even if you don't usually use packaged cake mix, it pays to keep this homemade mix on hand. It can be stored for 10 to 12 weeks and makes about 16 cups, enough for several cakes. Use it to create the delectable Spice Cake (page 116) and Chocolate Cake (page 117). Using those recipes as a guide, you can easily develop your own to make your family's favorite cakes.

1. In a large bowl, sift together the flour, sugar, baking powder and salt, then stir until well blended.
2. Add the vegetable shortening and, using a pastry blender tool or two knives, "cut" the shortening into the flour mixture, until it resembles very coarse crumbs.
3. Place the mix in a large, airtight container or a self-sealing plastic bag. Label, date and store the mix in a cool, dry place or in the refrigerator for 10 to 12 weeks.

Make your own real vanilla extract

Every kitchen needs a bottle of vanilla extract, so why not make your own? Vanilla is one of the most used flavorings, but as you know, real vanilla extract is not an inexpensive purchase. While imitation vanilla extract is less expensive, you pay the price in the loss of that real vanilla flavor.

1. Place a vanilla bean in a small, clean screw-top jar.
2. Pour 3 tablespoons plain vodka over the vanilla bean. Close the lid tightly and let the mixture stand for about 4 weeks.
3. Discard the vanilla bean from the infused vodka before using the extract.

Pasta

Simple Fresh Pasta

3 eggs
2 cups (300 g) plain flour

Makes 4 to 6 servings of spaghetti or linguini, or enough sheets for a large lasagna

Fresh pasta is quite easy to make, cooks more quickly than dried pasta, and is light and delicious. There are three steps to making fresh pasta: (1) mixing together a dough; (2) rolling the dough out and cutting it; and (3) cooking it. You can mix the dough by hand or in a food processor. This is the simplest recipe. The eggs provide enough moisture to form a dough.

1. In a large bowl, beat the eggs. Sift in the flour, stirring constantly, until a soft dough forms.
2. On a lightly floured surface, knead the dough until it is smooth and elastic.
3. Roll out and cut the dough by hand or with a pasta machine (see Rolling and Cutting Fresh Pasta, opposite).
4. To cook, bring a large pot of lightly salted water to a boil. Add the pasta. Fresh pasta cooks very quickly—thin strands may be cooked by the time they float to the surface of the water; other varieties will cook in about 1 to 2 minutes, while ravioli will cook in 6 minutes.

Luxury Fresh Pasta

2 cups (300 g) plain flour
2 large eggs
2 teaspoons olive oil
2 tablespoons water
½ teaspoon salt

Makes 4 to 6 servings of spaghetti or linguini, or enough sheets for a large lasagna

This dough contains olive oil and water, which makes it a little easier to handle.

1. On a lightly floured surface, pour the flour in a mound. Using your hands, make a well in the center of the mound.
2. In a small bowl, stir together the eggs, olive oil and water. Slowly pour the egg mixture into the flour well; sprinkle with the salt.
3. Carefully push the flour from around the edges into the well, stirring with your fingers to form a batter. Continue adding flour to the well until the mixture forms a soft dough.
4. Knead the dough for at least 5 minutes, until it is smooth and elastic. Cover the dough with an inverted bowl or plastic wrap, then let it rest for 1 hour before rolling.
5. Roll out and cut the dough by hand or with a pasta machine (see Rolling and Cutting Fresh Pasta, opposite).
6. To cook, bring a large pot of lightly salted water to a boil. Add the pasta. Fresh pasta cooks very quickly—thin strands may be cooked by the time they float to the surface of the water; other varieties will cook in about 1 to 2 minutes, while ravioli will cook in 6 minutes.

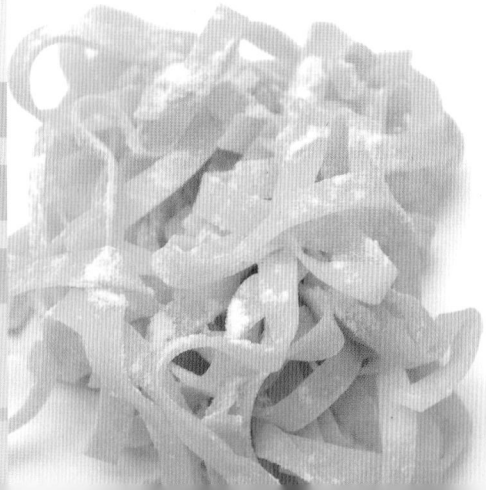

Rolling and cutting fresh pasta

It's easy to make pasta either by hand or with a pasta machine.

❖ **By hand** On a lightly floured surface, using a long, thin rolling pin, roll out one piece of dough to a 1/16-inch-thick, 20 x 14-inch rectangle. Lightly flour the top of the dough to prevent sticking. Fold the rectangle of dough in half lengthwise, then fold it again; you should have a 5 x 14-inch rectangle—do not press the dough together. Using a very sharp knife or pastry wheel—and a ruler or straightedge if needed—cut the sheet of dough into strips. Carefully unfold the strips and either hang them gently on a drying rack or lay them flat on dish towels. Let dry for 1 to 2 hours. Fresh pasta must air-dry before cooking or it will become gluey when boiled.

❖ **Using a pasta machine** Following the manufacturer's directions, pass the dough several times through the machine's rollers to knead it and make it elastic. With each pass, set the rollers closer together, until the pasta is thin enough to cut. Set the machine to cut the desired shapes and cut. Let the pasta dry on a drying rack or flat on dish towels for 1 to 2 hours.

Superfast Fresh Pasta

2¼ cups (335 g) plain flour
2 eggs
¼ cup (125 ml) water
1 tablespoon olive oil
1 teaspoon salt

Makes 4 to 6 servings of spaghetti or linguini, or enough sheets for a large lasagna

You can make quick work of mixing pasta dough if you use a food processor instead of your hands.

1. Fit a food processor with a plastic dough blade or a metal chopping blade. Add all the ingredients and process for 20 to 30 seconds, until the dough rides up in the center.
2. On a lightly floured surface, knead the dough for about 5 minutes, until it is smooth and elastic. Cover the dough with plastic wrap and let it sit for 30 minutes before rolling.
3. Roll out and cut the dough by hand or with a pasta machine (see Rolling and Cutting Fresh Pasta, above).
4. To cook, bring a large pot of lightly salted water to the boil. Add the pasta. Fresh pasta cooks very quickly—thin strands may be cooked by the time they float to the surface of the water; other varieties will cook in about 1 to 2 minutes, while ravioli will cook in 6 minutes.

Storing fresh pasta

Let the pasta dry for several hours, or until it is dry but not brittle. For long strands of pasta (fettuccine or linguini, for example), when the dough has dried slightly but is still pliable, gently wrap a loose bunch around your fingers to form a "nest." Place the nest in a cool, dry place to dry completely. For large lasagna sheets, allow each to dry completely. Then stack the pieces between sheets of parchment paper. Store cut pasta in self-sealing plastic bags or airtight containers in the refrigerator for up to 1 week, or freeze for up to 1 month.

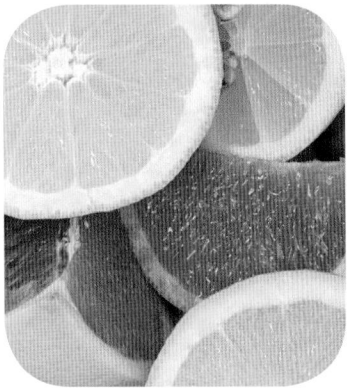

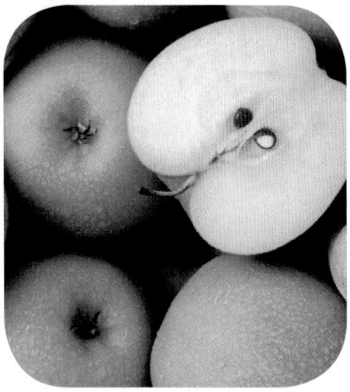

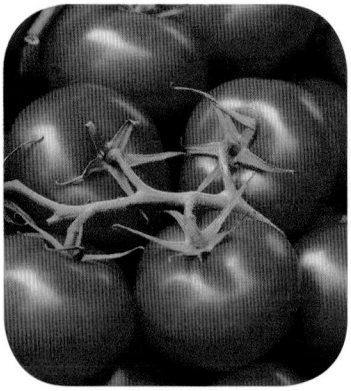

Pickles and Relishes

Dill Pickles ❖ Sweet Pickles ❖ Pickled Gherkins ❖ Chili Jam ❖ Pickle Relish ❖ Tomato Relish ❖ Pickled Cauliflower Florets ❖ Pickled Onions ❖ Red Onion Relish ❖ Pickled Spiced Plums ❖ Roasted Red Bell Peppers in Oil ❖ Oven-Dried Tomatoes

Chutneys

Mango Chutney ❖ Spicy Tomato Chutney ❖ Green Tomato Chutney ❖ Lemon Lime Chutney

Jams, Jellies and Marmalades

Dried-Apricot Jam ❖ Lemony Fig Jam ❖ Pear Jam ❖ Peach Jam ❖ Melon Ginger Jam ❖ Strawberry Jam ❖ Three-Berry Jam ❖ Apple Ginger Jelly ❖ Grape Jelly ❖ Mint Jelly ❖ Seville Orange Marmalade ❖ Citrus Marmalade

Frozen Vegetables

Asparagus ❖ Beets ❖ Bell Peppers ❖ Broad and Lima Beans ❖ Broccoli and Cauliflower ❖ Brussels Sprouts ❖ Carrots ❖ Green Beans ❖ Mushrooms ❖ Peas ❖ Pumpkin and Sweet Potato ❖ Sweet Corn ❖ Mixed Vegetables

Frozen Fruit

Apples ❖ Apricots ❖ Blackberries ❖ Blueberries ❖ Cherries ❖ Mangoes ❖ Peaches and Plums ❖ Raspberries ❖ Red Currants and Black Currants ❖ Strawberries

Pickled, Preserved and Frozen Foods

Whether you grow your own fruit and vegetables or like to buy produce when it's in season and at its best, the recipes in this chapter will help you take advantage of nature's seasonal abundance.

Tomatoes, bell peppers, cucumbers, corn, peaches and other fresh produce flood fruit stands, roadside stalls and supermarket shelves when they are at their seasonal peak and, following the simple law of supply and demand, the price is at its lowest. Indeed, you can often get a case of tomatoes or peaches for what you would pay for a handful at another time of year.

If you buy fresh vegetables and fruit at their peak and when their prices are most reasonable, you can freeze them and enjoy them throughout the year. All the instructions you need are in this chapter. Freezing is incredibly simple. With only a bit more effort, you can make your own unbelievably tasty pickles, relishes and chutneys. And if you also make your own jellies and jams, you will not only save money, but also have ready-made presents for friends and neighbors as well.

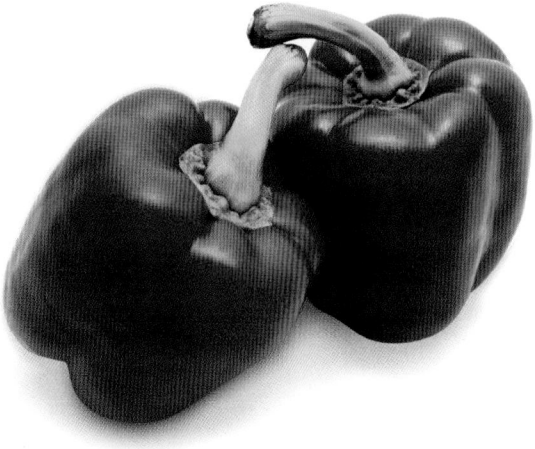

Pickles and Relishes

Dill Pickles

4 lb (1.8 kg) small to medium (4–5 inches/10–13 cm long) pickling cucumbers
4 cloves garlic
8 sprigs fresh dill
4 teaspoons mustard seeds
3 tablespoons salt
1 tablespoon sugar
1½ cups (375 ml) vinegar

FOR THE SOAKING BRINE
⅓ cup (100 g) salt
8 cups (2 liters) hot water

Makes 2 quart (2 liter) jars

Enjoy these as a snack, on an antipasto platter or sliced in hamburgers.

1 Scrub the cucumbers. To make the soaking brine, combine the salt and water in a large, nonreactive bowl. Stir until the salt has dissolved completely. Add the cucumbers to the brine and leave to soak overnight.
2 Drain the cucumbers and discard the soaking brine. Pack the cucumbers, standing on end, into two sterilized 1-quart canning jars. In each jar, place 2 garlic cloves, 4 dill sprigs and 2 teaspoons mustard seeds.
3 In a large, nonreactive saucepan, combine the 3 tablespoons salt, the sugar, vinegar and 3 cups (750 ml) water, then bring the mixture to a boil. Pour the hot brine over the cucumbers in the jars, dividing it equally.
4 Wipe the rims, cover and process for 20 minutes in boiling water (see Safe Bottling and Preserving, page 72). When cool, label, date and store in a cool, dark place for 4 to 6 weeks. Once a jar has been opened, store in the refrigerator.

Sweet Pickles

30 small to medium pickling cucumbers, scrubbed and thinly sliced
8 large onions, halved lengthwise and thinly sliced crosswise
1 red bell pepper, chopped
½ cup (150 g) pickling salt
4 cups (about 800 g) crushed ice
4 cups (1 liter) white vinegar
4½ cups (1 kg) sugar
2 tablespoons mustard seeds
2 teaspoons celery seeds
1 tablespoon ground turmeric
1 teaspoon ground ginger
1 teaspoon black peppercorns

Makes 8 pint (500 ml) jars

These pickles go well with corned beef sandwiches. It's best to use pickling salt; it keeps the pickles green, while natural anticaking agents keep the liquid clear.

1 In a very large colander set over a larger bowl or saucepan, combine the cucumber slices, onions and bell peppers. Sprinkle the mixture with the pickling salt and toss well. Cover the vegetables with a 2-inch layer of crushed ice. Refrigerate for 3 to 4 hours, adding more ice as needed.
2 In a very large, heavy, nonreactive saucepan, bring the vinegar, sugar, mustard seeds, celery seeds, turmeric, ginger and peppercorns to a boil over medium heat. Boil for 10 minutes, then stir in the cucumber mixture and return just to a boil.
3 Ladle the vegetables and liquid into eight sterilized 1-pint canning jars, leaving a ¼-inch space between the top of the pickles and the rim of the jar. Run a long, thin spatula around the inside of the jars to release any trapped air bubbles.
4 Wipe the rims, cover and process for 10 minutes in boiling water (see Safe Bottling and Preserving, page 72). When cool, label, date and store in a cool, dark place for 4 to 6 weeks. Once a jar has been opened, store in the refrigerator.

Pickled Gherkins

10 dozen (600 g) French gherkins or baby pickling cucumbers, scrubbed
1½ cups (450 g) pickling salt, plus 1–2 tablespoons extra, to taste
30 peppercorns—white, green or multicolored
6 small bay leaves
18 sprigs fresh tarragon
4–6 cups (1–1½ liters) white wine vinegar
4½ cups (1 kg) sugar

Makes about 6 half-pint (250 ml) jars

These tiny pickles, also called cornichons, are traditionally served with pâtés and terrines.

1 In a large, nonreactive bowl, sprinkle the gherkins with the 1½ cups salt. Loosely cover and let stand for 24 hours.
2 Drain the gherkins and discard the brine. Pack the gherkins, standing on end, into six warm, sterilized, widemouthed, half-pint canning jars, leaving a ¼-inch space at the top of the jar. In each jar, place 5 peppercorns, 1 bay leaf and 2 tarragon sprigs.
3 Meanwhile, in a large, heavy, nonreactive saucepan, combine the vinegar, sugar and remaining tarragon sprigs. Bring the mixture to a boil over high heat. Pour the mixture over the gherkins to cover. Cover the jars and stand overnight.
4 Drain the vinegar from the jars into a large, nonreactive saucepan. Stir in the remaining salt and, over high heat, bring the mixture to a boil. Remove the pan from the heat and let the brine cool. Pour the cooled brine over the pickles in the jars, dividing it equally.
5 Wipe the rims, cover and process for 15 minutes in boiling water (see Safe Bottling and Preserving, page 72). When cool, label, date and store in a cool, dark place for 4 to 6 weeks. Once a jar has been opened, store in the refrigerator.

Chili Jam

9 oz (250 g) bell peppers, halved, cored and seeded
2½ long red chile peppers, like cayenne, roughly chopped
¼ cup (60 ml) olive oil
1 small onion, finely chopped
2 cloves garlic, finely chopped
1 tablespoon grated palm sugar
1 tablespoon fish sauce
2 teaspoons tamarind paste
1 tablespoon finely chopped fresh coriander leaves
1 tablespoon finely chopped fresh mint

Makes about 1 cup (300 g)

Serve a bowl of this tasty savory jam with barbecued food or a dollop on a pan-fried chicken breast.

1 Place the bell peppers under a hot broiler, skin side up, for about 10 minutes, until the skins are charred. Transfer the hot bell peppers to a large heatproof bowl, cover with plastic wrap and cool for about 10 minutes, until safe to handle. Peel off the skins, then roughly chop the flesh. In a food processor, puree the bell peppers and chile peppers until smooth.
2 In a small saucepan, heat the oil over medium heat. Add the onion and cook for 1 to 2 minutes, until softened. Add the garlic and cook for 30 seconds.
3 Add the bell pepper–chili mixture, palm sugar, fish sauce and tamarind, then cook for 10 minutes over low heat, stirring occasionally. Stir the coriander and mint through, then let cool to room temperature; use immediately or store in an airtight container in the refrigerator for up to 2 weeks.

Pickle Relish

4 medium cucumbers, unpeeled and finely chopped
2 large red bell peppers, cored, seeded and chopped
2 large green bell peppers, cored, seeded and chopped
1 medium yellow onion, chopped
1 tablespoon ground turmeric
½ cup (150 g) kosher salt
6 cups (1½ liters) water
2 cinnamon sticks, broken in half
1 tablespoon mustard seed's
2 teaspoons whole allspice
1 teaspoon whole cloves
2 cups (440 g) sugar
2 cups (500 ml) cider vinegar

Makes 8 half-pint (250 ml) jars

The word "relish" says it all—savor the flavor—and put it on your hot dog or a ham sandwich. This luscious recipe is most inexpensive, and jars of pickle relish make fine gifts

1. In a large, heavy, nonreactive saucepan or Dutch oven, combine the cucumbers, bell peppers and onion; sprinkle the turmeric over all the vegetables. In a large bowl, dissolve the salt in the water to make a brine. Pour the brine over the vegetables, loosely cover the saucepan and let stand for 6 to 8 hours. Drain the vegetables, rinse well several times and return the vegetables to the saucepan.
2. Cut a 4-inch square of cheesecloth. Place the cinnamon sticks, mustard seeds, allspice and cloves in the center of the cloth, bring the corners together to make a bag and secure with kitchen string, Add the spice bag to the saucepan along with the sugar and cider vinegar. Over high heat, bring the mixture to a rolling boil and cook until the sugar is completely dissolved. Reduce the heat to medium and boil gently, uncovered, for 10 minutes. Remove and discard the spice bag.
3. Spoon the relish into eight warm, sterilized jars, leaving a ¼-inch space between the top of the relish and the rim of the jar. Wipe the rims, cover and process for 10 minutes in boiling water (see Safe Bottling and Preserving, page 72). Cool and test for airtight seals. Label, date and store in a cool, dark place for 4 to 6 weeks. Once a jar has been opened, store the relish in the refrigerator.

In preserving, acid content is crucial

Jams, jellies, marmalades, chutneys and pickles—basically any fruit, mixture or preserve with a high enough acid content to inhibit the growth of microorganisms—can be safely bottled with a hot-water bath (page 72). Low-acid vegetables—every type other than tomatoes, which are actually a fruit—should be frozen for storage or bottled with a pressure cooker unless you are pickling them. Pickling vegetables in vinegar adds enough acidity to allow for safe hot-water processing.

Tomato Relish

4½ lb (2 kg) tomatoes, skinned and finely chopped
3 large onions, finely chopped
1½ tablespoons salt
3 large celery stalks, finely chopped
1 red bell pepper, finely chopped
2¼ cups (500 g) sugar
1 tablespoon mustard seeds
1¾ cups (440 ml) vinegar

Makes 4 half-pint (250 ml) jars

Use this versatile relish to accompany cold meats or salad, or spread it on sandwiches.

1 In a bowl, combine the tomatoes and onions, then sprinkle with the salt and leave overnight. The next day, pour the mixture into a colander and leave to drain for 5 to 6 hours.
2 In a bowl, combine the celery, bell pepper, sugar, mustard seeds and vinegar. Stir in the tomato mixture. Spoon the relish into four warm, sterilized, widemouthed, half-pint jars. Label, date and store in the refrigerator for up to 1 month.

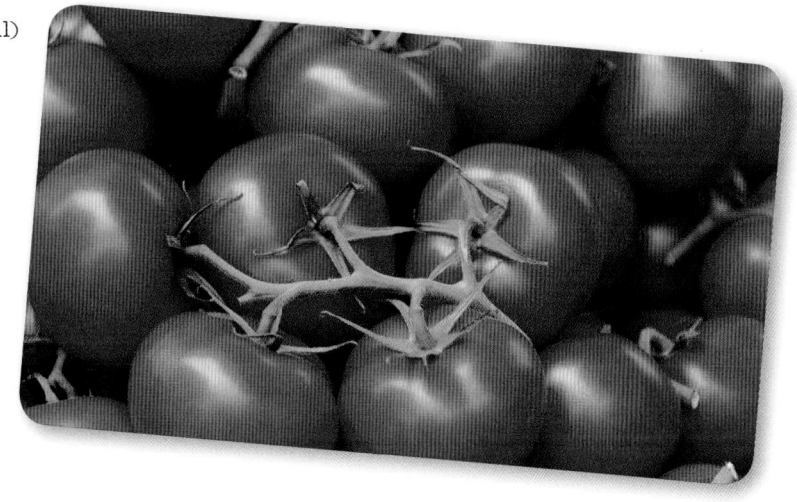

Pickled Cauliflower Florets

1 large cauliflower, cut into florets
white vinegar, to cover the cauliflower
1 tablespoon salt
1 tablespoon white peppercorns
1 tablespoon light brown sugar
1 bell pepper, finely sliced
6 small dried red chile peppers

Makes 2 quart (1 liter) jars

This is a traditional addition to any antipasto plate.

1 In a large, nonreactive saucepan or stockpot, place the cauliflower florets and pour in enough vinegar to cover. Add the salt, peppercorns and sugar and bring the mixture to a boil over high heat.
2 Add the bell pepper and boil for 1 minute. Using a slotted spoon, transfer the cauliflower to two warm, sterilized, widemouthed, 1-quart jars, reserving the brine. Pack the cauliflower firmly into the jars, dividing the bell pepper strips between them. Add 3 chile peppers to each jar.
3 Pour the hot brine over the vegetables in the jars until the cauliflower is completely covered, leaving a ¼-inch space between the top of the brine and the rim of the jars. Wipe the rims, cover and process for 20 minutes in boiling water (see Safe Bottling and Preserving, page 72). Cool, label, date and store in a cool, dark place for 4 to 6 weeks; the cauliflower will be ready to eat in 2 weeks. Once a jar has been opened, store in the refrigerator.

Pickled Onions

4 lb (1.8 kg) small white pickling onions
½ cup (150 g) pickling salt
8 black peppercorns
4 red chiles (wear gloves when handling; they burn)
4 bay leaves
4 cups (1 liter) cider vinegar

Makes 4 pint (500 ml) jars

These yummy onions are a tasty appetizer or a match for blue cheese.

1 Place the onions in a large, heatproof, nonreactive bowl. Pour enough boiling water over them to cover. Let stand for 5 minutes, then drain. Trim the root end and the crowns of the onions; the peels should slip off easily. Do not remove too many onion layers.
2 Place the peeled onions in a large bowl and cover with cold water. Add the salt and mix well, then let stand overnight.
3 Drain the onions. Using a large slotted spoon, transfer the onions to four warm, sterilized, widemouthed, 1-pint jars. To each jar, add 2 peppercorns, 1 red chile and 1 bay leaf.
4 In a large, nonreactive saucepan, bring the vinegar to a boil over high heat. Immediately pour the hot vinegar over the onions in the jars to cover them, leaving a ⅛-inch space between the top of the vinegar and the rim of the jars.
5 Wipe the rims, cover and process for 10 minutes in boiling water (see Safe Bottling and Preserving, page 72). Cool, label, date and store in a cool, dark place; the onions will be ready to eat in 4 weeks. Once a jar has been opened, store in the refrigerator.

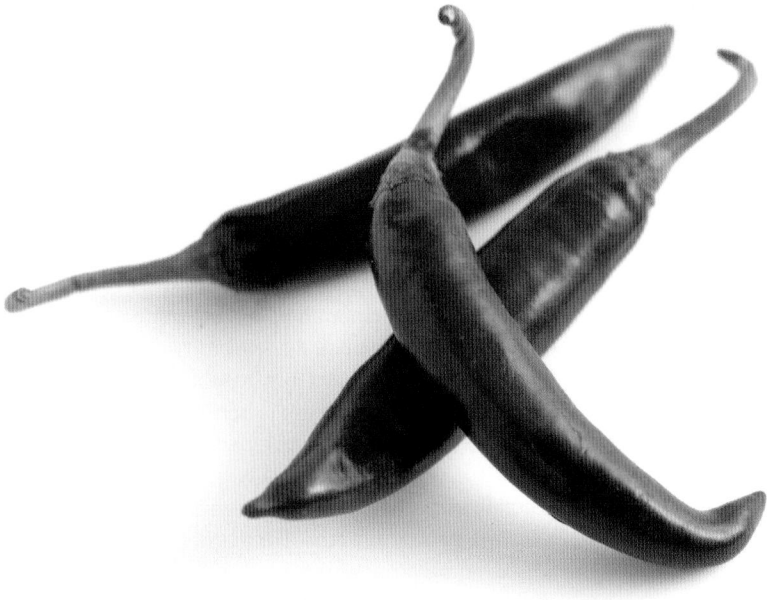

Red Onion Relish

¼ cup (60 ml) olive oil
2 lb (900 g) red onions, sliced
½ cup (110 g) sugar
1 teaspoon salt
½ teaspoon freshly ground black pepper
4 tablespoons balsamic or sherry vinegar
1 cup (250 ml) red wine

Makes 2 half-pint (250 ml) jars

A noteworthy accompaniment to almost any variety of cheese, this red onion treat is cheaper and tastier when made at home.

1. In a large, nonreactive saucepan, heat the olive oil over medium heat. Add the onions and cook for about 20 minutes, stirring occasionally.
2. Stir the sugar, salt and pepper into the onions. Reduce the heat to low, cover the saucepan, and cook very gently for 10 minutes; if the heat is too high, use a heat diffuser.
3. Add the vinegar and wine, then cook, uncovered and stirring at regular intervals, for 20 to 30 minutes, until the mixture has the consistency of chutney. Skim off and discard any foam that forms during cooking.
4. Ladle the relish into two warm, sterilized, widemouthed, half-pint jars, leaving a ¼-inch space between the top of the relish and the rim of the jar.
5. Wipe the rims, cover and process for 10 minutes in boiling water (see Safe Bottling and Preserving, page 72). Cool, label, date and store in a cool, dark place; the onion relish will be ready to eat in 4 weeks. Once a jar has been opened, store in the refrigerator.

Pickled Spiced Plums

1⅔ cups (360 g) sugar
1 cup (250 ml) cider vinegar
4 cinnamon sticks, broken
1 tablespoon whole cloves
1 tablespoon black peppercorns
2–3 strips orange zest
2 lb (900 g) small, firm red or purple plums, scrubbed

Makes 2 quart (1 liter) jars

Enjoy the enticing spices of these aromatic plums—the perfect partner to roast pork or lamb.

1. In a saucepan, combine the sugar and 2⅔ cups (670 ml) water. Bring to a boil over medium-high heat, stirring to dissolve the sugar. Reduce the heat and simmer for 10 minutes.
2. Stir in the vinegar, cinnamon sticks, cloves, peppercorns and orange zest. Cover the pan and gently simmer for 15 minutes.
3. Using a sterilized skewer, prick each plum in several places. Divide the plums between two warm, sterilized, widemouthed, 1-quart jars. Pour the hot, spiced syrup over the plums to cover them, leaving a ¼-inch space between the top of the syrup and the rim of the jars.
4. Wipe the rims of the jars, cover and process for 25 minutes in boiling water (see Safe Bottling and Preserving, page 72). Cool, label, date and store in a cool, dark place; the plums will be ready to eat in 4 weeks. Once a jar has been opened, store in the refrigerator.

Safe bottling and preserving

Pickling and preserving your food extends its shelf-life by ridding it of microorganisms and discouraging their growth. A simple way to do this is with a "hot-water bath," where food is processed at a high enough temperature for a long enough time to knock out bugs. To prevent a fresh batch of bugs creeping in, it is essential that our freshly preserved or pickled goods go straight into jars that have just been sterilized, which again is very easy to do. You can buy preserving kits or put one together yourself. Here's what you need to do.

❖ **You will need:**

- 1 large, deep, heavy, nonreactive saucepan or stockpot with a tight-fitting lid
- 1 wire rack or basket to fit the saucepan
- Glass jars and lids (the jars and metal screw bands to hold the lids in place can be reused; new lids must be used every time)
- Tongs (to transfer hot jars)
- Additional wire racks for cooling the jars

❖ **Here is how to proceed:**

1 Start by sterilizing all the jars. Wash them in hot, soapy water, rinse thoroughly and place in a saucepan of boiling water that covers the jars by 1 inch; boil for 10 minutes. Remove the saucepan from the heat, but let the jars sit in the water until ready to use.

2 Prepare the lids following the manufacturer's directions.

3 Once the food is cooked, remove the cooking saucepan from the heat. Carefully remove the jars from the hot water and place on a wooden chopping board (placing them straight on a cold workbench could cause them to crack). Ladle the food into the warm, clean jars, leaving a ⅛ to ¼-inch space between the top of the food and the rim of the jar as specified in the recipe. Run a sterilized spatula around the inside of the jar to remove any large air bubbles.

4 Using a clean, damp cloth, wipe the rims of each jar. Following the manufacturer's directions, apply the lids and screw bands.

5 Place a wire rack in the processing saucepan and fill halfway with hot water. Place the filled jars on the rack, then add boiling water (pour around the jars, not directly on them) until they are covered by at least 1 inch of boiling water. Cover the saucepan. Set the saucepan over high heat and bring the water to a boil; begin timing when the water comes to a rolling boil. Process for the time specified in the recipe.

6 When the processing time has been reached, use the tongs to transfer the jars from the saucepan to a second wire rack and let the jars cool completely; be sure to leave space between the jars on the rack. Let the jars stand for 12 to 24 hours.

7 Gently press the center of each lid: if the depression in the center holds, the seal is good, so you can remove the screw band and store the jar; if the depression does not hold, the seal is not good and you should store the jar in the refrigerator and use the food immediately.

8 Label and date each jar. Store in a dark, cool (40°F to 60°F) storage space; check the seals periodically and just before opening. Any jar that leaks, or food that smells or looks questionable when opened, should be discarded. Never taste food to check for freshness.

Roasted Red Bell Peppers in Oil

4 lb (1.8 kg/about 8 medium) firm red bell peppers, halved, cored and seeded
2 tablespoons coriander seeds
1 tablespoon peppercorns
5 cloves garlic
5 bay leaves
olive oil, to cover

Makes 3 half-pint (250 ml) jars

Colorful and luscious, these bell peppers are a must for any antipasto platter and make a superb snack on crusty bread.

1 Place the bell peppers on a broiler pan or heavy-duty baking sheet, skin side up. Set the pan 2 to 3 inches from a preheated broiler and broil 8 to 10 minutes, turning the peppers every few minutes so their skins blacken evenly. Transfer the hot bell peppers to a large heatproof bowl, cover with plastic wrap and cool for about 10 minutes, until safe to handle. Peel the skins, then thickly slice the bell peppers.

2 Transfer the bell peppers to three warm, sterilized, widemouthed, half-pint jars, dividing them equally. Add some of the coriander seeds, peppercorns, garlic and bay leaves to each jar, dividing them equally and arranging bell peppers and spices attractively.

3 Pour olive oil into each jar to cover the bell peppers, leaving a ¼-inch space between the top of the oil and the rim of the jars. Using a sterilized skewer, expel any air bubbles from the oil. Wipe the rims of the jars, cover and store in the refrigerator for up to 1 month; the bell peppers will be ready to eat within a few days.

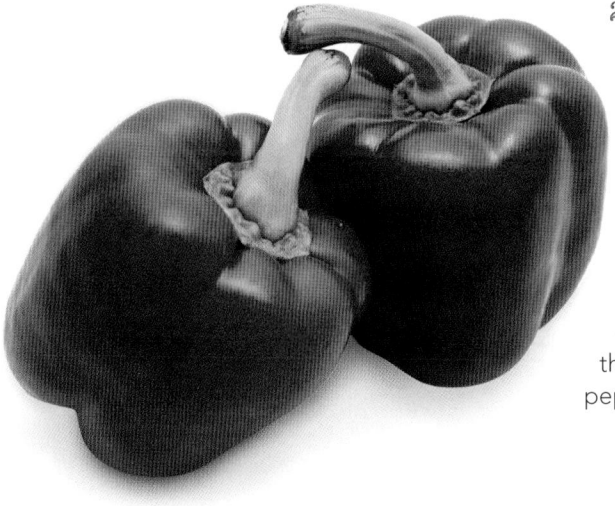

Oven-Dried Tomatoes

2 lb (1.8 kg) Italian plum or large cherry tomatoes, halved
¼ cup (75 g) pickling salt
¼ teaspoon freshly ground black pepper
2 tablespoons dried marjoram
olive oil, to cover

Makes 2 half-pint (500 ml) jars

Oven drying is an easy, relatively quick way to preserve garden-fresh tomatoes.

1 Preheat the oven to very low, just below 200°F.

2 Using a teaspoon, remove the seeds but not the fibrous tissue from the tomato halves. Line a baking sheet with foil. Place the tomatoes, cut side up, on the baking sheet and sprinkle them with the salt, pepper and marjoram. Place the baking sheet in the oven and bake for 12 to 24 hours; check periodically to be sure the tomatoes are drying, not cooking. As they dry, the tomatoes will slowly darken and wrinkle. Small tomatoes may take only 12 hours to dry; large tomatoes may take as long as 24 hours.

3 Spoon the tomatoes into two warm, sterilized, half-pint jars. Pour olive oil over the tomatoes to cover, leaving a ¼-inch space between the top of the oil and the rim of the jar. Wipe the rims of the jars, cover and cool. Label, date and store in the refrigerator for up to 1 month.

Chutneys

Mango Chutney

5 lb (2.25 kg) green mangoes (4–5), pitted, peeled and chopped
1 teaspoon pickling salt
1¼ cups (310 ml) cider vinegar
1¼ cups (310 ml) nonalcoholic apple cider, or apple juice
1 tablespoon chopped fresh ginger
2 teaspoons ground cayenne pepper
1 large onion, chopped
1½ cups (345 g) firmly packed dark brown sugar

Makes 6 half-pint (250 ml) jars

The pungent flavor of fresh ginger and the heat of cayenne pepper combine in this classic companion to spicy curries.

1 In a large, nonmetallic bowl, sprinkle the mangoes with the salt. Set aside for 24 hours.
2 Rinse the mangoes under cold, running water, then drain thoroughly and place in a very large, heavy, nonreactive saucepan. Add the vinegar, apple cider, ginger, cayenne pepper, onion and sugar. Simmer the mixture, uncovered, over low heat for 30 to 40 minutes.
3 Spoon the chutney into six warm, sterilized, widemouthed, half-pint jars, leaving a ¼-inch space between the top of the chutney and the rim of the jar. Wipe the rims, cover the jars and process for 10 minutes in boiling water (see Safe Bottling and Preserving, page 72). Cool, label, date and store in a cool, dark place; the chutney will be ready to eat in 4 weeks. Once a jar has been opened, store in the refrigerator.

Spicy Tomato Chutney

5 lb (2.25 kg) tomatoes
5 onions, chopped
3 cloves garlic, crushed
2 tablespoons mustard powder
1 tablespoon salt
1 tablespoon chopped fresh ginger
1 tablespoon cumin seeds
2 teaspoons ground turmeric
1 teaspoon mustard seeds
1 teaspoon ground cayenne pepper
1 cup (250 ml) cider vinegar

Makes 8 half-pint (250 ml) jars

Turmeric, cumin, mustard and cayenne pepper all add spice to this intense, easy-to-make chutney. Stir a dollop into curry as it is cooking to add even more flavor, then serve the chutney on the side for extra spice.

1 In a very large, heavy, nonreactive saucepan, combine all the ingredients. Bring the mixture to a boil over medium-high heat; reduce the heat to low and gently simmer, uncovered and stirring occasionally, for 50 to 60 minutes, until thickened.
2 Spoon the chutney into eight warm, sterilized, widemouthed half-pint jars, leaving a ¼-inch space between the top of the chutney and the rim of the jar. Wipe the rims, cover the jars and process for 10 minutes in boiling water (see Safe Bottling and Preserving, page 72). Cool, label, date and store in a cool, dark place; the chutney will be ready to eat in 4 weeks. Once a jar has been opened, store in the refrigerator.

Green Tomato Chutney

4 lb (1.8 kg) green tomatoes, chopped
2 onions, chopped
1 large green apple, peeled, cored and chopped
¾ cup (90 g) raisins
1 teaspoon salt
1 teaspoon ground allspice
1 teaspoon curry powder
½ teaspoon ground cayenne pepper
1 cup (230 g) firmly packed brown sugar
2 cups (500 ml) cider vinegar

Makes 6 half-pint (250 ml) jars

If it looks like all your tomatoes will ripen at once, harvest some green ones now and put up a few jars of this tasty condiment.

1. In a very large, heavy, nonreactive saucepan, combine all the ingredients. Over low heat, bring the mixture to a simmer and gently cook, uncovered, for about 45 minutes, until thickened. Stir occasionally to prevent the chutney burning; remove from the heat if the chutney begins to dry out.
2. Spoon the chutney into six warm, sterilized, widemouthed, half-pint jars, leaving a ¼-inch space between the top of the chutney and the rim of the jar. Wipe the rims, cover the jars and process for 10 minutes in boiling water (see Safe Bottling and Preserving, page 72). Cool, label, date and store in a cool, dark place; the chutney will be ready to eat in 4 weeks. Once a jar has been opened, store in the refrigerator.

Lemon Lime Chutney

4 large lemons, washed and wiped
2 limes, washed and wiped
2 onions, chopped
1 teaspoon salt
2½ cups (625 ml) cider vinegar
¾ cup (90 g) raisins
1 tablespoon mustard seeds
1 teaspoon ground ginger
½ teaspoon ground cayenne pepper
2 cups (440 g) sugar

Makes 5 half-pint (250 ml) jars

This citrus sensation is superb with mildly spiced couscous and lamb. It's an expensive luxury when store-bought, but an inexpensive treat when you make it at home.

1. Finely chop the whole lemons and limes, including the skin, and remove any seeds. In a large bowl, combine the chopped lemons, limes and onions. Sprinkle the mixture with the salt, then set aside for 12 hours.
2. Pour the lemon mixture and all the juices into a large, heavy, nonreactive saucepan. Bring the mixture to a simmer over medium heat, then gently cook, uncovered, until the fruit is soft. Stir in the vinegar, raisins, mustard seeds, ginger, cayenne pepper and sugar. Increase the heat and bring the mixture to a boil; reduce the heat and simmer, uncovered, for about 45 minutes, until thickened.
3. Spoon the chutney into five warm, sterilized, widemouthed, half-pint jars, leaving a ¼-inch space between the top of the chutney and the rim of the jar. Wipe the rims, cover and process for 10 minutes in boiling water (see Safe Bottling and Preserving, page 72). Cool, label, date and store the jars in a cool, dark place; the chutney will be ready to eat in 4 weeks. Once a jar has been opened, store in the refrigerator.

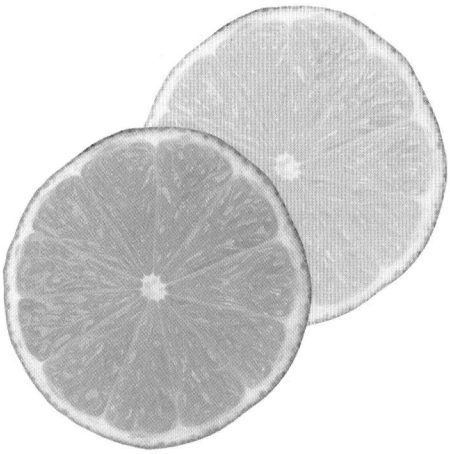

Jams, Jellies and Marmalades

Dried-Apricot Jam

2½ cups (450 g) dried apricots
3½ cups (875 ml) orange juice
¾ cup (165 g) sugar
1 tablespoon lemon juice
½ teaspoon ground cinnamon
¼ teaspoon ground ginger

Makes 4 half-pint (250 ml) jars

Buy dried apricots in bulk at health food stores, or look for them on sale and stock up. Using dried apricots intensifies the flavor, giving you a superior jam at a reasonable price.

1. In a very large, heavy, nonreactive saucepan or stockpot, combine the apricots, orange juice and sugar. Bring the mixture to a boil over medium-high heat; reduce the heat, cover the saucepan and simmer for 30 minutes.
2. Stir in the lemon juice, cinnamon and ginger. Remove the pan from the heat and let the mixture cool to room temperature.
3. Transfer the mixture to a food processor or blender and puree. Spoon the puree into four warm, sterilized, widemouthed, half-pint jars, leaving a ¼-inch space between the top of the jam and the rim of the jar. Wipe the rims, cover and process for 10 minutes in boiling water (see Safe Bottling and Preserving, page 72). Cool, label, date and store in a cool, dark place; the jam will be ready to eat in 2 weeks. Once a jar has been opened, store in the refrigerator.

The trio of good jamming ingredients

To make a great jam, jelly or marmalade, you need three components to work in harmony: acid, pectin and sugar. If the proportions of each or any one of these is off, you may not be happy with the results.

❖ **Acid** Added to the mixture as citrus juice (usually lemon) or tartaric acid, this improves both the taste and appearance of the finished product, and in conjunction with pectin, helps the mixture to jell.

❖ **Pectin** Most fruits contain some amount of pectin naturally and it is released when the fruit is boiled, but not all fruits are created equal. Apples are known for their pectin, so they are sometimes added in one form or another to fruits that are lower in pectin to help them jell. Currants and red plums are also high-pectin fruits; moderate-pectin fruits include apricots, blueberries, peaches and raspberries. Pectin is also found in peels (particularly citrus) and seeds, so these are sometimes included in part of a recipe to release their pectin during cooking. Pectin is also available in powdered form (check out health food stores and larger supermarkets) and in liquid form in some countries. If you make jams regularly, it is prudent to keep some pectin on hand, just in case your jam, marmalade or jelly is not setting. Always follow the manufacturer's directions carefully.

❖ **Sugar** Another factor in jelling, sugar also helps to preserve the fruit. It really brings out the flavor of the fruit, in addition to adding sweetness and countering any bitterness.

Lemony Fig Jam

2¾ cups (500 g) dried figs, washed and roughly chopped
3 cups (660 g) sugar
zest and juice of 2 lemons
½ cup (80 g) pine nuts, lightly toasted

Makes 3 half-pint (250 ml) jars

The tart lemons set off the sweet figs in this distinctively different jam. It makes a lovely gift without needing to go to an expensive food specialty store.

1. In a bowl, combine the figs and 4 cups (1 liter) water. Cover and let stand for 12 hours or overnight.
2. Transfer the figs and soaking water to a very large, heavy, nonreactive saucepan or stockpot. Bring the mixture to a boil over high heat; reduce the heat to low and simmer for 35 minutes.
3. Add the sugar, lemon zest and juice, and stir until the sugar has dissolved. Return the mixture to a boil, then reduce the heat slightly and cook for 10 to 15 minutes, until the jam thickens. Using a slotted spoon, skim off any foam that rises to the surface. Add the pine nuts and stir until well combined.
4. Remove the saucepan from the heat and stir to distribute the fruit and nuts evenly. Spoon the hot jam into three warm, sterilized, widemouthed, half-pint jars, leaving a ¼-inch space between the top of the jam and the rim of the jar. Wipe the rims, cover and process for 10 minutes in boiling water (see Safe Bottling and Preserving, page 72). Cool, label, date and store in a cool, dark place; the jam will be ready to eat in 2 weeks. Once a jar has been opened, store in the refrigerator.

Pear Jam

8 cups (about 2.5 kg) peeled, cored and chopped pears
4 cups (880 g) sugar
1 teaspoon ground cinnamon
¼ teaspoon ground cloves

Makes 6 half-pint (250 ml) jars

Jazzed up with cinnamon and cloves, this spicy jam can be made for very little money and doesn't require any pectin to thicken it.

1. In a very large, heavy, nonreactive saucepan or stockpot, combine all the ingredients. Simmer the mixture, uncovered, over medium-low heat for 1½ to 2 hours, until thickened. Occasionally stir the mixture while it cooks, increasing the frequency of stirring as the mixture thickens.
2. Remove the saucepan from the heat; skim off any foam that rises to the surface. Spoon the hot jam into six warm, sterilized, widemouthed, half-pint jars, leaving a ¼-inch space between the top of the jam and the rim of the jar. Wipe the rims, cover and process for 10 minutes in boiling water (see Safe Bottling and Preserving, page 72). Cool, label, date and store in a cool, dark place. Once a jar has been opened, store in the refrigerator.

Peach Jam

2½ lb (1 kg) peaches (about 4)
3 strips (½ x 2 inches) orange zest
⅔ cup (170 ml) fresh orange juice
⅔ cup (170 ml) unsweetened white grape juice
⅔ cup (155 g) firmly packed light brown sugar
1 tablespoon lemon juice
¼ teaspoon ground ginger

Makes 6 half-pint (250 ml) jars

The natural sweetness of peaches means you don't need to add much sugar. Peaches are cheap in summer, so buy them in season and put up enough jars for the year.

1 In a very large, heavy, nonreactive saucepan or stockpot, bring 8 to 10 cups (2 to 2.5 liters) water to a boil over medium-high heat. Add the peaches, two at a time, and boil for 30 seconds. Using a slotted spoon, transfer the peaches to a colander and rinse with cold water; the skins should slide off easily. Peel, pit and roughly chop the peaches.
2 Place the chopped peaches in a large, heavy, nonreactive saucepan or stockpot with the orange zest and juice, grape juice, sugar, lemon juice and ginger. Slowly bring the mixture to a boil over medium heat. Boil, stirring frequently, for about 30 minutes, until the jam thickens.
3 Remove the saucepan from the heat and stir to distribute the fruit evenly; skim off any foam that rises to the surface, then remove and discard the orange zest. Spoon the hot jam into six warm, sterilized, widemouthed, half-pint jars, leaving a ¼-inch space between the top of the jam and the rim of the jar. Wipe the rims, cover and process for 10 minutes in boiling water (see Safe Bottling and Preserving, page 72). Cool, label, date and store in a cool, dark place. Once a jar has been opened, store in the refrigerator.

Melon Ginger Jam

6¼ cups (1 kg) peeled, seeded and finely chopped jam melon
1 cup (220 g) glacé ginger, diced, or ½ cup (100 g) peeled, finely chopped fresh ginger
4½ cups (1 kg) sugar
juice of 6 lemons
¼ teaspoon ground cayenne pepper

Makes 4 half-pint (250 ml) jars

This recipe uses the low-sugar jam melon, the variety traditionally used in jam rather than eaten fresh. You won't often find these in stores, but you can grow it from seed; alternatively, use casaba or honeydew melon.

1 In a nonreactive bowl, combine the melon, ginger and sugar, then leave overnight.
2 Place the melon mixture in a very large, heavy, nonreactive saucepan or stockpot and boil until it is transparent. Add the lemon juice and cayenne pepper, then continue to boil for 5 to 10 minutes, until the jam reaches the jelling point (see Has It Jelled Yet? page 81). Using a slotted spoon, skim off any foam that rises to the surface.
3 Remove the saucepan from the heat. Spoon the hot jam into four warm, sterilized, widemouthed, half-pint jars, leaving a ¼-inch space between the top of the jam and the rim. Wipe the rims, cover and process for 10 minutes in boiling water (see Safe Bottling and Preserving, page 72). Cool, label, date and store in a cool, dark place; the jam will be ready to eat in 2 weeks. Once a jar has been opened, store in the refrigerator.

Strawberry Jam

4 cups (600 g) strawberries, washed and hulled
¼ cup (60 ml) lemon juice
1 package (about 1¾ oz/50 g) powdered fruit pectin
7 cups (1.5 kg) sugar

Makes 8 half-pint (250 ml) jars

The price of this dainty fruit goes way down in summer. Look for the ripest, reddest berries for the best flavor.

1. Place the strawberries in a bowl and crush them, using a potato masher. You should have about 4 cups of crushed berries.
2. Transfer the crushed berries to a very large, heavy, nonreactive saucepan or stockpot and add the lemon juice. Stir in the pectin, checking the manufacturer's directions to make sure that one package of pectin is appropriate for 4 cups of strawberries. Bring the mixture to a boil over high heat, stirring occasionally, then add the sugar and stir until dissolved. Boil, stirring constantly, for 1 minute.
3. Remove the saucepan from the heat. Using a slotted spoon, skim off any foam that rises to the surface.
4. Spoon the hot jam into eight warm, sterilized, widemouthed, half-pint jars, leaving a ¼-inch space between the top of the jam and the rim of the jar. Wipe the rims, cover and process for 10 minutes in boiling water (see Safe Bottling and Preserving, page 72). Cool, label, date and store in a cool, dark place; the jam will be ready to eat in 2 weeks. Once a jar has been opened, store in the refrigerator.

Three-Berry Jam

4 cups (620 g) blueberries, fresh or frozen
2½ cups (310 g) raspberries, fresh or frozen
2½ cups (375 g) strawberries, fresh or frozen
¼ cup (60 ml) lemon juice
2 packages (1¾ oz/50 g each) powdered fruit pectin
11 cups (2.4 kg) sugar

Makes 6 pint (500 ml) jars

This sweet salute to summer makes the most of berries in season. Combining three berries makes a deliciously different jam that is so much cheaper than store-bought.

1. In a very large, heavy, nonreactive saucepan or stockpot, combine the blueberries, raspberries, strawberries and lemon juice. Slightly crush the fruit using the back of a wooden spoon. Stir in the pectin, checking the manufacturer's directions to ensure that two packages of pectin are appropriate for the quantity and type of berries. Bring the mixture to a boil over high heat, stirring constantly.
2. Add the sugar, return the mixture to a boil, then boil for 1 minute, stirring constantly. Remove the saucepan from the heat; skim off any foam that rises to the surface.
3. Spoon the hot jam into six warm, sterilized, widemouthed, pint jars, leaving a ¼-inch space between the top of the jam and the rim of the jar. Wipe the rims, cover and process for 15 minutes in boiling water (see Safe Bottling and Preserving, page 72). Cool, label, date and store in a cool, dark place. Once a jar has been opened, store in the refrigerator.

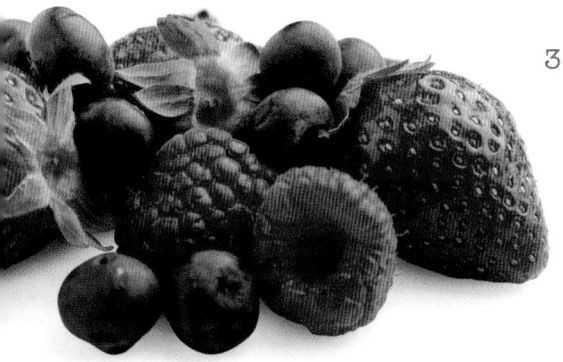

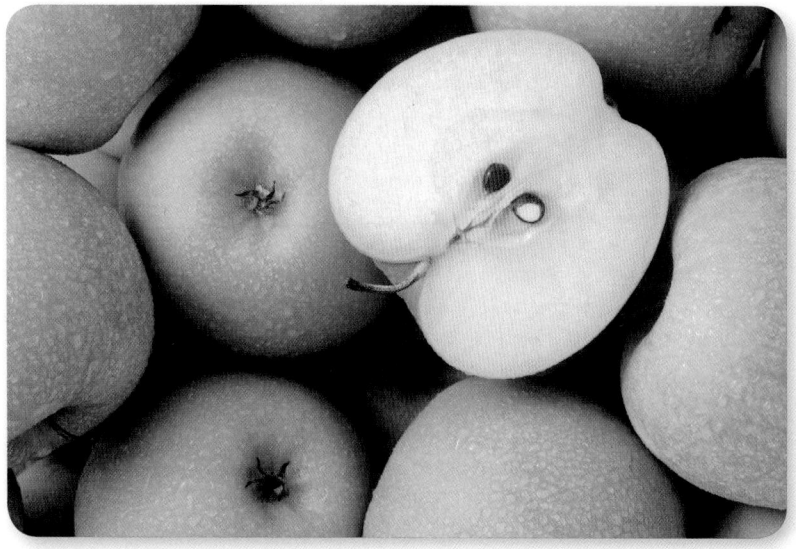

Apple Ginger Jelly

5 lb (2.5 kg) green apples (8–10), roughly chopped, core and peel intact
½ cup (125 ml) lemon juice
1 inch (3 cm) piece fresh ginger, peeled and bruised
sugar

Makes 5 half-pint (250 ml) jars

Although you remove the solids later, the naturally rich pectin in the apple seeds means you don't need to add commercial pectin to this delicious jelly.

1 In a very large, heavy, nonreactive saucepan or stockpot, combine the apples, lemon juice, ginger and 6 cups (1.5 liters) water. Bring the mixture to a simmer over medium heat, then simmer for 25 to 30 minutes, until the fruit is very soft.
2 Strain the apple mixture through a wet jelly bag overnight (see A Bag to Give You Perfectly Clear Jelly, page 82).
3 Measure the juice; to each 1 cup (250 ml) juice, you'll need ¾ cup (165 g) sugar. In a large, nonreactive saucepan over medium-high heat, bring the apple juice to a boil; add the appropriate amount of sugar and stir until the sugar has dissolved. Slightly reduce the heat and gently boil the mixture for 5 to 10 minutes, until the jelly reaches the jelling point (see Has It Jelled Yet?, opposite). Using a slotted spoon, skim off any foam that rises to the surface.
4 Remove the saucepan from the heat. Spoon the hot jelly into five warm, sterilized, widemouthed, half-pint jars, leaving a ¼-inch space between the top of the jelly and the rim of the jar. Wipe the rims, cover and process for 10 minutes in boiling water (see Safe Bottling and Preserving, page 72). Cool, label, date and store in a cool, dark place; the jelly will be ready to eat in 2 weeks. Once a jar has been opened, store in the refrigerator.

Grape Jelly

3 pounds Concord grapes
3¼ cups water
¾ cup sugar for every 1 cup juice

Makes about 8 half-pint (250 ml) jars

Peanut butter's best friend, grape jelly is a childhood favorite. Look for Concord grapes in season (September and October).

1. Wash the grapes and remove them from the stems. In a heavy, nonreactive saucepan, combine the grapes and water. Using a potato masher, crush the grapes. Over moderately high heat, bring the mixture to a boil; cover the saucepan, and cook for 10 to 15 minutes. Remove the saucepan from the heat and let the mixture cool to room temperature.
2. Strain the grape mixture through a wet jelly bag overnight (see A Bag to Give You Perfectly Clear Jelly, page 82).
3. Measure the juice left after the straining; this will determine how much sugar to add. In a large, nonreactive saucepan over medium-high heat, bring the grape juice to a boil; add the appropriate amount of sugar and stir until the sugar has dissolved. Increase the heat and boil rapidly until the jelly reaches the jelling point (see Has It Jelled Yet? below), about 12 to 16 minutes. Using a slotted spoon, skim off and discard any foam that rises to the surface.
4. Remove the saucepan from the heat. Spoon the hot jelly into 4 warm, sterilized, widemouthed, half-pint jars, leaving a ¼-inch space between the top of the jelly and the rim of the jar.Wipe the rims, cover, and process for 10 minutes in boiling water (see Safe Bottling and Preserving, page 72). Dry, label and date. Store the jars of jelly in a cool, dark place; the jelly will be ready to eat in 2 weeks. Once a jar has been opened, store the jelly in the refrigerator.

Has it jelled yet?

The crucial moment in jam- and jelly-making is the temperature at which the mixture jells and no longer needs to be cooked. To determine that "jelling point," most cooking experts recommend that you use a candy thermometer, but the plate method works well, too.

❖ **Thermometer** Determine the jelling point for your altitude. Hold a candy thermometer vertically in a pot of boiling water. Read the temperature at eye level and add 8°F for the jelling point. From sea level to about 1,000 feet above, the boiling point should be 212°F and the jelling point is 220°F.

❖ **Plate method** At the point indicated in the recipe, remove the saucepan from the heat and drop a teaspoonful of the jam or jelly onto a small, cold plate. Lightly press the jam or jelly with a fingertip—the surface should wrinkle, which indicates that it has begun to jell. If the jam or jelly is still too liquid or does not pass the press test, return the saucepan to the heat and cook a few minutes longer, then retest.

Mint Jelly

1 cup (20 g) tightly packed fresh mint leaves
½ cup (125 ml) cider vinegar
3½ cups (770 g) sugar
1 package (about 1¾ oz/50 g) powdered pectin
5 drops green food coloring

Makes 3 or 4 half-pint (250 ml) jars

The classic, emerald-green accompaniment to lamb, this jelly makes an eye-catching gift. You can make your own very inexpensively, particularly if you have a patch of mint.

1 Wash the mint, remove the stems and coarsely chop the leaves. Place in a very large, heavy, nonreactive saucepan or stockpot with the vinegar, sugar and 1 cup (250 ml) water. Stir in the pectin, checking the manufacturer's directions to make sure that one package of pectin is appropriate for this quantity of jelly.
2 Over high heat, bring the mixture to a boil, stirring constantly. Remove the saucepan from the heat and add the food coloring. Place back over the heat, return to a boil, then boil for 30 seconds. Remove from the heat and strain the mixture through two layers of cheesecloth.
3 Spoon the hot jelly into three or four warm, sterilized, widemouthed, half-pint jars, leaving a ¼-inch space between the top of the jelly and the rim of the jar. Wipe the rims, cover and process for 10 minutes in boiling water (see Safe Bottling and Preserving, page 72). Cool, label, date and store in a cool, dark place. Once a jar has been opened, store in the refrigerator.

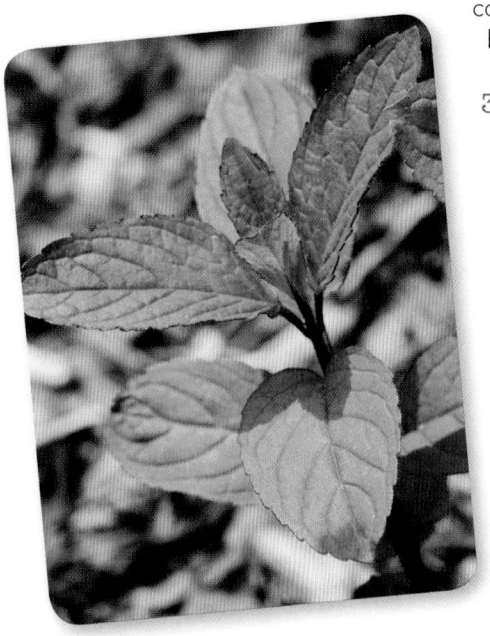

A bag to give you perfectly clear jelly

Jelly is meant to be crystal clear, unlike jams and marmalades, so removing even the tiniest solid particles is crucial to achieving perfect results. Fortunately, there is equipment to facilitate the desired finished product: a jelly bag.

Cone-shaped with a hanging handle, a jelly bag forces the solids out of the jelly mixture over a period of time (generally 12 hours or overnight). After boiling the fruit with the liquid, dampen the jelly bag and hang it over a large, nonreactive bowl or saucepan. Pour the boiled fruit and liquid through, then let it stand for the specified amount of time. The weight of the fruit solids will be enough to press down and push out the liquid; don't squeeze the bag to extrude more liquid or you may make the jelly cloudy.

How to make perfect marmalade

A dose of patience and careful attention to stirring are the two qualities needed to make marmalade—the first so you don't try to hurry the process, and the second to avoid scorching the fruit or syrup and tainting the finished taste. Unlike clear jelly, or thicker jam with pureed or chunks of fruit, marmalade is a thick syrup with bits of fruit that are cooked until they are almost translucent.

Seville Orange Marmalade

2 lb (1 kg, 4–6) Seville oranges, washed
juice of 3 lemons
8 cups (1.8 kg) sugar
¼ cup (90 ml) Scotch whisky (optional)

Makes 8 half-pint (250 ml) jars

This is what most people think of when they hear the word "marmalade." If Seville oranges are difficult to find, substitute any firm, thin-skinned variety, such as Valencia. Here, the pectin in the orange seeds helps the marmalade set.

1. Using a sharp knife, cut the oranges crosswise into thin slices, catching any juice and reserving the seeds. Combine the oranges with their juice in a large bowl with 4 cups (1 liter) water. Tie the reserved seeds in a bag of cheesecloth and add it to the bowl. Cover the bowl and let the orange mixture stand in a cool place for 18 hours.
2. Transfer the orange mixture to a very large, heavy, nonreactive saucepan or stockpot and add the lemon juice. Simmer the mixture, uncovered, over medium-low heat for 20 to 30 minutes, until the orange zest is tender.
3. Add the sugar and stir until it has dissolved. Bring the mixture to a boil and cook for 30 to 40 minutes, until the marmalade has reached the jelling point (see Has It Jelled Yet?, page 81). Using a slotted spoon, skim off any foam that rises to the surface.
4. Remove the saucepan from the heat, then stir to distribute the fruit evenly. Spoon the hot marmalade into eight warm, sterilized, widemouthed, half-pint jars, leaving a ¼-inch space between the top of the marmalade and the rim of the jar. Wipe the rims, cover and process for 10 minutes in boiling water (see Safe Bottling and Preserving, page 72). Cool, label, date and store in a cool, dark place; the marmalade will be ready to eat in 2 weeks. Once a jar has been opened, store in the refrigerator.

Citrus Marmalade

1 large grapefruit, washed
1 large orange, washed
1 large lemon, washed
12 cups (2.6 kg) sugar

Makes 8 half-pint (250 ml) jars

Popularity and tradition marry in this bright marmalade, composed of grapefruit, orange and lemon. Be sure to leave enough time, as it needs to stand for two 12-hour (or overnight) periods for the flavors to develop.

1 Using a sharp knife, cut the grapefruit, orange and lemon crosswise into thin slices, then cut each slice into quarters. Remove the seeds and tie in a bag of cheesecloth.
2 Combine the fruit, bag of seeds and 3 cups (750 ml) water in a very large, heavy, nonreactive saucepan or stockpot. Bring the mixture to a boil and cook for 10 minutes. Remove the saucepan from the heat, cover and let stand in a cool place for 12 hours.
3 Return the mixture to a boil over high heat; reduce the heat to medium and cook for about 40 minutes, until the zests are tender. Remove the pan from the heat, cover and let stand in a cool place for a further 12 hours.
4 Reheat the mixture over medium heat. Add the sugar and stir until the sugar has dissolved. Return the mixture to a boil and cook for 20 to 30 minutes, until the marmalade has reached the jelling point (see Has It Jelled Yet?, page 81). Using a slotted spoon, skim off any foam that rises to the surface.
5 Remove the saucepan from the heat, then stir to distribute the fruit evenly. Spoon the hot marmalade into eight warm, sterilized, widemouthed, half-pint jars, leaving a ¼-inch space between the top of the marmalade and the rim of the jar. Wipe the rims, cover and process for 10 minutes in boiling water (see Safe Bottling and Preserving, page 72). Cool, label, date and store in a cool, dark place; the marmalade will be ready to eat in 2 weeks. Once a jar has been opened, store in the refrigerator.

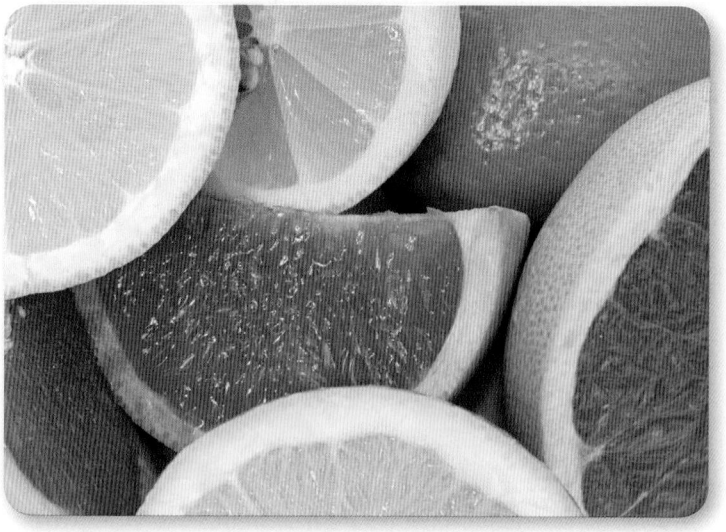

Frozen Vegetables

Freeze vegetables in self-sealing freezer bags that you have labeled and dated with a permanent marker; be sure to expel any excess air from the bag before sealing. Once the vegetables have thawed, do not refreeze.

Asparagus

2½–3 lb (1–1.3 kg) fresh yields 4 cups frozen

Wash, trim and cut into 2-inch pieces. Sort the asparagus according to the thickness of the spears; water-blanch thin spears for 2 minutes and thick spears for 4 minutes. Rinse briefly under cold water and drain thoroughly. Pack, seal, label, date and freeze.

Beets

2½–3 lb (1–1.3 kg) fresh yields 4 cups frozen

Wash and trim, leaving 1-inch stems (be careful not to pierce the skins). Sort according to size and cook small beets in boiling water for 25 to 30 minutes and large ones for 45 to 50 minutes, until tender when pierced with a fork. Drain and cool. Peel off the skins and slice or cube the flesh, as desired. Pack, seal, label, date and freeze.

Bell Peppers

3 lb (1.3 kg) fresh yields 4 cups frozen

Cut out the stems and any seeds. Halve or cut the bell peppers into slices or rings. Blanch the halves for 2 minutes and slices and rings for 1 minute. Cool quickly and drain thoroughly. Pack, seal, label, date and freeze.

How to blanch vegetables

You can blanch vegetables with either boiling water or steam. Which method you use—and the time required to do it—depends on the vegetable involved.

❖ **Water-blanching** Bring at least 12 cups (3 liters) water to a boil in a large saucepan. Place 1 pound prepared vegetable pieces in a wire-mesh basket and plunge into the boiling water. When the water returns to a boil, cook the vegetables for the time required. Lift the basket and place it into a large bowl of cold or ice water to cool; change the water or add ice to keep the water cold. Drain completely.

❖ **Steam-blanching** Place the prepared vegetables in a single layer inside a steamer basket in a large saucepan containing 2 inches of boiling water. Cover and steam the vegetables for the time required. Cool, but don't rinse the vegetables.

Broad and Lima Beans

2½ lb (1 kg) fresh yields 4 cups frozen

Shell young, tender beans and discard any damaged ones. Water-blanch small beans for 1 minute, medium beans for 2 minutes and large beans for 3 minutes. Cool quickly and drain thoroughly. Pack, seal, label, date and freeze.

Broccoli and Cauliflower

2–2½ lb (900 g–1 kg) fresh yields 4 cups frozen

Wash and peel the stalks if woody. Cut the stalks and florets into 1½-inch pieces. Steam-blanch for 5 minutes. Cool quickly and drain thoroughly. Pack, seal, label, date and freeze.

Brussels Sprouts

2–2½ lb (900 g–1 kg) fresh yields 4 cups frozen

Trim off coarse leaves and stems, then sort by size. Water-blanch small sprouts for 3 minutes, large sprouts for 5 minutes. Cool quickly and drain thoroughly. Pack, seal, label, date and freeze.

Carrots

2½–3 lb (1–1.3 kg) fresh yields 4 cups frozen

Wash, trim and, if desired, cut into 2-inch pieces or 2-inch slices. Blanch whole carrots for 5 minutes, slices for 2 minutes. Rinse briefly under cold water and drain thoroughly. Pack, seal, label, date and freeze.

Green Beans

1½–2½ lb (800 g–1 kg) fresh yields 4 cups frozen

Wash, then trim tops and any blemishes. Small green beans may be water-blanched whole; cut the larger beans into 2-inch pieces. Blanch whole beans for 3 minutes, pieces for 2 minutes. Cool quickly and drain thoroughly. Pack, seal, label, date and freeze.

Mushrooms

1–2½ lb (450 g–1 kg) fresh yields 4 cups frozen

Wipe with a damp cloth to remove any dirt; do not peel or rinse.
Button varieties: Spread whole, raw mushrooms on a baking tray and place in the freezer. When they are hard, pack, seal, label, date and freeze.
Wild mushrooms (portobello, shiitake): Slice and sauté in butter. Pour the mushrooms with the cooking liquid into individual bags. Seal, label, date and freeze.

Peas

2½ lb (1 kg) fresh yields 4 cups frozen

Peas: Shell the peas, discarding any damaged ones; water-blanch for 1½ minutes. Cool quickly and drain thoroughly. Pack, seal, label, date and freeze.
Sugar snap or snow peas: String the pods and water-blanch for 2 minutes. Cool quickly and drain thoroughly. Pack, seal, label, date and freeze.

Pumpkin and Sweet Potato

3 lb (1.3 kg) fresh yields 4 cups frozen puree

Wash, peel and cut in half; remove any seeds and strings. Cut into slices or cubes, then steam-blanch until tender. Mash and let cool completely. Pack in plastic dishes (leaving a ½-inch space at the top), then seal, label, date and freeze.

Sweet Corn

2½ lb (1 kg) fresh kernels yields 4 cups frozen

Ears: Use young cobs only; remove the husks and silks. Water-blanch for 4 minutes. Cool quickly and drain well. Individually wrap each ear in freezer paper or foil, molding it to the shape of the ear, so it is airtight. Pack several together in a freezer bag, expelling as much air as possible.
Kernels: Blanch the ears as above and cool completely. Using a very sharp knife, cut the kernels off the cobs and separate into meal-sized portions. Pack, seal, label, date and freeze.

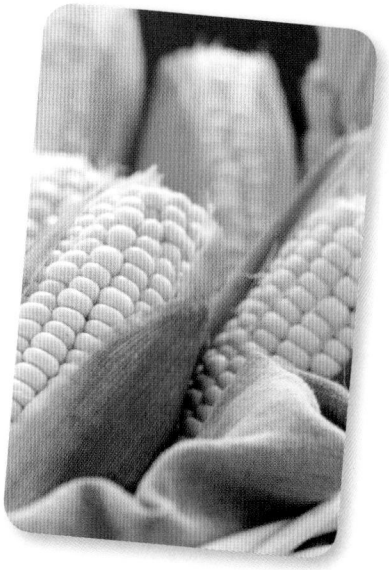

Mixed Vegetables

Mix together family favorites, such as peas and corn, peas and beans, or a stir-fry such as broccoli, carrot, baby corn, beans, mushrooms and red bell pepper.

Chop larger vegetables or cut them into bite-sized pieces. Blanch according to directions for each individual vegetable, noting that a shorter blanching time may be required for smaller piece size. When they are cool, mix the vegetables and pack in plastic freezer bags in meal-sized quantities. Seal, label, date and freeze.

Frozen Fruit

Use only unblemished fruit and keep the handling time to a minimum (fruit tends to brown when handled). To stop cut fruit from turning brown, follow the "dipping" instructions. Be sure to expel any excess air before sealing the freezer bags. Thaw frozen fruit in the bag in the refrigerator for several hours, or place the bag in a bowl of cool water for 30 minutes.

Apples

2½–3 lb (1–1.3 kg) fresh yields 4 cups prepared

Peel, core and slice the apples. Dip and drain the slices thoroughly. Arrange in a single layer on a rimmed tray and freeze until just firm. Pack, seal, label, date and freeze.

Apricots

1¼–1½ lb (600–700 g) fresh yields 4 cups prepared

Halve and pit the apricots, then slice if desired. Dip and drain the halves or slices thoroughly. Arrange in a single layer on a rimmed tray and freeze until just firm. Pack, seal, label, date and freeze.

Blackberries

1 lb (450 g) fresh yields 4 cups prepared

Remove the stems and leaves. Dip and drain the berries thoroughly. Arrange in a single layer on a rimmed tray and freeze until just firm. Pack, seal, label, date and freeze.

Blueberries

1–1½ lb (450–700 g) fresh yields 4 cups prepared

Remove any stems. Dip and drain the berries thoroughly. Arrange in a single layer on a rimmed tray and freeze until just firm. Pack, seal, label, date and freeze.

Cherries

2–3 lb (900 g–1.3 kg) fresh yields 4 cups prepared

Stem and pit the cherries. Dip and drain thoroughly. Arrange in a single layer on a rimmed tray and freeze until just firm. Pack, seal, label, date and freeze.

Mangoes

2½–3 lb (1–1.3 kg) fresh yields 4 cups prepared

Halve and pit the mangoes, then slice if desired. Dip and drain the halves or slices thoroughly. Arrange in a single layer on a rimmed tray and freeze until just firm. Pack, seal, label, date and freeze.

Peaches and Plums

2–3 lb (900 g–1.3 kg) fresh yields 4 cups prepared

Halve and pit the fruit, then slice, if desired. Dip and drain the slices or halves thoroughly. Arrange in a single layer on a rimmed tray and freeze until just firm. Pack, seal, label, date and freeze.

Raspberries

1 lb (450 g) fresh yields 4 cups prepared

Remove the stems and leaves. Dip and drain the berries thoroughly. Arrange in a single layer on a rimmed tray and freeze until just firm. Pack, seal, label, date and freeze.

Red Currants and Black Currants

1–1½ lb (450–700 g) fresh yields 4 cups prepared

Remove any stems. Dip and drain the currants thoroughly. Arrange in a single layer on a rimmed tray and freeze until just firm. Pack, seal, label, date and freeze.

Strawberries

1¼ lb (600 g) fresh yields 4 cups prepared

Remove the leaves and hull the strawberries; slice or leave whole. Dip and drain the berries thoroughly. Arrange in a single layer on a rimmed tray and freeze until just firm. Pack, seal, label, date and freeze.

How to prepare fruit for freezing

"Dipping" cut fruit before freezing stops it from browning. When working, keep fresh fruit in a bowl of acidulated water (about 8 cups/2 liters water with 1½ tablespoons of lemon juice or mild vinegar added). After dipping, drain the fruit on paper towels to remove as much moisture as possible. This prevents ice from forming around the pieces and stops them from sticking together.

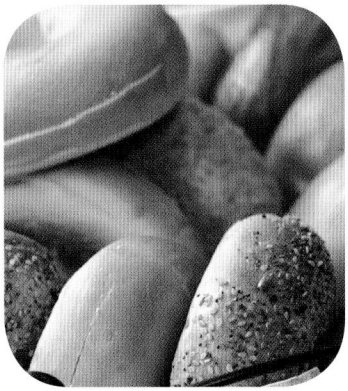

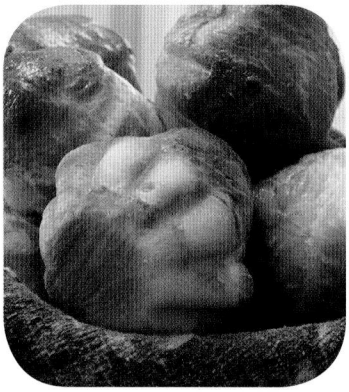

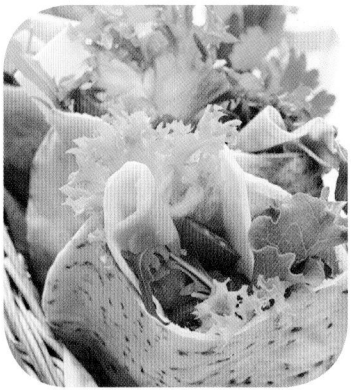

Quick Breads

Beer Bread ❖ Savory Zucchini Bread ❖ Corn Bread ❖ Cheese and Parsley Bread ❖ Irish Soda Bread ❖ Olive and Sun-Dried Tomato Bread ❖ Sesame Pumpkin Bread ❖ Banana Nut Bread ❖ Carrot Bread ❖ Pecan Bread ❖ Sweet Zucchini Bread

Yeast Breads

French Bread ❖ Multigrain Bread ❖ Soy and Linseed Bread ❖ Focaccia ❖ Challah ❖ Brioche ❖ Cinnamon-Raisin Swirl Bread ❖ Pita Bread ❖ Sourdough Bread

Muffins

Apple and Raisin Muffins ❖ Chocolate Chip Muffins ❖ Blueberry Muffins ❖ Bran Muffins ❖ Herb and Bacon Muffins ❖ Cranberry Cheddar Muffins

Rolls

Potato Dinner Rolls ❖ Bagels ❖ Crescent Rolls ❖ Cinnamon Rolls ❖ Hot Cross Buns ❖ Sticky Buns

Cakes

Spice Cake ❖ Chocolate Cake ❖ Devil's Food Cake ❖ Angel Cake ❖ Butter Cake ❖ Banana Cake ❖ Orange Cake ❖ Cheesecake with Strawberry Glaze ❖ Cupcakes ❖ Vanilla Icing ❖ Chocolate Ganache Icing ❖ Chocolate Buttercream Icing ❖ Simple Glaze Icing ❖ Cream Cheese Icing

Pies and Meringues

Basic Double Crust Pie Pastry ❖ Basic Single Crust Pie Pastry ❖ Puff Pastry ❖ Shortcrust Pastry ❖ Custard Pie ❖ Perfect Apple Pie ❖ Meringue Shells ❖ Pavlova

Cookies, Slices and Brownies

Chocolate Chip Cookies ❖ Oatmeal Cookies ❖ Peanut Butter Cookies ❖ Coconut Macaroons ❖ Gingersnaps ❖ Blondies ❖ Shortbread ❖ Sugar Cookies ❖ Brownies ❖ Graham Crackers

Baked Goods You Can Make

Nothing can compare to the aroma—or taste—of freshly baked bread from your own kitchen. But with the abundance of supermarket bread, it is not a pleasure that we encounter that often anymore.

The sad truth of the matter is that many of those packaged and wrapped breads, rolls, muffins, cakes, pies and cookies that you find in the typical supermarket may be made from bleached flour—flour that has been stripped of most of its healthy nutrients and fiber. These have often been replaced with additives and preservatives to give the product a longer shelf life.

If your baking has been limited to the occasional pie or birthday cake, you will be pleasantly surprised at how easy, fast and economical it is to make your own everyday baked goods such as bread, rolls and muffins. You will discover not only how much better they taste, but also the enormous variety of savory and sweet baked bread products you can serve, fresh and additive-free, to your family. The same is true of the really sweet baked goodies—there's an ample selection of cakes, pies and cookies on the following pages. Some of the cakes can be made in almost no time using the cake mix from Chapter 1, and you can make pies with handmade pastry that is flaky, with a rich flavor that complements any filling.

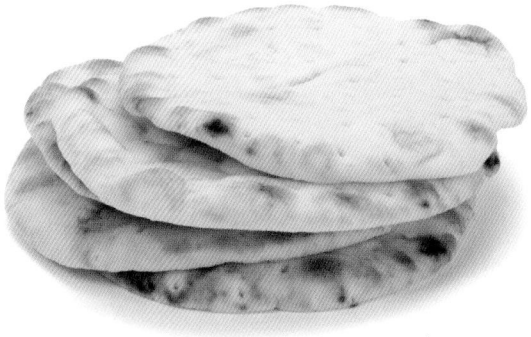

Quick Breads

Beer Bread

2½ cups (375 g) plain flour
2 tablespoons sugar
2 teaspoons baking powder
1 teaspoon salt
1 cup (250 ml) beer
¼ cup (60 g) plus 2 tablespoons butter, melted

Makes 1 loaf

The type of beer used will affect the flavor of the bread. Use a light lager for a mild taste—or be bold with a stout (such as Guinness) for a richer, darker flavor.

1. Preheat the oven to 350°F. Lightly grease an 8 x 14-inch loaf pan and line it with parchment paper.
2. In a large bowl, sift together the flour, sugar, baking powder and salt. Add the beer and the ¼ cup (60 g) melted butter, and stir until a soft dough forms.
3. Spoon the dough into the loaf pan and brush the remaining 2 tablespoons of melted butter over the top of the loaf. Bake until the loaf is golden brown and sounds hollow when tapped, 40 to 45 minutes. Turn the loaf out onto a wire rack to cool.

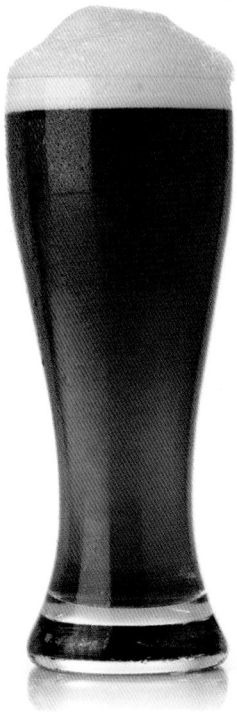

Savory Zucchini Bread

2 cups (300 g) plain flour
1 teaspoon baking powder
1 tablespoon sugar
1 teaspoon salt
⅓ cup (90 g) butter, chopped
1 cup (125 g) grated sharp cheddar
1 cup (250 ml) milk
1 large egg
1 cup (135 g) grated zucchini, squeezed dry in a dish towel to remove excess moisture
1 tablespoon grated onion
1 teaspoon Dijon mustard

Makes 1 loaf

Use this recipe to make a loaf or muffins—either version is a splendid backdrop to cream cheese, smoked salmon and a few capers. Toasted slices of this bread are delicious with a hearty soup.

1. Preheat the oven to 375°F. Lightly grease an 8 x 4-inch loaf pan.
2. In a large bowl, sift together the flour, baking powder, sugar and salt. Using a pastry blender or two knives, cut in the butter until the mixture resembles coarse crumbs. Stir in the cheese.
3. In a bowl, combine the milk and egg, and beat until well blended. Stir in the zucchini, onion and mustard. Add the milk mixture to the dry ingredients. Using a fork, stir just until all the ingredients are moistened and the dough holds together; do not overmix or the bread may be too heavy.
4. Spoon the dough into the loaf pan. Bake until the bread is well risen and brown and a toothpick inserted into the center of the loaf comes out clean, 40 to 45 minutes.
5. Transfer to a wire rack to cool in the pan for 10 minutes, then remove the bread from the pan and let it cool completely.

Corn Bread

1½ cups (225 g) plain flour
1¼ cups (185 g) cornmeal
4 teaspoons baking powder
2 tablespoons sugar
1 teaspoon salt
1 egg
1¼ cups (310 ml) cold milk
¼ cup (60 ml) vegetable oil

Makes 1 loaf (about 9 squares)

This beautiful yellow bread is a wholesome and tasty addition to any meal.

1 Preheat the oven to 400°F. Lightly grease an 8-inch square baking pan.
2 In a large bowl, sift together the dry ingredients. In a smaller bowl, combine the egg, milk and oil, then beat until well blended. Make a well in the center of the dry ingredients. Pour in the milk mixture all at once and, using a fork, stir just until the wet and dry ingredients are blended—do not overmix.
3 Pour the batter into the baking pan and bake until the bread pulls away slightly from the sides of the pan and is lightly browned, 20 to 25 minutes.
4 Transfer the pan to a wire rack and let the bread cool for 10 minutes. Cut into large squares and serve warm.

VARIATION

Corn muffins: Prepare the batter as above, but pour into well-greased or paper-lined muffin cups. Bake until the muffins are lightly browned and springy to the touch, 17 to 20 minutes.

Cheese and Parsley Bread

2 cups (300 g) whole wheat flour
1 teaspoon baking powder
1 teaspoon baking soda
¾ cup (90 g) grated cheddar or ¼ cup (25 g) grated Parmesan cheese
¼ cup (5 g) fresh parsley
1 teaspoon salt
¾ cup (185 ml) milk or buttermilk

Makes 1 loaf (8 wedges)

Golden, crusty, savory—this loaf is essentially a big scone and totally irresistible. Quick breads such as this are best eaten on the day they are made.

1 Preheat the oven to 450°F. In a food processor, place the flour, baking powder, baking soda, all but 1 tablespoon of the cheese, the parsley and salt. Process until the cheese crumbles into the flour and the parsley is finely chopped.
2 Add the milk or buttermilk all at once, and process just until a soft dough forms, about 5 seconds.
3 Lightly flour a work surface and a baking sheet. Turn the dough out onto the work surface and knead gently. Transfer to the baking sheet and form into a round loaf. Using a sharp knife, cut the dough almost through into 8 wedge-shaped pieces. Sprinkle the wedges with the remaining tablespoon of cheese.
4 Bake until the loaf is puffed and brown, 20 to 25 minutes. Remove the loaf from the oven, wrap it in a clean lint-free dish towel, and let it cool slightly. Cut through the marked wedges of the bread to serve.

Irish Soda Bread

4 cups (600 g) plain flour
3 tablespoons sugar
3 teaspoons baking powder
1 teaspoon salt
¾ teaspoon baking soda
⅓ cup (90 g) cold butter or margarine
1½ cups (225 g) currants or raisins
1 tablespoon caraway seeds
2 eggs, lightly beaten
1½ cups (375 ml) buttermilk

Makes 1 loaf

This easy-to-make bread can be topped with a sprinkling of seeds or oatmeal and is a wonderful accompaniment to stews and hearty soups.

1 Preheat the oven to 350°F. In a large bowl, sift together the flour, sugar, baking powder, salt and baking soda. Using a pastry blender or two knives, cut in the butter until the mixture resembles coarse crumbs. Stir in the currants or raisins and caraway seeds.
2 Set aside 1 tablespoon of the beaten egg. In a bowl, combine the buttermilk and remaining eggs and stir until well blended. Make a well in the center of the flour mixture. Pour the buttermilk mixture into the well and stir just until the flour is moistened and a sticky dough forms.
3 Flour a work surface well. Turn the dough out onto the work surface and, using well-floured hands, knead about 10 times. Shape the dough into a round loaf.
4 Lightly grease a 9-inch round baking pan. Place the loaf in the pan. Using a sharp knife, cut a cross, ¼-inch deep, in the top center of the loaf. Brush the loaf with the reserved egg.
5 Bake until a toothpick inserted near the center of the loaf comes out clean, about 1 hour and 20 minutes. If the top of the loaf browns too quickly, cover loosely with foil for the final 20 minutes of baking time. Transfer to a wire rack and cool in the pan for 10 minutes, then turn out the loaf and leave on the rack to cool completely.

If you run out of buttermilk

If a recipe calls for 1 cup (250 ml) buttermilk and you don't have any on hand, pour 1 tablespoon white vinegar or lemon juice into a 1 cup (250 ml) measure and add enough regular milk to make 1 cup. Or simply substitute 1 cup (250 g) natural yogurt.

Yeast Breads

French Bread

¼ oz (7 g) package dry yeast
1½ cups (375 ml) warm water (about 110°F–115°F)
1 tablespoon sugar
2 teaspoons salt
1 tablespoon butter, melted
4 cups (600 g) plain flour, plus extra for sprinkling
cornmeal, for sprinkling

Makes 2 loaves

Many meals can be finished off with a loaf of French bread to sop up the gravy, hold the cheese or complement the salad. Nothing is better, but unfortunately, nothing goes stale more quickly, so making your own not only saves money but also ensures a fresh, crusty loaf. Unusually, this recipe doesn't require kneading.

1. In a large bowl, combine the yeast with ½ cup (125 ml) of the water and stir until the yeast is dissolved. Add the sugar, salt, butter and remaining water and stir until all the ingredients are well blended. Add the flour and stir until the dough is smooth; do not knead. Cover the bowl and let the dough rise in a warm place until doubled in size, about 1 hour.
2. Lightly flour a work surface. Divide the dough in half; let the dough rest again for 10 minutes. Using a lightly floured rolling pin, roll one dough half into a 10 x 8-inch rectangle. Beginning on a long side, roll up the dough, jelly-roll-fashion; pinch the edges to seal the loaf. Repeat with the remaining dough half.
3. Lightly grease a baking sheet and sprinkle it with cornmeal. Place the loaves, seam side down, on the baking sheet; sprinkle the tops with additional cornmeal. Cover the loaves and let them rise in a warm place until doubled in size, about 45 minutes.
4. Preheat the oven to 400°F. Using a sharp knife, make five diagonal cuts across the top of each loaf. Bake the loaves until lightly browned, 20 to 30 minutes. Transfer the loaves to wire racks to cool.

Making yeast breads is easier than you think

One of the absolute best aromas in the world is that of fresh home-baked bread. You may have shied away from yeast breads in the past, thinking that yeast would be difficult to work with. Not at all. Just follow the package directions and you'll be turning out perfect loaves in no time. If you enjoy the aroma and the price of homemade bread but time is a factor, you may want to invest in a bread machine. Most recipes can be converted for a machine.

Multigrain Bread

2 teaspoons sugar
½ cup (125 ml) lukewarm water (about 105°F–115°F)
two ¼ oz (7 g) packages dry yeast
1¼–1½ cups (185–225 g) plain flour, plus extra for sprinkling
1 cup (150 g) whole wheat flour
1 cup (100 g) rye flour
⅓ cup (50 g) sifted stone-ground yellow or white cornmeal
¼ cup (20 g) wheat bran
¼ cup (25 g) wheat germ
1 cup (250 ml) buttermilk or natural yogurt
3 tablespoons butter, melted
1½ teaspoons salt

Makes 1 loaf

Whole wheat flour, rye flour, stone-ground cornmeal, wheat bran, wheat germ and buttermilk form this hearty, wholesome bread that your family will rave about. Your wallet will be pretty happy with it, too.

1 In a large bowl, combine the sugar, water and yeast. Stir until the solids are dissolved. Let stand until the mixture is bubbly, about 10 minutes.
2 In another large bowl, combine 1¼ cups (185 g) of the plain flour with the whole wheat and rye flours, cornmeal, wheat bran and wheat germ.
3 Place the buttermilk, butter and salt in a small saucepan and gently heat until the mixture is lukewarm.
4 Pour the buttermilk mixture into the yeast mixture. Using a wooden spoon or an electric mixer with the dough hook attached, beat at medium speed, adding the flour mixture 1 cup at a time, until the dough is soft but manageable; beat in the remaining ¼ cup (35 g) of plain flour if needed to reach the desired consistency. Continue to beat until the dough is smooth and elastic, 7 to 8 minutes. If mixing by hand, knead on a floured work surface for 8 to 10 minutes.
5 Generously butter a large bowl. Shape the dough into a ball and place it in the bowl, turning it until it is completely coated with butter. Cover the bowl with a dish towel and let the dough rise in a warm place until doubled in size, 1½ to 2 hours.
6 Lightly grease a 9 x 5 x 3-inch loaf pan; lightly flour a work surface. Punch down the dough and turn it out onto the work surface. Knead gently for 2 minutes. Shape the dough into a loaf, place it in the loaf pan, cover and leave to rise again until doubled in size, about 1 hour.
7 Preheat the oven to 375°F. Bake until the loaf is golden brown and sounds hollow when tapped, 40 to 45 minutes. Transfer the pan to a wire rack and let the bread cool for 10 minutes. Using a knife, loosen the edges of the bread from the sides of the pan and turn the loaf out onto the wire rack to cool completely.

Soy and Linseed Bread

3⅓ cups (500 g) finely milled bread flour, plus extra for kneading
1 teaspoon salt
2 teaspoons superfine sugar
2 teaspoons instant dry yeast
1½ cups (375 ml) warm water
2 cans (14 oz/400 g) soybeans, drained
2 tablespoons linseeds
2 teaspoons milk

Makes 1 loaf

Soybeans and linseeds are said to be great for women's health. Add them to your diet with this chewy loaf.

1 Sift 3 cups (450 g) of the flour into a bowl. Stir in the salt, sugar and yeast. Make a well in the center, add the warm water and mix to form a soft dough. Turn the dough out onto a lightly floured surface and knead for 10 minutes, incorporating the remaining flour, until smooth and elastic.
2 Place the dough in a lightly oiled bowl and cover with lightly greased plastic wrap. Let the dough rise in a warm place until doubled in size, about 1 hour.
3 Preheat the oven to 375°F and grease a large baking sheet. Punch the dough down and turn it out onto a lightly floured surface. Add the soybeans and linseeds and knead into the dough until well combined. Shape the dough into a 6 x 10-inch oval, place on the baking sheet and cut shallow slits across the top at 2-inch intervals. Brush with milk. Bake for 30 minutes, or until golden brown and hollow when tapped on top. Leave on the sheet for 5 minutes, then transfer to a wire rack to cool.

Focaccia

¼ oz (7 g) package dry yeast
¼ teaspoon sugar
2 cups (500 ml) warm water (about 105°F–110°F)
4½–5½ cups (675–825 g) bread flour or plain flour
¼ cup (60 ml) olive oil, plus extra for drizzling
1 tablespoon salt
tiny sprigs fresh rosemary
sea salt

Makes 2 loaves

This chewy Italian bread can be topped with vegetables, grilled meats, cold cuts, cheese—or just olive oil.

1 In a small bowl, combine the yeast, sugar and water. Stir until the solids are dissolved. Let stand until the mixture is bubbly, about 10 minutes.
2 Pour 4½ cups (675 g) of the flour into a large bowl and make a well in the center. Pour the yeast mixture, oil and salt into the well, then stir until well blended. Add additional flour as needed to reach the desired consistency.
3 Lightly flour a work surface; lightly coat a large bowl with olive oil. Turn the dough out onto the work surface and knead until smooth, about 10 minutes. Place the dough in the bowl, turning it to coat with the oil. Cover the bowl with lightly oiled plastic wrap and set in a warm place to rise for 1 hour.
4 Lightly grease two baking sheets. Divide the dough in half and spread them on the sheets. With your fingers, press down and outward until each is a round loaf about ½-inch thick. Cover with lightly oiled plastic wrap and let rise for 10 to 20 minutes.
5 With your fingers, press the loaves down and out again. Cover again and let the loaves rise for 30 minutes.
6 Preheat the oven to 425°F. With your fingers, indent the loaves all over. Press a sprig of rosemary into each dent, drizzle with oil, then sprinkle with salt. Bake until firm and golden, about 25 minutes. Serve warm.

Challah

two ¼ oz (7 g) packages dry yeast
1 cup (250 ml) warm water (about 110°F–115°F)
½ cup (125 ml) vegetable oil
⅓ cup (75 g) sugar
1 tablespoon salt
5 eggs
6–6½ cups (900–975 g) plain flour
1 tablespoon sesame or poppy seeds (optional)

Makes 2 loaves

The traditional bread of the Jewish Sabbath, this attractive loaf is braided and given a shiny coating of egg wash.

1 In a large bowl, combine the yeast and the warm water and stir until the yeast has dissolved. Add the oil, sugar, salt, 4 eggs and 4 cups (600 g) of the flour. Beat until all the ingredients are well blended and the consistency is smooth. Stir in enough of the remaining flour to form a firm dough.
2 Lightly flour a work surface. Turn the dough out onto the work surface and knead until firm and elastic, 6 to 8 minutes. Lightly grease a large bowl with butter or oil, place the dough in the bowl and turn it to coat the entire ball. Cover the bowl and let the dough rise in a warm place until doubled in size, about 1 hour.
3 Punch down the dough, turn it out onto another floured work surface, and divide in half. Divide each portion into thirds, then roll each piece into a rope about 15 inches long.
4 Lightly grease a baking sheet. Place three dough ropes on the sheet, pinching them together at one end. Braid the ropes together and pinch the opposite ends to seal them, then tuck the pinched ends under at both ends. Repeat with the remaining dough ropes to make a second loaf. Cover the loaves with a dish towel and let rise again until doubled in size, about 1 hour.
5 Preheat the oven to 350°F. In a small bowl, beat the remaining egg with 1 teaspoon cold water. Brush the egg mixture over the loaves. If desired, sprinkle the loaves with the sesame or poppy seeds. Bake until golden brown, 30 to 35 minutes. Transfer the loaves to wire racks and let them cool completely.

Take a mix-and-match approach to gift baskets

When pondering gift-giving with your own homemade items, take a tip from those high-end catalogues and pair natural partners in an attractive package—breads with jams, jellies or marmalades; pasta with homemade sauces; cookies with cocoa, coffee or tea blends; muesli with fresh-baked muffins; canned fruit with a dessert sauce; soup with hearty rolls; pita breads with hummus. Whenever you browse through a garage sale, look for baskets, saucepans, ceramic or porcelain bowls and other fun packaging for your personalized gifts.

Brioche

2⅓ cups (350 g) plain flour
½ teaspoon salt
3½ oz (100 g) butter, softened
1 teaspoon dry yeast
⅓ cup (80 ml) lukewarm milk
3 eggs
1½ tablespoons sugar
1 egg yolk, for brushing

Makes 20 brioche

Sweet and buttery, these French breakfast rolls are beautiful to look at and delicious to eat. Although they require a little bit of work, the result is spectacular.

1 If you have them, grease individual fluted brioche pans generously with butter. Otherwise, use two standard muffin pans.
2 Place the flour, salt and butter in a bowl. In a small bowl, sprinkle the yeast over the milk and stir until dissolved. Whisk in the eggs and sugar, then add to the flour mixture. Knead for 5 minutes using the dough hook of an electric mixer until the dough no longer sticks to the side of the bowl. (This dough is wet and sticky; an electric mixer makes the task of kneading much easier than if you try to work with your hands.)
3 Cover the dough and leave to rise in a cool place for 2 hours; it must not get too warm. Knead for 5 minutes, then cover and leave to rise again for 30 to 50 minutes, until doubled in size.
4 Turn the dough out onto a lightly floured work surface and shape into a cylinder. Slice into 25 pieces. Shape 20 pieces into balls and press them into the pans.
5 Using an index finger, make a deep hole in the center of each of the 20 balls. Cut each remaining piece of dough into four, then shape into small balls. Pull a pointed cone of dough up from each one and push the point deep into the holes made in the large dough balls.
6 Beat the egg yolk with 2 tablespoons water and brush over the brioche. Cover with a dish towel and leave for 30 minutes, until doubled in size.
7 Preheat the oven to 425°F. Bake the brioche for 15 to 20 minutes, or until golden; they should slip out of the pans easily when they are done. Transfer to wire racks to cool.

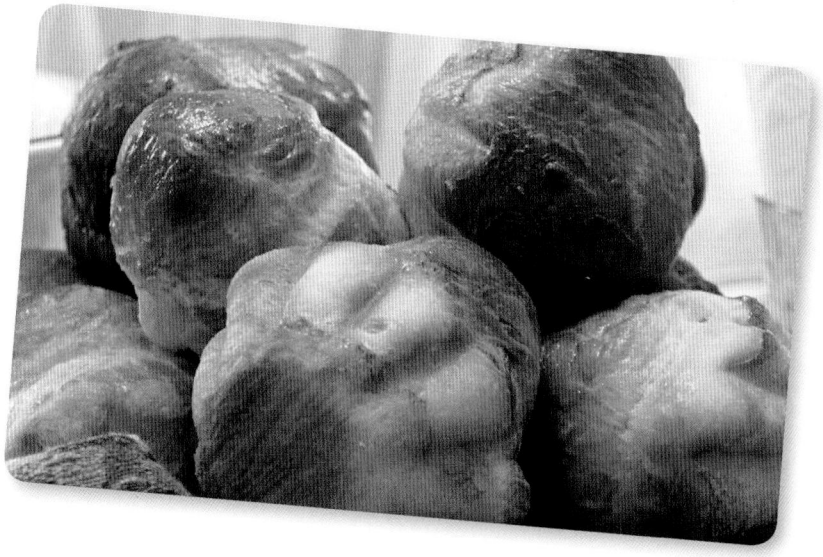

Cinnamon-Raisin Swirl Bread

1 cup (250 ml) lukewarm milk (about 105°F–115°F)
two ¼ oz (7 g) packages dry yeast
1½ tablespoons sugar
2¼ cups (625 ml) lukewarm water (about 105°F–115°F)
5 tablespoons (75 g) butter or margarine, melted
2 teaspoons salt
6–6½ cups (900–975 g) plain flour
1 cup (125 g) seedless raisins, soaked in hot water for 15–30 minutes, drained well

CINNAMON SWIRL FILLING
½ cup (110 g) sugar
1 tablespoon ground cinnamon
3 tablespoons butter or margarine, melted

ICING
2 cups (250 g) sifted confectioners' sugar
2 tablespoons water

Makes 2 loaves

This beautiful bread—spiraled with cinnamon, thick with raisins and drizzled with icing—is a treat for all the senses and will fill your house with a delicious aroma as it bakes.

1 In a large bowl, combine the milk, yeast and 1 teaspoon of the sugar. Stir until the solids are dissolved. Let stand until the mixture is bubbly, about 10 minutes. In a bowl, combine 1¼ cups (310 ml) of the warm water, 4 tablespoons of the butter, the salt and the remaining sugar. Stir the butter mixture into the yeast mixture.
2 Using a wooden spoon or an electric mixer with a dough hook attached, beat in the flour, 1 cup (150 g) at a time, until a soft dough forms. Continue to beat at medium speed until the dough is elastic, 7 to 8 minutes. If mixing by hand, knead on a floured work surface for 8 to 10 minutes.
3 Pour the remaining butter into a large bowl. Shape the dough into a ball and place in the bowl, turning it to completely coat it with butter. Cover the bowl with a dish towel and let the dough rise in a warm place until doubled in size, about 1 hour.
4 Lightly butter two 9 x 5 x 3-inch loaf pans. Lightly flour a work surface. Punch down the dough and turn it out onto the work surface. Knead the dough gently for 2 minutes. Divide the dough in half, cover and rest for 5 to 10 minutes. Working with one half at a time and using a rolling pin, roll each portion into a 9 x 15-inch rectangle. Sprinkle half the raisins over each portion of the dough and gently knead until evenly distributed. Cover the dough and rest for 10 minutes.
5 For the filling, combine the sugar, cinnamon and 2 tablespoons of the butter in a small bowl and stir until well blended. Using a rolling pin on a floured surface, again roll each dough half into a 9 x 15-inch rectangle. Spread each half with half the filling. Beginning on a short side, roll up the dough, jelly-roll fashion, to make a loaf; repeat with the remaining dough. Place the loaves, seam side down, in the loaf pans, cover with a dish towel and let rise for 1 hour.
6 Preheat the oven to 400°F. Brush the tops of the loaves with the remaining tablespoon of butter. Bake until the bread is brown and sounds hollow when tapped, 35 to 40 minutes. Transfer the pans to wire racks and let the bread cool for 10 minutes. Using a knife, loosen the edges of the bread from the sides of the pans, turn out the bread and leave on the wire racks to cool.
7 For the icing, combine the confectioners' sugar and water in a small bowl and stir until smooth. Brush, pour or drizzle the icing over the cooled loaves.

Pita Bread

1½ cups (375 ml) warm water (about 105°F–110°F)
1 teaspoon dry yeast
1 teaspoon sugar
3 cups (450 g) bread flour or plain flour
1 heaped teaspoon salt
1½ teaspoons olive oil, plus extra for drizzling
3 tablespoons finely chopped fresh herbs, such as thyme, rosemary, coriander or parsley (optional)

Makes 4 pita breads

This popular staple of Middle Eastern and Mediterranean cuisine is a wonderfully versatile bread. You can stuff the pockets with almost anything you can think of to make a sandwich; slice the bread into triangles, toast it and serve with any dip; or even top it with tomato paste, marinated vegetables and mozzarella for a variation on pizza.

1 In a large bowl, combine the water and yeast; stir until the yeast has dissolved. Add the sugar and 1½ cups (225 g) of the flour. Using the paddle attachment of an electric mixer, stir until well blended. Cover the bowl with lightly oiled plastic wrap and let the dough rise in a warm place until doubled in size, about 2 hours.
2 Add the salt, olive oil and remaining flour. Again using the paddle attachment, beat the mixture until it is smooth and elastic, 5 to 10 minutes.
3 Lightly flour a work surface and lightly oil a large bowl. Turn the dough out onto the work surface and knead until smooth and elastic, 10 to 12 minutes. Place the dough in the bowl, turning it to completely coat it with the oil. Cover the bowl with lightly oiled plastic wrap and let the dough rise in a warm place for 1½ hours.
4 Preheat the oven to 475°F. Line a baking sheet with parchment paper or foil.
5 Lightly flour the work surface again and turn out the dough. Divide the dough into four balls. Using a rolling pin, roll each ball into a circle about ½ inch thick and 6 inches in diameter. Place on the baking sheet, lightly brush each one with oil and, if desired, sprinkle with herbs. Bake until the pita breads are golden, about 8 minutes. Transfer to wire racks to cool.

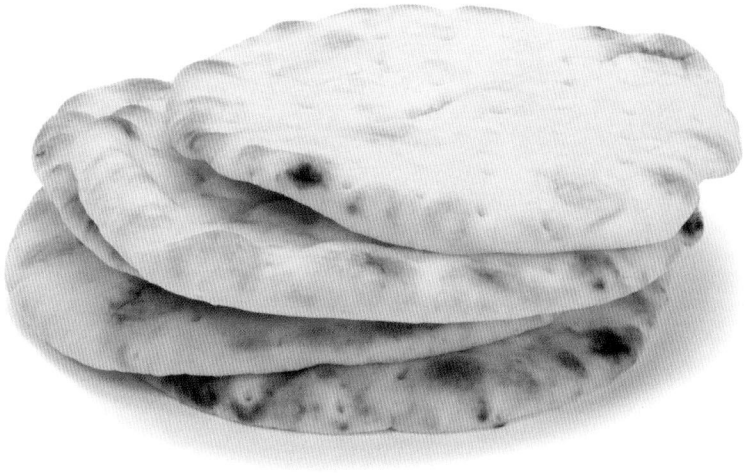

Sourdough Bread

STARTER
2 cups (500 ml) lukewarm water (about 105°F–115°F)
¼ oz (7 g) package dry yeast
1½ cups (225 g) bread flour

DOUGH
1½ cups starter (see above)
2 tablespoons sugar
1 tablespoon salt
5–6 cups (750–900 g) bread flour
4 tablespoons (½ stick/80 g) butter, melted

Makes 2 loaves

The starter is essential to the chewy texture and signature flavor of sourdough bread. Once you have a starter, you use some for each loaf you bake, but continue to feed the starter to keep it going—an endless supply for a sensational bread.

1 Combine the starter ingredients in a glass or ceramic bowl and whisk until well blended. Cover the bowl loosely with waxed paper and set in a warm place for 12 hours or overnight.
2 To prepare the dough, combine the starter in a large bowl with the sugar, salt, 2½ cups (375 g) of the flour and 1 cup (250 ml) water. Using a wooden spoon or the paddle attachment of an electric mixer, beat the dough at medium speed until smooth, about 15 seconds.
3 If using an electric mixer, remove the paddle and attach a dough hook. Add ¼ cup (60 ml) of the melted butter and 2½ cups (375 g) of the remaining flour, ½ cup (75 g) at a time. Continue beating for about 10 minutes, adding an extra ½ to 1 cup (75 to 150 g) of flour, if necessary, to make a smooth and elastic dough. (If mixing by hand, you will probably have to knead in the last of the flour.)
4 Generously butter a large bowl. Using your hands, shape the dough into a ball and place in the bowl, turning it to completely coat it with the butter. Cover the bowl with a dish towel and let the dough rise in a warm place until doubled in size, 1 to 1½ hours. Punch down the dough, cover again and allow to rise for 1½ hours longer.
5 Lightly flour a work surface and lightly grease two 8-inch-round cake or springform pans. Punch down the dough again and turn out onto the work surface. Knead lightly until the dough is smooth, 2 to 3 minutes. Divide the dough in half and roll each half into a ball. Place one ball in each pan, cover both with a dish towel and let rise again until the dough is doubled in size, 45 minutes to 1 hour.
6 Preheat the oven to 350°F. Brush the loaves with the remaining melted butter. Using a sharp knife, cut a diagonal slash across the top of each loaf. Bake until the loaves are richly golden and sound hollow when tapped, 45 to 50 minutes. Transfer to a wire rack to cool.

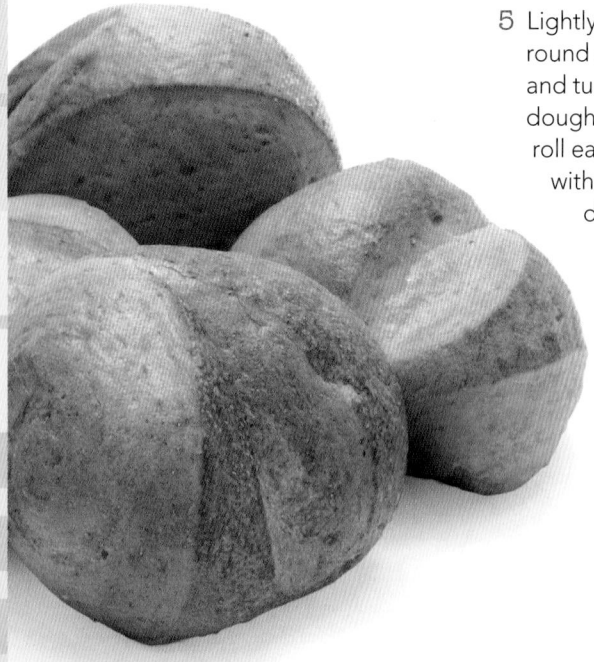

Muffins

Apple and Raisin Muffins

2 cups (300 g) plain flour
3 teaspoons baking powder
1 teaspoon salt
½ teaspoon ground cinnamon
¼ teaspoon ground nutmeg
¾ cup (150 g) peeled, grated apple
⅓ cup (40 g) golden seedless raisins
⅔ cup (155 g) firmly packed light brown sugar
¼ cup (30 g) chopped walnuts or pecans
2 eggs, well beaten
⅔ cup (170 ml) milk
¼ cup (60 ml) vegetable oil
1 cup (75 g) corn, bran or wheat flakes cereal

Makes 12 muffins

Grated apple is the sweetener in these muffins, which reduces the need for added sugar and lets the natural flavors stand out.

1 Preheat the oven to 400°F. Lightly grease a standard 12-cup muffin pan or line with paper baking cups.
2 In a large bowl, combine the flour, baking powder, salt, cinnamon and nutmeg. Add the apple, raisins, sugar and nuts and stir until well blended. Make a well in the center.
3 In a small bowl, combine the eggs, milk and oil. Mix well, then pour into the dry ingredients. Using a fork, stir just until the dry ingredients are moistened. Do not overmix; the batter should be lumpy. Fold in the cereal.
4 Spoon the batter into the prepared muffin cups, filling them two-thirds full. Bake until the muffins are puffed and browned, 15 to 20 minutes. Transfer the pan to a wire rack and let the muffins cool for 5 minutes. Turn the muffins out (you may need to run a knife around the edges to loosen them). Serve warm.

Chocolate Chip Muffins

2 cups (300 g) plain flour
3 teaspoons baking powder
½ teaspoon baking soda
½ cup (95 g) soft brown sugar
1 large egg
1 cup (250 ml) milk
¼ cup (60 g) unsalted butter, melted and cooled
⅔ cup (100 g) dark, milk or white chocolate chips

Makes 12 muffins

Melt-and-mix recipes such as these muffins are among the easiest baked goods you can make.

1 Preheat the oven to 400°F. Lightly grease a standard 12-cup muffin pan or line with paper baking cups.
2 Sift the dry ingredients into a large bowl and make a well in the center.
3 Beat together the egg and milk and add to the dry ingredients with the melted butter. Lightly stir the mixture together with a fork, being careful not to overmix. Fold in the chocolate chips.
4 Fill the prepared muffin cups three-quarters full, then bake for about 20 minutes, until the muffins are well risen, golden brown and cooked through. Transfer the pan to a wire rack and let the muffins cool for 5 minutes. Turn the muffins out (you may need to run a knife around the edges to loosen them). Serve warm or cool.

Blueberry Muffins

1½ cups (235 g) fresh blueberries or thawed frozen blueberries
3 cups (450 g) plain flour
1 tablespoon baking powder
½ teaspoon baking soda
1 teaspoon salt
¾ cup (165 g) sugar, plus extra for sprinkling
¼ cup (60 g) butter, melted
2 eggs, lightly beaten
1 cup (250 ml) buttermilk or natural yogurt
1½ teaspoons vanilla extract

Makes 12 muffins

You don't need to wait until blueberries are in season to make these muffins. Frozen berries work just as well and are often more economical.

1 Preheat the oven to 400°F. Lightly grease a standard 12-cup muffin pan or line with paper baking cups.
2 In a bowl, toss the blueberries with 2 tablespoons of the flour until completely coated. Put the remaining flour in a large bowl with the baking powder, baking soda, salt and sugar; stir to blend, then make a well in the center.
3 In a small bowl, combine the butter, eggs, buttermilk or yogurt and vanilla. Mix well, then pour into the dry ingredients. Using a fork, stir just until the dry ingredients are moistened. Do not overmix; the batter should be lumpy. Fold in the blueberries.
4 Spoon the batter into the prepared muffin cups, filling them two-thirds full; sprinkle the muffin tops with a little extra sugar. Bake until the muffins are golden, 20 to 25 minutes. Transfer the pan to a wire rack and let the muffins cool for 5 minutes. Turn the muffins out (you may need to run a knife around the edges to loosen them). Serve warm or cool.

Bran Muffins

1 cup (125 g) raisins
1¼ cups (185 g) plain flour
1 tablespoon baking powder
⅓ cup (75 g) sugar
1 teaspoon cinnamon
½ teaspoon salt
1 cup (70 g) bran cereal (not flakes)
1 cup (250 ml) milk
1 egg
¼ cup (60 ml) vegetable oil

Makes 12 muffins

These low-fat, high-fiber muffins are excellent for a healthy breakfast.

1 Preheat the oven to 400°F. Lightly grease a standard 12-cup muffin pan or line with paper baking cups.
2 In a bowl, toss the raisins with 2 tablespoons of the flour until completely coated. Put the remaining flour in a bowl with the baking powder, sugar, cinnamon and salt. Stir until well blended.
3 In a large bowl, combine the bran cereal and milk; let the mixture stand for 2 minutes. Add the egg and oil and stir until well blended. Add the dry ingredients to the bran mixture and, using a fork, stir just until the dry ingredients are moistened; do not overmix. Fold in the raisins.
4 Spoon the batter into the prepared muffin cups, filling them two-thirds full. Bake until the muffins are golden brown, 18 to 20 minutes. Transfer the pan to a wire rack and let the muffins cool for 5 minutes. Turn the muffins out (you may need to run a knife around the edges to loosen them). Serve warm or cool.

Herb and Bacon Muffins

1¾ cups (260 g) plain flour
2 teaspoons baking powder
½ teaspoon salt
3 tablespoons chopped fresh herbs
¼ cup (25 g) grated Parmesan cheese
1 tablespoon sugar
2 slices rindless bacon, cooked and cut into small bits
1 egg, beaten
1 cup (250 ml) milk
¼ cup (½ stick/60 g) butter, melted

Makes 12 regular muffins or 24 mini muffins

You can add whatever herbs you fancy to this muffin recipe—fresh thyme, basil or marjoram would be superb.

1 Preheat the oven to 400°F. Lightly grease a standard 12-cup or 24-cup mini muffin pan or line with paper baking cups.
2 In a large bowl, sift together the flour, baking powder and salt. Add the herbs, cheese, sugar and bacon and stir until well blended, then make a well in the center.
3 In a small bowl, combine the egg, milk and butter. Mix well, then pour into the dry ingredients. Using a fork, stir just until the dry ingredients are moistened. Do not overmix; the batter should be lumpy.
4 Spoon the batter into the prepared muffin cups, filling them two-thirds full. Bake until the muffins are browned: 15 to 20 minutes for regular muffins and 12 to 15 minutes for mini muffins. Transfer the pan to a wire rack and let the muffins cool for 5 minutes. Turn the muffins out (you may need to run a knife around the edges to loosen them). Serve warm.

Cranberry Cheddar Muffins

2 cups (300 g) plain flour
⅔ cup (155 g) firmly packed light brown sugar
½ cup (60 g) finely grated cheddar
2½ teaspoons baking powder
½ teaspoon baking soda
½ teaspoon salt
¼ teaspoon ground allspice or mixed spice
pinch of ground cayenne pepper
1¼ cups (310 ml) buttermilk or natural yogurt
¼ cup (½ stick/60 g) butter, melted
1 egg, separated
1 cup (155 g) washed fresh or unthawed frozen cranberries

Makes 12 muffins

Savory muffins make a substantial breakfast or snack on their own or an unusual accompaniment to serve with soup or roast poultry.

1 Preheat the oven to 400°F. Lightly grease a standard 12-cup muffin pan or line with paper baking cups.
2 In a large bowl, combine the flour, sugar, cheese, baking powder, baking soda, salt and spices. Stir until well blended, then make a well in the center.
3 In a small bowl, whisk together the buttermilk or yogurt, butter and egg yolk. In another small bowl, beat the egg white until soft peaks form.
4 Pour the buttermilk mixture into the dry ingredients. Using a fork, stir just until the dry ingredients are moistened. Do not overmix; the batter should be lumpy. Fold in the egg white and cranberries.
5 Spoon the batter into the prepared muffin cups, filling them three-quarters full. Bake until a toothpick inserted in a muffin comes out clean, about 20 minutes. Transfer the pan to a wire rack and let the muffins cool for 5 minutes. Turn the muffins out (you may need to run a knife around the edges to loosen them). Serve warm or cool.

Rolls

Potato Dinner Rolls

2 tablespoons sugar
½ cup (125 ml) lukewarm water (about 105°F–115°F)
two ¼ oz (7 g) packages dry yeast
1 cup (250 ml) milk
2 teaspoons salt
½ cup (125 g) butter, melted, plus 3 tablespoons extra
1 large all-purpose potato, peeled, diced and boiled, then pushed through a fine sieve or a potato ricer
6½–7 cups (about 1 kg) plain flour
1 egg, lightly beaten

Makes 64 rolls

These classic homemade rolls will melt in your mouth. The secret is the potato.

1 In a small bowl, combine the sugar, water and yeast and stir until the solids are dissolved. Let stand until the mixture is bubbly, about 10 minutes.
2 In a small saucepan over medium-high heat, bring the milk and 1 cup (250 ml) water to a boil. Pour into a large heatproof bowl, stir in the salt and ¼ cup (60 ml) of the melted butter and let cool for 10 minutes. Using a wooden spoon or electric mixer with a paddle attachment, add the potato, 2 cups (300 g) of the flour and the egg, beating at medium speed for 1 minute after each addition. Add the yeast mixture and beat for 1 minute longer.
3 If using the mixer, remove the paddle and attach a dough hook. Add another 4½ cups (675 g) flour and beat for 3 to 5 minutes, until a soft, manageable dough forms, then continue adding the flour, ¼ to ½ cup (35 to 75 g) at a time, as needed to reach the desired consistency.
4 Generously butter a large bowl. Using your hands, shape the dough into a ball and place in the bowl, turning it to completely coat it with the butter. Cover the bowl with a dish towel and let the dough rise in a warm place until doubled in size, about 50 minutes.
5 Lightly flour a work surface; lightly grease six baking sheets (or bake the rolls in batches). Punch down the dough and turn out onto the work surface. Divide the dough into four equal portions. Using a rolling pin, roll each dough portion one at a time into an 8 x 10-inch rectangle about ¼-inch thick. Using a floured 2½-inch biscuit cutter, cut out 12 rounds. Gather the scraps together and reroll; cut out four more rounds.
6 Brush each dough round with melted butter. Using the blunt side of a knife, crease each circle along the diameter and fold, stretching the top half so it covers the bottom half. Pinch the edges to seal.
7 Arrange the rolls on the baking sheets and brush the tops with the remaining butter. Cover with a dish towel and let rise for 30 minutes.
8 Preheat the oven to 350°F. Bake the rolls until golden brown, about 30 minutes. Serve immediately or cool on wire racks.

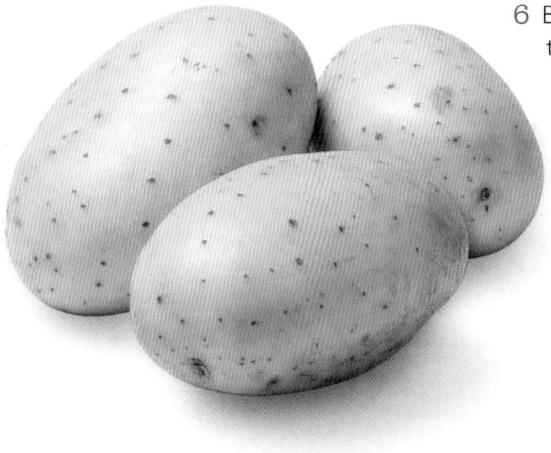

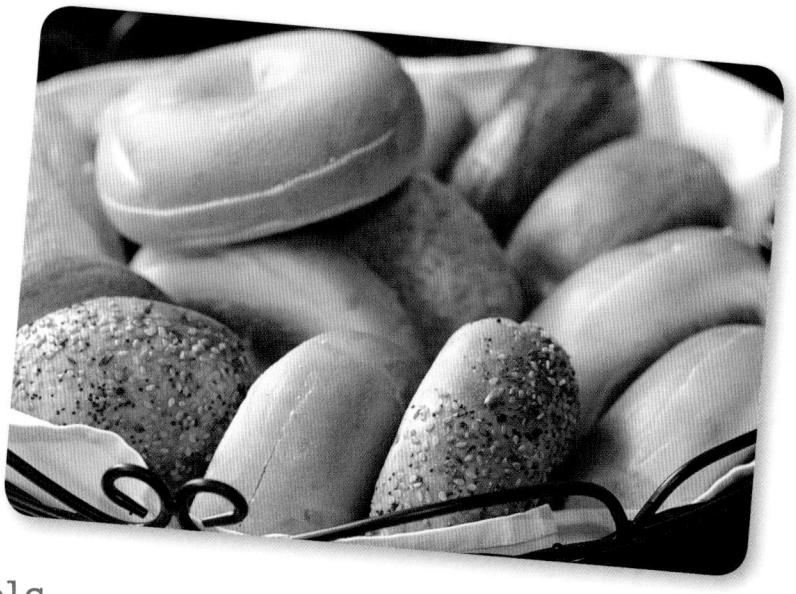

Bagels

1¾ cups (260 g) white bread flour
1¾ cups (175 g) rye flour
1½ teaspoons salt
¼ oz (7 g) package dry yeast
1 teaspoon caraway seeds
3 eggs
1 teaspoon treacle, molasses, or corn syrup
2 teaspoons sunflower oil

Makes 12 bagels

These little bread rings, Jewish in origin, are delicious teamed with savory fixings such as smoked salmon and cream cheese, or egg salad. The double cooking method gives bagels their unique softness and slightly chewy crust.

1 Place all the flour in a large mixing bowl and stir in the salt, yeast and caraway seeds. Make a well in the center.
2 Lightly whisk 2 eggs with the treacle and oil, and pour into the well in the flour. Add ¾ cup (200 ml) lukewarm water and mix to a soft dough.
3 Turn out onto a lightly floured surface and knead for 10 minutes, or until smooth and elastic. Place the dough in a large greased bowl, cover with a damp dish towel and leave to rise in a warm place until doubled in size, about 40 minutes.
4 Turn the dough out onto the floured work surface and knead lightly, then divide into 12 equal pieces. Form each into a sausage 8 inches long, then shape it into a ring. Dampen the ends with a little water, slightly overlap them, then gently pinch together to seal.
5 Arrange the bagels on a lightly oiled baking sheet, cover with oiled plastic wrap and leave to rise in a warm place for 20 minutes, or until slightly puffy.
6 Preheat the oven to 400°F. Bring a large saucepan of lightly salted water to a boil. Drop the bagels into the water, one at a time, and poach for 20 seconds. Lift them out with a large slotted spoon and return to the baking sheet.
7 Lightly beat the remaining egg and brush it over the bagels. Bake for 14 to 15 minutes, or until well risen and golden brown. Transfer to a wire rack to cool. Store in an airtight container for up to 3 days.

Crescent Rolls

¼ (7 g) package dry yeast
¼ cup (60 ml) warm water (110°F–115°F)
1 tablespoon plus ½ cup (110g) sugar
¾ cup (200 ml) warm milk (110°F–115°F)
3 eggs, lightly beaten
½ cup (1 stick/125g) butter or margarine, softened
1 teaspoon salt
5–5½ cups (750–825g) plain flour
Additional butter or margarine, melted

Makes 24 rolls

Don't spend your money on store-bought tubes. These homemade crescent rolls taste much better, have incredible texture and are not at all difficult to prepare.

1 In a large bowl, combine the yeast and water, and stir until the yeast is dissolved. Add 1 tablespoon sugar, and let the mixture stand until bubbly, about 5 minutes.
2 Add the milk, eggs, butter or margarine, salt and ½ cup sugar. Stir until all the ingredients are well blended. Add 5 cups flour, 1 cup at a time, stirring after each addition until the mixture forms a stiff dough; add as much of the remaining ½ cup of flour as you need to reach the desired consistency
3 Butter a large bowl well; lightly flour a work surface. Turn out the dough onto the work surface and knead until the dough is smooth and elastic, 6 to 8 minutes. Using your hands, shape the dough into a ball and place in the prepared bowl, turning it to completely coat the surface of the dough with butter. Cover the bowl with a dish towel and set in a warm, draft-free place to rise until doubled in size, about 1½ hours.
4 Reflour the work surface and lightly grease two baking sheets. Punch down the dough and divide it into thirds; work with one portion at a time. Place one dough portion on the work surface. Using a rolling pin, roll out the dough into a 12-inch-diameter circle. Using a sharp knife or pizza cutter, cut the circle into eight wedges. Brush the wedges with some melted butter. Starting at the wide end, roll up each wedge. Place each wedge on the baking sheet, 2 inches apart, with the small point tucked underneath and slightly bend the wedge to form a crescent shape. Repeat with the remaining dough. Cover the crescents with a dish towel and let rise in a warm place until doubled in size, about 30 minutes.
5 Preheat the oven to 375°F. Bake until the crescents are golden brown, 10 to 12 minutes. Remove the crescents to wire racks and cool slightly.

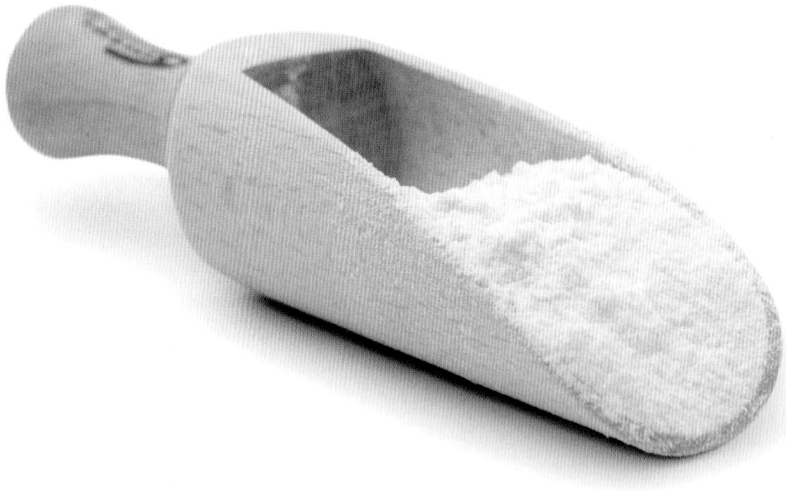

Cinnamon Rolls

¼ oz (7 g) package dry yeast
1 cup (250 ml) warm milk (about 110°F–115°F)
½ cup (110 g) sugar
⅓ cup (80 g) butter, melted
2 eggs
1 teaspoon salt
4–4½ cups (600–675 g) plain flour

CINNAMON FILLING
¾ cup (165 g) firmly packed brown sugar
2 tablespoons ground cinnamon
¼ cup (½ stick/60 g) butter, melted

CREAM CHEESE ICING
½ cup (½ stick/125 g) butter, softened
1½ cups (185 g) confectioners' sugar
¼ cup (60 g) cream cheese, softened
½ teaspoon vanilla extract
pinch of salt

Makes 16 rolls

Your whole house will be infused with the aroma of these sweet delicacies as they're baking. Cream cheese icing is the perfect finishing touch.

1 In a large bowl, combine the yeast and the milk; stir until the yeast has completely dissolved. Add the sugar, butter, eggs, salt and 2 cups (300 g) of the flour and beat until smooth. Stir in enough of the remaining flour to form a soft, sticky dough.
2 Lightly flour a work surface; lightly butter a large bowl. Turn the dough out onto the work surface and knead until smooth and elastic, 6 to 8 minutes. Place the dough in the bowl, turning it to completely coat it with butter. Cover the bowl with a dish towel and let the dough rise in a warm place until doubled in size, about 1 hour.
3 For the filling, mix the sugar and cinnamon in a small bowl until well blended. Lightly grease two 13 x 9 x 2-inch baking sheets; reflour the work surface.
4 Punch down the dough and turn out onto the work surface. Divide the dough in half. Using a rolling pin, roll each half into an 11 x 8-inch rectangle. Brush each rectangle with some of the melted butter. Sprinkle half the filling over each rectangle, leaving a ½-inch border around all the edges. Starting from a long side, roll up each rectangle jelly-roll-fashion, then pinch the seams together to seal. Using a sharp knife, cut each roll into eight slices. Place the slices, cut side down, on the baking sheets. Cover the sheets and let the dough rise again until doubled in size, about 1 hour.
5 Preheat the oven to 350°F. Bake the rolls until golden brown, 20 to 25 minutes. Transfer the sheets to wire racks and let the rolls cool for 5 to 10 minutes.
6 In a small bowl, beat all the icing ingredients together until smooth. Ice the warm rolls and serve.

Hot Cross Buns

two ¼ oz (7 g) packages dry yeast
2 cups (500 ml) warm milk (about 110°F–115°F)
⅓ cup (80 g) butter, softened
2 eggs, lightly beaten
¼ cup (55 g) sugar
1½ teaspoons salt
6–7 cups (900 g–1 kg) plain flour
½ cup (60 g) raisins
½ cup (75 g) dried currants
1 teaspoon ground cinnamon
¼ teaspoon ground allspice or mixed spice
1 egg yolk

ICING
2 cups (250 g) sifted confectioners' sugar
2 tablespoons water

Makes 30 buns

This traditional Easter morning bun is just sweet enough and loaded with dried fruit.

1 In a large bowl, combine the yeast and milk and stir until the yeast has dissolved. Add the butter, eggs, sugar and salt, then stir until well blended.
2 In a bowl, combine 3 cups (450 g) of the flour, the raisins, currants, cinnamon and allspice. Add the flour mixture to the yeast mixture and stir until well blended. Add enough of the remaining flour to form a soft dough.
3 Lightly flour a work surface; generously butter a large bowl. Turn the dough out onto the work surface and knead until smooth and elastic, 6 to 8 minutes. Place the dough in the bowl, turning it to coat it completely with butter. Cover the bowl with a dish towel and let the dough rise in a warm place until doubled in size, about 1 hour.
4 Lightly grease three baking sheets. Punch down the dough. Pinch off enough to form a ball about 1½ to 2 inches in diameter. Repeat with the remaining dough, placing the dough balls 2 inches apart on the baking sheets. Using a sharp knife, cut a cross on top of each dough ball. Cover with a dish towel and allow to rise again until doubled in size, about 30 minutes.
5 Preheat the oven to 375°F. Whisk the egg yolk with 2 tablespoons water, then brush over the risen buns. Bake the buns until golden brown, 15 to 20 minutes. Transfer the buns to wire racks to cool.
6 In a small bowl, combine the icing ingredients and stir until smooth. Place the icing in a piping bag, or place in a self-sealing plastic bag and snip off one corner. Pipe a cross in the cuts on top of each bun. Serve warm.

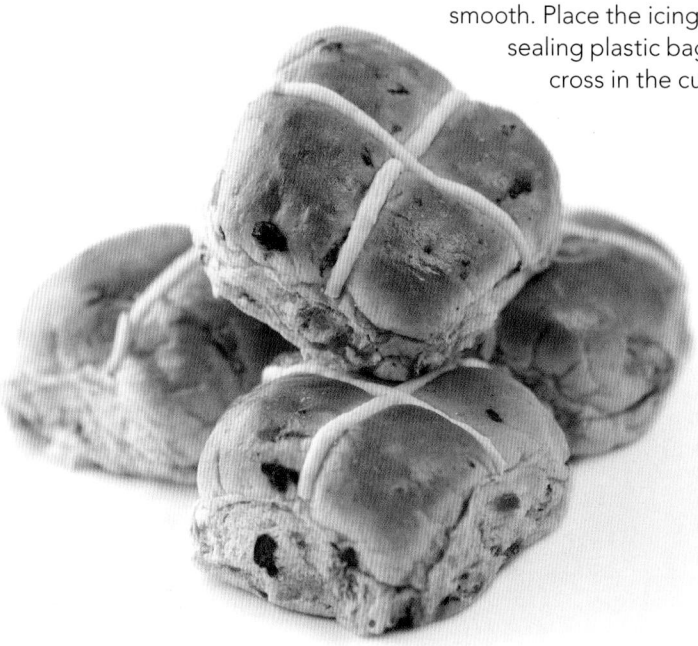

Sticky Buns

2 tablespoons sugar
½ cup (125 ml) lukewarm water (about 105°F–115°F)
two ¼ oz (7 g) packages dry yeast
1 cup (250 ml) milk
2 teaspoons salt
½ cup (1 stick/125 g) butter, melted, plus 3 tablespoons extra
1 large all-purpose potato, peeled, diced and boiled, then pushed through a fine sieve or a potato ricer
6½–7 cups (about 1 kg) plain flour
1 egg, lightly beaten

FILLING
½ cup (115 g) firmly packed light brown sugar
½ cup (125 ml) light corn syrup (optional)
2 teaspoons ground cinnamon
1 cup (250 g) softened butter, plus extra melted butter for brushing
2 cups (240 g) chopped pecans

Makes 30 buns

A nutty variation on the cinnamon roll, these gooey, sticky treats are sensational.

1 In a small bowl, combine the sugar, warm water and yeast; stir until the solids are completely dissolved. Let stand until the mixture is bubbly, about 10 minutes.
2 In a small saucepan over medium-high heat, bring the milk and 1 cup (250 ml) water to a boil. Pour into a large heatproof bowl, stir in the salt and ¼ cup (60 ml) of the melted butter and let cool for 10 minutes. Using a wooden spoon or electric mixer with a paddle attachment, add the potato, 2 cups (300 g) of the flour and the egg, beating at medium speed for 1 minute after each addition. Add the yeast mixture and beat for 1 minute longer.
3 If using the mixer, remove the paddle and attach a dough hook. Add 4½ cups (675 g) of the remaining flour and beat for 3 to 5 minutes, until a soft, manageable dough forms, then continue adding the flour, ¼ to ½ cup (35 to 75 g) at a time, as needed to reach the desired consistency.
4 Generously butter a large bowl. Using your hands, shape the dough into a ball and place in the bowl, turning it to completely coat it with the butter. Cover the bowl with a dish towel and let the dough rise in a warm place until doubled in size, about 50 minutes.
5 Lightly flour a work surface; lightly grease six baking sheets (or bake the rolls in batches). Punch down the dough and turn out onto the work surface. Divide the dough in half. Using a rolling pin, roll each dough half into a 15 x 12-inch rectangle about ¼-inch thick.
6 For the filling, combine the sugar, corn syrup (if using), cinnamon and butter in a small bowl and mix well. Spread half the filling over each rectangle, leaving a ½-inch border around all the edges. Sprinkle each rectangle with half the pecans. Lightly grease a 15 x 10-inch jelly-roll pan.
7 Starting from a long side, roll up each rectangle in jelly-roll-fashion, then pinch the seams together to seal; place seam side down. Using a sharp knife, cut each roll into fifteen 1-inch slices. Arrange the slices, not touching, in the jelly-roll pan. Cover with a dish towel and leave to rise for 20 minutes.
8 Preheat the oven to 350°F. Bake the buns until golden brown, about 40 minutes. Brush the buns with a little melted butter and bake for 5 minutes longer. Serve warm.

Cakes

Spice Cake

5 cups (950 g) Basic Cake Mix (page 61)
1¼ teaspoons ground nutmeg
1¼ teaspoons ground cinnamon
½ teaspoon ground cloves
¼ cup (60 g) butter
½ cup (125 g) sour cream or natural yogurt
2 eggs, lightly beaten

Makes 1 sheet cake

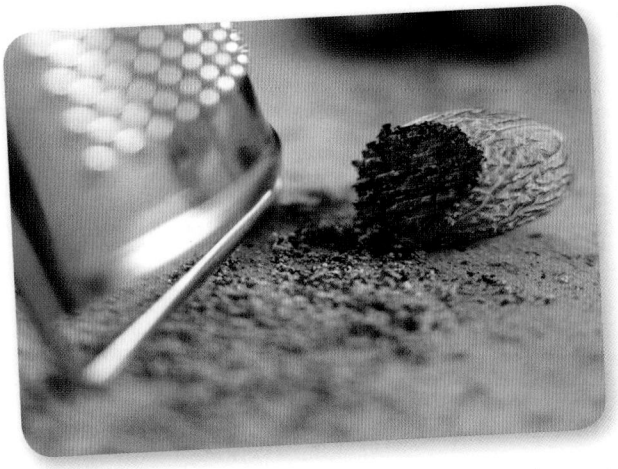

Inviting on its own, this spice-filled cake is also wonderful with Chocolate Buttercream Icing (page 122). Much less expensive than a bakery cake, it is also tastier. This cake and the one that follows are outstanding examples of what you can do with the Basic Cake Mix from page 61.

1 Preheat the oven to 375°F. Generously grease a 13 x 9 x 2-inch baking pan.
2 In a large heatproof bowl, combine the cake mix, nutmeg, cinnamon and cloves; stir to distribute the spices evenly.
3 In a small saucepan over medium-high heat, combine the butter and 1 cup (250 ml) water. Bring the mixture to a boil, then add to the cake mixture. Beat with a wooden spoon or electric beaters until well blended.
4 Stir in the sour cream and eggs; beat until they are well incorporated and no streaks of white remain.
5 Pour the batter into the baking pan. Bake until a toothpick inserted into the center of the cake comes out clean and the top of the cake springs back when lightly touched, about 40 minutes. Transfer the pan to a wire rack and let the cake cool completely before turning out.

Chocolate Cake

3⅓ cups (625 g) Basic Cake Mix (page 61)
½ cup (60 g) cocoa powder
1 cup (250 ml) milk
2 eggs, lightly beaten
3 tablespoons butter, melted

Makes 12 servings

If you like chocolate, this cake is guaranteed to please both your guests and your budget.

1 Preheat the oven to 375°F. Lightly grease and flour two 8-inch round cake pans.
2 In a large bowl, combine the cake mix and cocoa. Add half the milk, then beat for 2 minutes on medium speed, using electric beaters. Add the remaining milk, the eggs and butter, then beat for 2 minutes longer.
3 Divide the batter equally between the cake pans. Bake the cakes until a toothpick inserted into the center comes out clean and the top of the cake springs back when lightly touched, about 25 minutes.
4 Transfer the cake pans to wire racks and leave for 10 minutes to cool slightly. Run a knife around the edge of each cake to loosen it from the side of the pan, then carefully invert the pan and remove the cake. Set the cakes on the wire racks and let them cool completely. Fill and ice as desired.

Devil's Food Cake

1 tablespoon unsweetened cocoa powder
2 cups (300 g) sifted cake flour
1½ teaspoons baking soda
1 teaspoon salt
½ teaspoon baking powder
1½ cups (330 g) sugar
1 cup (250 ml) buttermilk, at room temperature
½ cup (1 stick/125 g) butter or margarine, softened
1 teaspoon vanilla extract
3 eggs, at room temperature
3 ounces (90 g) semisweet chocolate, melted

Makes 1 layer cake or 12 servings

This is a one-bowl cake—meant to be beaten with an electric mixer so all the ingredients are in an order to prevent overmixing. Devil's food cake has a beguiling, bitter chocolate flavor that is moister and more distinctive in homemade versions.

1 Preheat the oven to 350°F. Lightly grease two 8-inch round cake pans, dust with the cocoa, divided equally; tap out any excess powder
2 In a large bowl, combine the flour, baking soda, salt, baking powder, sugar, buttermilk, butter, vanilla, eggs and chocolate, being careful to add the ingredients in the order listed. Using an electric mixer at low speed, beat all the ingredients for 1 minute, using a spatula to scrape down the sides of the bowl occasionally. Increase the speed to medium-high, and beat for 2 minutes longer, scraping the sides of the bowl twice.
3 Pour the batter into the prepared cake pans. Bake until a toothpick inserted into the center of the cake layers comes out clean, about 30 minutes. Remove the pans to wire racks and let the cake layers cool for 10 minutes.Turn each layer out of its cake pan, then set the layers back on the wire racks to cool completely. Fill and frost as desired.

Angel Cake

1½ cups (375 ml) egg whites (about 15 eggs)
1½ teaspoons cream of tartar
¼ teaspoon salt
1½ cups (330 g) sugar
1 cup (150 g) sifted plain flour or cake flour
2 teaspoons vanilla extract
¼ teaspoon almond extract

Makes 12 servings

Aptly named indeed, this cake is so light and airy that you'll swear it will float away if you don't eat it quickly. It's also free of any fat and can be the base for many a light, luscious dessert. Suspending the cake upside down while it cools helps to create the cake's light texture.

1 Place the oven rack in the lowest possible position. Preheat the oven to 325°F; set out a 10-inch tube pan.
2 In a large bowl, combine the egg whites, cream of tartar and salt. Beat until frothy, using electric beaters on medium speed. Gradually add the sugar, 2 tablespoons at a time, beating constantly. Increase the speed to high and continue beating until the mixture forms very soft peaks.
3 Fold the flour, ¼ cup (35 g) at a time, into the egg whites, then fold in the vanilla and almond extracts.
4 Spoon the batter into the ungreased tube pan and gently smooth the top with a spatula. Cut the spatula through the batter once to break and release any large air bubbles.
5 Bake until the top of the cake springs back when lightly touched, 50 to 60 minutes. Invert the tube pan with the central tube over the neck of a large bottle and let the cake cool completely. Using a knife, loosen the edges of the cake from the sides of the pan, then turn the cake out onto a cake plate.

Butter Cake

¾ cup (185 g) unsalted butter
1 cup (230 g) superfine sugar
3 large eggs
2 cups (300 g) self-rising flour
¼ cup (60 ml) milk

Makes 8 servings

This is a dependable basic cake that will come in handy for all sorts of occasions.

1 Preheat the oven to 350°F. Grease a deep 8-inch round cake pan and line the base with parchment paper.
2 Beat the butter until very soft, using electric beaters. Add the sugar and continue beating until the mixture is light, pale and fluffy.
3 Beat in the eggs gradually, adding a teaspoon of flour with each addition to prevent curdling. Fold in the rest of the flour alternately with milk, adding about a third at a time.
4 Pour the batter into the cake pan and bake for 50 to 60 minutes, or until a toothpick inserted in the center of the cake comes out clean.
5 Transfer the pan to a wire rack and let the cake cool for a few minutes, then turn out onto a wire rack to cool completely.

Banana Cake

2 large, ripe bananas, about 14 oz (400 g) in total
2 cups (300 g) self-rising flour
1 teaspoon baking powder
¼ cup (55 g) firmly packed soft brown sugar
⅓ cup (80 ml) sunflower oil
⅓ cup (80 ml) low-fat milk
2 eggs
1 cup (125 g) golden seedless raisins

Makes 8 servings

Quick and easy to prepare, this cake makes a healthy snack for hungry children or a handy addition to lunch boxes. And it's a great way to use up bananas that have been sitting in the fruit bowl for too long.

1 Preheat the oven to 350°F. Grease a deep 9-inch round cake pan and line the base with parchment paper. Peel the bananas, then mash in a small bowl with a fork.
2 Sift the flour and baking powder into a large bowl and stir in the sugar. In a separate bowl, mix together the oil, milk and eggs, then add to the flour mixture. Stir in the raisins and mashed bananas.
3 Pour the batter into the cake pan and bake for 50 to 55 minutes, until the cake is well risen and a toothpick inserted in the center comes out clean. Transfer the pan to a wire rack and let the cake cool for 15 minutes. Run a knife around the edge of the cake to loosen it, then turn it out onto a wire rack to cool completely. The cake can be kept in an airtight container for up to 4 days.

Orange Cake

3 eggs, separated, plus 1 egg yolk
7 oz (200 g) butter, softened
1 cup (230 g) superfine sugar
2 teaspoons grated orange zest
1½ cups (225 g) plain flour
3 teaspoons baking powder

GLAZE
½ cup (125 ml) orange juice
¼ cup (60 ml) orange liqueur
½ cup (110 g) sugar
1 teaspoon grated orange zest

Makes 8 servings

Store this cake in an airtight container and let it stand for a couple of days before eating it. You'll be rewarded with a full orange flavor.

1 Preheat the oven to 350°F. Grease a 9-inch springform pan and line it with parchment paper.
2 Beat the egg whites until stiff. Combine the 4 egg yolks, butter, sugar and orange zest in a bowl, then beat using electric beaters until the mixture is light and fluffy, about 5 minutes.
3 Sift the flour and baking powder, then stir into the butter mixture about a tablespoon at a time. Fold the egg white into the mixture with a metal spoon.
4 Pour the batter into the cake pan and smooth the top. Bake for 35 to 40 minutes, or until golden brown. Remove the cake from the oven, but leave it in the pan.
5 Stir the glaze ingredients in a small saucepan over low heat until the sugar has dissolved. Prick the hot cake a few times with a fork and drizzle with the glaze. Transfer the pan to a wire rack and let the cake cool completely before removing the outer ring of the pan.

Cheesecake with Strawberry Glaze

CRUST
1¼ cups (155 g) crumbled store-bought or homemade Graham Crackers (page 133)
⅓ cup (90 g) butter or margarine, melted
¼ cup (55 g) sugar

FILLING
three 8 oz (250 g) packages cream cheese
1 cup (220 g) sugar
3 eggs
1 cup (250 g) sour cream

STRAWBERRY GLAZE
¼ cup (80 g) strawberry jam
1 tablespoon water
1 pint (500 g) fresh strawberries, hulled and thinly sliced

Makes 6 to 8 servings

Depending on availability, you can substitute raspberries, blackberries or blueberries in this recipe. Whatever you choose, you will have a dessert to rival an expensive bakery or deli cheesecake.

1 Preheat the oven to 325°F. Combine the crust ingredients in a bowl and toss using a fork until well blended. Press the crust mixture firmly over the base of a 9-inch springform pan.
2 For the filling, combine the cream cheese and sugar in a food processor or blender and pulse until well blended and smooth. With the motor running, add the eggs one at a time. Scrape down the sides of the bowl, add the sour cream and process until the mixture is smooth and well blended.
3 Pour the mixture into the cake pan and bake until the filling is only slightly wobbly in the middle, about 50 minutes (it will firm up as it cools). Transfer the pan to a wire rack and let the cheesecake cool to room temperature. Remove the sides of the pan before glazing the cheesecake.
4 For the glaze, combine the jam and water in a small saucepan and bring to a boil over medium-high heat. Remove from the heat and let the glaze cool slightly.
5 Brush the cheesecake with about one-third of the glaze. Beginning along an outside edge of the cake, arrange the strawberry slices in overlapping concentric circles over the cheesecake. Brush the remaining glaze lightly over the strawberries.

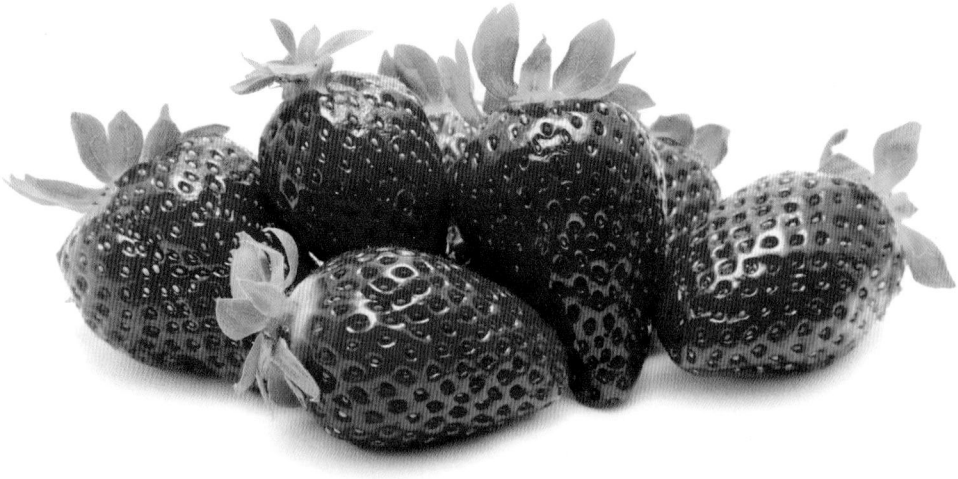

Cupcakes

8 oz (225 g) butter, softened
1 cup (230 g) superfine sugar
1 teaspoon vanilla extract
4 large eggs
1⅔ cups (250 g) self-rising flour
1 tablespoon milk

ICING
½ cup (125 g) butter, softened
2 cups (250 g) confectioners' sugar
2 tablespoons milk
food coloring (optional)

Makes 12

The icing on cupcakes isn't just to make them look pretty and add extra flavor; it also keeps them fresh.

1 Preheat the oven to 350°F. In a large bowl, cream the butter and sugar until pale and fluffy, using electric beaters.
2 Add the vanilla, then add the eggs one at a time, mixing well after each addition.
3 Sift the flour into the mixture. Using a plastic spatula or wooden spoon, fold in the flour and milk until combined.
4 Spoon the batter into 12 paper cupcake liners, filling them two-thirds full. Bake the cupcakes until golden, about 15 minutes. Turn the cupcakes out onto a wire rack to cool.
5 For the icing, beat the butter and confectioners' sugar in a bowl using electric beaters until well creamed, about 2 minutes. Add the milk and food coloring, if using, mixing until combined.
6 Ice the cooled cupcakes and decorate as desired.

Vanilla Icing

⅓ cup (90 g) butter or margarine, softened
4 cups (500 g) confectioners' sugar, sifted
¼ cup (60 ml) light cream
2 teaspoons vanilla extract
1–2 drops food coloring (optional)

Makes enough to fill and ice one 8- to 9-inch (20–23 cm) layer cake, 24 cupcakes or one 9 x 13-inch (33 x 23 cm) sheet cake

This classic icing is easy and cheap to make, luscious to eat and versatile.

1 In a bowl, beat the butter until light and fluffy, using electric beaters on moderately high speed.
2 Reduce the speed to medium, and alternately add the sugar and the cream, a little at a time, beating constantly. Add the vanilla and beat until the icing is creamy. If desired, add food coloring to tint the icing.

VARIATION
Orange Buttercream Icing: Add ¼ cup (60 ml) orange juice and 1 tablespoon finely grated orange zest.

Chocolate Ganache Icing

¼ cup (55 g) superfine sugar
2 oz (50 g) unsalted butter
2 cups (500 ml) light cream
2 tablespoons dark rum
1 lb (500 g) dark cooking chocolate, melted

Makes about 4 cups

Ganache is a decadent mixture of chocolate and cream that gives a rich and glossy icing—perfect for special-occasion cakes.

In a saucepan, combine the sugar, butter, cream and rum. Gently heat, stirring often, until the sugar has dissolved. Stir in the melted chocolate, then transfer to a bowl and chill the mixture for 30 minutes, or until set. Spread over the cooled cake.

Chocolate Buttercream Icing

⅓ cup (90 g) butter, softened
4 cups (500 g) confectioners' sugar, sifted
¼ cup (60 ml) light cream
2 teaspoons vanilla extract
3 oz (90 g) dark chocolate, melted, or ½ cup (60 g) sifted cocoa powder

Makes enough to fill and ice one 8- or 9-inch (20–23 cm) layer cake, 24 cupcakes or one 13 x 9 x 2-inch (33 x 23 cm) sheet cake

This is the icing that kids like to lick out of the bowl. Inexpensive and easy to make, it is delicious.

1 In a bowl, beat the butter until light and fluffy, using electric beaters on moderately high speed.
2 Reduce the speed to medium, and alternately add the sugar and the cream, a little at a time, beating constantly. Add the vanilla and melted chocolate or cocoa powder and beat until the icing is creamy.

Simple Glaze Icing

¾ cup (90 g) confectioners' sugar
1 tablespoon warm water, or as needed
food coloring (optional)

Makes enough to cover an 8-inch (20 cm) cake

This simplest of all icings is economical to make and can be spread, drizzled or piped, depending on how thick you make it.

Sift the confectioners' sugar into a bowl and gradually mix in enough water to make a smooth icing of the desired consistency. Add food coloring, if using, a drop at a time, until the required depth of color is reached. Spread over the cooled cake.

Cream Cheese Icing

2½ oz (75 g) cream cheese, softened
1 oz (30 g) butter, softened
1½ cups (185 g) confectioners' sugar
finely grated zest of 1 lemon
1 tablespoon lemon juice

Makes enough to cover an 8-inch (20 cm) cake

This soft, rich, lemony icing is the classic topping for carrot cake, but also goes well with other well-flavored, dense-textured cakes.

In a large bowl, combine all the ingredients. Beat with a wooden spoon until smooth. Spread over the cooled cake.

Pies and Meringues

Basic Double Crust Pie Pastry

2¼ cups (335 g) flour
½ teaspoon salt
½ cup (1 stick/125 g) cold butter, chopped
¼ cup (60 g) vegetable shortening
5–6 tablespoons iced water

Makes enough for an 8- or 9-inch (20–23 cm) double crust pie

Sweet and savory pies are among the most popular items in the frozen food section of any supermarket, and sweet pies appear in every bakery section. (You'll find recipes for main-dish pies starting on page 176 and ones for sweet pies on page 125.) Don't waste your cash on ready-made piecrust. It's quick and easy, and if you know a few tricks, it will turn out light and flaky every time. Here is the basic recipe for a pie that has a top crust as well as a bottom one.

1 In a large bowl, sift together the flour and salt. Using a pastry blender or two knives, cut in the butter and shortening until the mixture resembles coarse bread crumbs.
2 Add the iced water, 1 tablespoon at a time, stirring the mixture with a fork to incorporate the water into the dough. Add water only until the dough begins to hold together. Handling the dough as little as possible, divide it in half, shape each half into a ball and wrap each ball in plastic wrap. Chill the dough balls for at least 1 hour before using.
3 For the bottom crust, place one ball of dough on a lightly floured board or pastry cloth. Flatten the ball slightly; then, using a lightly floured rolling pin, roll from the center outward in all directions. Make the dough circle large enough to cover the bottom and sides of a pie plate plus about 1 inch more.
4 For the top crust, place the remaining ball of dough on the lightly floured surface and flatten slightly. Roll the dough from the center outward in all directions until the circle is large enough to cover the pie plate plus about a ½-inch margin.

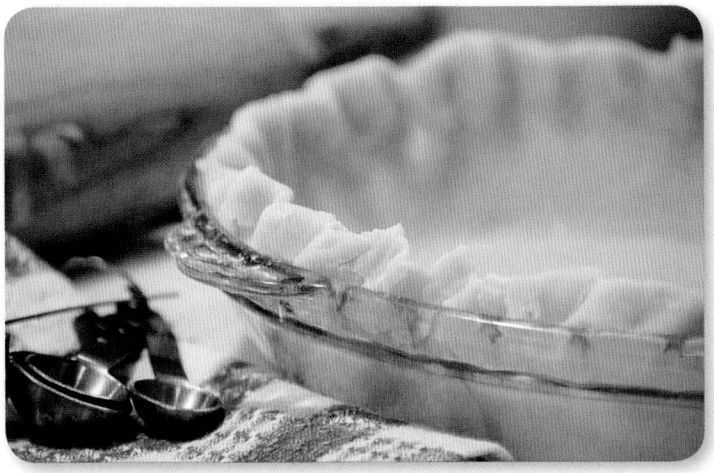

Basic Single Crust Pie Pastry

1½ cups (225 g) plain flour
¼ teaspoon salt
½ cup (125 g) cold butter, chopped
3 tablespoons (60 g) vegetable shortening
3–4 tablespoons iced water

Makes enough for an 8- to 9-inch (20–23 cm) single crust pie

Use this recipe when you are making an open-faced pie or tart, such as one with a meringue or crumble topping.

1 In a large bowl, sift together the flour and salt. Using a pastry blender or two knives, cut in the butter and shortening until the mixture resembles coarse bread crumbs.
2 Add the iced water, 1 tablespoon at a time, stirring the mixture with a fork to incorporate the water into the dough. Add only enough water for the dough to hold together. Handling the dough as little as possible, shape it into a ball and wrap it in plastic wrap. Chill the dough ball for at least 1 hour before using.
3 Place the dough on a lightly floured board or pastry cloth. Flatten the ball slightly; then, using a lightly floured rolling pin, roll from the center of the ball outward in all directions. Make the dough circle large enough to cover the bottom and sides of a pie plate plus about 1 inch more. Drape carefully over a pie plate, fold over the outer edge and trim or crimp it with your fingers to make a decorative edge. Fill and bake according to the pie recipe.
4 For a prebaked pie shell, preheat the oven to 375°F. Place the pie shell on a baking sheet and prick the bottom. Line the bottom with two layers of foil and add dried beans or pastry beads to weigh it down, otherwise the base will puff up during cooking. Bake 10 to 15 minutes, or until golden brown.

Puff Pastry

2½ cups (375 g) plain flour
⅔ cup (160 g) butter, chopped
¾ cup (185 ml) chilled water
4½ oz (125 g) vegetable shortening

Makes enough for a 8- or 9-inch (20–23 cm) pie

This airy, crisp and flaky pastry can be used for the top crust on pies, for sausage rolls, or to make delicate pastries such as mille-feuille.

1 Sift the flour into a bowl and rub in half the butter. Add the water and mix to a soft dough. On a lightly floured surface, roll the dough into a rectangle about ¼-inch thick. Dot half the remaining butter over the top two-thirds of the rectangle, then fold the bottom third up and over the center third. Then bring the top third down so that it covers the bottom third. Press edges together with the rolling pin.
2 Give the dough a quarter turn to the left so that the side joins are to the bottom and top. Roll out again into a rectangle ¼-inch thick. Dot vegetable shortening over the top two-thirds of the pastry; fold and turn as before. Repeat, using the remaining butter. Wrap in plastic wrap and chill for 30 minutes.
3 Roll out and bake as directed in the recipe.

Shortcrust Pastry

¾ cup (185 g) unsalted butter, chilled and diced
1⅔ cups (250 g) plain flour
pinch of salt
3 tablespoons iced water

Makes enough to line a 9- or 10-inch (22–26 cm) loose-based flan pan

This is the classic crisp pastry for pies and tarts. The trick is to handle it as little as possible (using a food processor helps) and to chill it both before and after rolling it out.

1 Place the butter, flour and salt in a bowl. Rub in the butter with your fingertips until the mixture resembles coarse bread crumbs. Alternatively, combine in a food processor and pulse until the mixture resembles coarse bread crumbs.
2 Add 2 tablespoons of the water and cut in with two knives or a pastry blender, or pulse if using a food processor, just until the mixture comes together, adding a little more water as necessary. Do not overmix.
3 Turn the dough out onto a lightly floured work surface and knead just enough to bring it together into a ball. Shape the dough into a round. Flatten it a little, cover with plastic wrap and place in the refrigerator for at least 30 minutes, or preferably overnight.
4 Roll out the dough on a lightly floured work surface to about ¼-inch thick and use it to line an ungreased flan pan, pie plate or tartlet pans.
5 Prick the pastry several times with a fork. Chill for 30 minutes; this helps stop the pastry from shrinking when it is baked.
6 Bake blind if instructed by the recipe.

Custard Pie

Basic Single Crust Pie Pastry (page 124)
4 eggs
2½ cups (625 ml) milk
½ cup (110 g) sugar
1 teaspoon vanilla extract
1 teaspoon almond extract
1 teaspoon salt
1 teaspoon ground nutmeg

Makes 6 to 8 servings

This creamy pie is never as good from a store as it is from your kitchen.

1 Preheat the oven to 400°F. Line a 9-inch pie plate with the piecrust; trim or turn under the edges of the dough and, if desired, form a decorative edge around the piecrust. Prick the bottom of the crust, line with foil or parchment paper, fill with dried beans or pastry beads and bake it for 10 minutes.
2 Meanwhile, in a large bowl, beat the eggs. Add the remaining ingredients and stir to blend well. Pour the filling into the piecrust, then cover the edges of the crust with pieces of foil.
3 Bake until a knife inserted near the center of the pie comes out clean, 20 to 25 minutes. Let the pie cool completely before serving; store in the refrigerator.

Perfect Apple Pie

Basic Double Crust Pie Pastry (page 123)
1 large egg, separated
4 tart apples, such as Granny Smith or Jonathan
4 sweet apples, such as golden delicious
2 tablespoons lemon juice
½ cup (115 g) firmly packed light brown sugar
½ cup (110 g) sugar
⅓ cup (50 g) sifted plain flour
¼ teaspoon ground cinnamon
⅛ teaspoon ground allspice
⅛ teaspoon grated nutmeg
2 tablespoons butter
1 tablespoon iced water

Makes 8 servings

Apple pie is a perennial favorite, and you will never enjoy a store-bought example again after you have tasted the homemade type.

1 Preheat the oven to 425°F. Line a 9-inch pie plate with the bottom piecrust, letting the edges hang over about 1 inch. In a cup, whisk the egg white until frothy and brush over the bottom crust; reserve the egg yolk for the top crust glaze. Roll out the remaining piecrust. Cover the top crust with plastic wrap until ready to use.
2 Peel, core and slice all the apples about ¼-inch thick, placing them in a large bowl. Sprinkle the apple slices with the lemon juice as you work to prevent browning. In a small bowl, combine the sugars, flour, cinnamon, allspice and nutmeg. Sprinkle the sugar mixture over the apple slices, tossing as you work to coat all the slices. Spoon the apple slices into the piecrust, mounding the slices higher in the center. Cut the butter into small pieces and scatter among the apple slices.
3 Using a pastry brush, moisten the edges of the bottom piecrust with a little water. Carefully transfer the top crust to cover the pie filling. Fold the top edges of the pastry over and under the bottom crust edges; pinch the edges together to seal. Cut slits or make decorative vents; if desired, form a decorative edge around the piecrust. In a small bowl, whisk the reserved egg yolk and cold water together. Brush the glaze over the top of the pie, avoiding the slits or decorative vents.
4 Bake the pie for 15 minutes; reduce the temperature to 375°F and bake until the filling is bubbly and the piecrust is golden brown, about 35 minutes more. If the crust edges are browning too quickly, cover them with pieces of foil. Place the pie on a rack to cool for at least 20 minutes before serving.

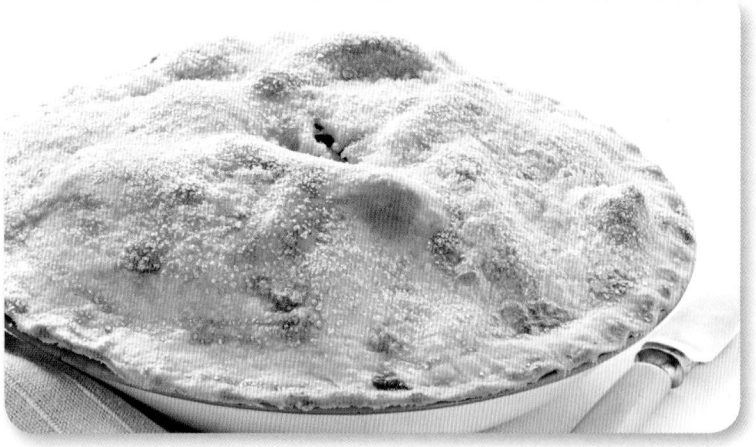

Meringue Shells

1 cup (250 ml) egg whites (10 large eggs)
¾ cup (165 g) sugar
½ cup (60 g) sifted confectioners' sugar

Makes 6 individual meringues or 1 meringue pie shell

The finished appearance of the meringue shells should be dry and crisp but not browned.

1. Preheat the oven to 250°F. Line a baking sheet with parchment paper.
2. In a large bowl with electric beaters on low, slowly beat the egg whites until frothy. Still beating on low, gradually add ½ cup (110 g) of the sugar until the egg whites look silvery. Increase the mixer speed to medium, and slowly add the remaining sugar, beating just until the egg whites form stiff peaks. Using a spatula, fold in the confectioners' sugar.
3. Fit a piping bag with a number 6 star tip, and fill the bag with the meringue. Pipe six coiled circles of meringue onto the baking sheet. Pipe a second-tier ring of meringue along the outer edge of each of the first circles. (If you don't have a piping bag and nozzle, spoon six mounds of meringue onto the baking sheet and, using the back of the spoon, press a hollow in the center of each mound to make a shell.)
4. Bake the meringues for 1 hour; turn off the oven but do not open the oven door. Let the meringues stand in the warm oven for 1 hour longer. Transfer the meringues to wire racks to cool.

SERVING SUGGESTION

Meringue Shells with Raspberry Sauce: Sweetly tart raspberries are the perfect foil for crisp meringue shells. Make ¾ cup (185 ml) Raspberry Sauce (page 59). Place each meringue on a plate. Spoon raspberry sauce into each shell and serve immediately.

Pavlova

Meringue Shells (above)
2 cups (500 ml) whipping cream
2 tablespoons sugar
fresh fruit, such as 1 quart (250 g) strawberries, trimmed and sliced; or 4 kiwis, peeled and sliced, plus the pulp from 4 passion fruit

Makes 12 servings

Legend has it that this resplendent dessert was concocted in honor of the celebrated ballerina Anna Pavlova.

1. Preheat the oven to 250°F. Line a 14-inch baking sheet with parchment paper. Spoon the meringue onto the baking sheet, forming a 12-inch round shape with slightly built-up edges. Bake for 1 hour; turn off the oven but do not open the oven door. Let the meringue stand in the warm oven for 1 hour longer. Transfer the meringue shell to a wire rack to cool.
2. In a large bowl, beat the whipping cream until it forms soft peaks, using electric beaters on moderately high speed. Gradually add the sugar, beating constantly until stiff peaks form.
3. Spoon the whipped cream into the meringue shell, mounding it decoratively. Arrange the fruit on top of the whipped cream and serve immediately.

Cookies, Slices and Brownies

Chocolate Chip Cookies

1 cup (250 g) butter, softened
¾ cup (165 g) sugar
¾ cup (165 g) firmly packed brown sugar
2 eggs
1 teaspoon vanilla extract
2¼ cups (335 g) plain flour
1 teaspoon salt
1 teaspoon baking soda
1 cup (170 g) dark chocolate chips
1 cup (125 g) chopped walnuts or pecans (optional)

Makes about 40 cookies

This American classic has been loved for generations. Although there are plenty of types to choose from in stores, homemade are just better.

1 Preheat the oven to 350°F; lightly grease two or more baking sheets.
2 In a bowl, beat the butter and sugars until well creamed, using electric beaters. Add the eggs one at a time, beating well after each addition. Add the vanilla and stir until well blended.
3 In a small bowl, combine the flour, salt and baking soda. Add the flour mixture to the butter mixture, stirring until well blended. Add the chocolate chips and nuts, if using, and stir until they are evenly distributed.
4 Using a tablespoon, drop the dough onto the baking sheets, spacing the mounds about 2 inches apart. Bake the cookies until golden brown, about 10 minutes. Transfer the cookies to wire racks to cool.

Oatmeal Cookies

1 cup (120 g) raisins
1 cup (250 ml) boiling water
¾ cup (185 g) shortening
1 cup (230 g) firmly packed light brown sugar
½ cup (110 g) granulated sugar
2 eggs
1 teaspoon vanilla extract
2½ cups (375 g) plain flour
1 teaspoon baking soda
1 teaspoon salt
1 teaspoon ground cinnamon
½ teaspoon baking powder
¼ teaspoon ground cloves
2 cups (200 g) quick-cooking oats

Makes 5 dozen cookies

One of America's favorite flavors in one of its favorite cookies is a perfect home-bake success. It is easy and delectable.

1 Preheat the oven to 375°F; set out two or more baking sheets.
2 In a small bowl, combine the raisins and the boiling water. Let stand until the raisins are plump, about 15 minutes. Drain the raisins, reserving the liquid. Add enough water to the raisin liquid to equal ½ cup (125 ml).
3 In a large bowl, combine the shortening, sugars, eggs and vanilla, and beat until the mixture is well creamed. Stir in the raisin liquid. Add the flour, baking soda, salt, cinnamon, baking powder and cloves, and stir until all the ingredients are well blended. Stir in the raisins and the oats.
4 Using a teaspoon, drop the dough onto the prepared sheets, spacing the cookies about 2 inches apart. Bake until the cookies are light brown, 10 to 12 minutes.Transfer the cookies to wire racks to cool completely

Peanut Butter Cookies

½ cup (125 g) butter or margarine, softened
½ cup (110 g) sugar, plus extra for decorating
½ cup (115 g) firmly packed brown sugar
½ cup (125 g) Peanut Butter (page 33)
1 egg
½ teaspoon vanilla extract
1¼ cups (185 g) plain flour
½ teaspoon baking soda
½ teaspoon baking powder

Makes 45 to 50 cookies

Homemade cookies are always so much better than commercial types. These appeal to children and adults alike and are easy to make and delectable.

1. In a large bowl, beat the butter and sugars until well creamed, using electric beaters. Add the peanut butter, egg and vanilla and beat until smooth.
2. In a small bowl, combine the flour, baking soda and baking powder. Add the flour mixture to the butter mixture and beat until well blended. Cover with plastic wrap and place in the refrigerator until the dough is chilled, about 1 hour.
3. Meanwhile, preheat the oven to 375°F. Set out two or more baking sheets.
4. Pinch off a walnut-sized portion of the chilled dough. Using floured hands, roll the dough into a 1-inch (3 cm) diameter ball and place on one of the baking sheets. Repeat with the remaining dough, spacing the balls about 2 inches (5 cm) apart. Using a fork dipped in sugar, flatten each dough ball by pressing the panes in a crisscross pattern on each cookie.
5. Bake until the cookies are set and lightly browned underneath, 10 to 12 minutes. Transfer the cookies to wire racks and leave to cool completely.

Coconut Macaroons

3 egg whites
1 cup (220 g) sugar
2½ cups (225 g) desiccated coconut
1 cup (160 g) macadamia nuts or almonds, finely chopped

Makes about 35 macaroons

Desiccated coconut makes for a delectable macaroon, which you can make better and more inexpensively than any manufacturer.

1. Preheat the oven to 350°F; lightly grease two baking sheets.
2. In a bowl, beat the egg whites until soft peaks form, using electric beaters on high. Gradually add the sugar, beating after each addition, until stiff, glossy peaks form. Fold in the coconut and nuts until well blended.
3. Using a tablespoon, scoop out a portion of the dough. Using damp hands, roll the dough into a ball and place on the baking sheets. Repeat with the remaining dough.
4. Bake the macaroons until lightly golden, 20 to 25 minutes. Transfer the macaroons to wire racks to cool completely. Store in an airtight container for 2 to 3 days.

Gingersnaps

¾ cup (185 g) vegetable shortening
½ cup (110 g) sugar, plus extra for rolling
½ cup (115 g) firmly packed brown sugar
1 egg
¼ cup (90 g) molasses
2 cups (300 g) plain flour
2 teaspoons baking soda
1½ teaspoons ground ginger
1 teaspoon ground cinnamon
½ teaspoon salt

Makes about 40 cookies

The warm tang of ginger infuses each bite of these old-fashioned favorites. As they bake, the spicy aroma will warm the kitchen.

1 Preheat the oven to 350°F; lightly grease two or more baking sheets.
2 In a large bowl, beat the shortening and sugars until well creamed, using electric beaters. Add the egg and molasses and beat until well blended.
3 In a small bowl, combine the flour, baking soda, ginger, cinnamon and salt. Gradually add the flour mixture to the butter mixture, beating after each addition, until well blended.
4 Place some additional sugar in a small bowl. Pinch off a walnut-sized portion of the dough. Using your hands, roll the portion into a ball, then roll the ball in the sugar and place it on one of the baking sheets. Repeat with the remaining dough, spacing the balls about 2 inches apart.
5 Bake the cookies until lightly browned and crinkly, 12 to 15 minutes. Transfer the cookies to a wire rack and leave to cool completely.

Blondies

¾ cup (185 g) butter, softened
1½ cups (330 g) sugar
3 eggs
2 teaspoons vanilla extract
1¾ cups (260 g) plain flour
1 teaspoon baking powder
½ teaspoon salt
2 cups (250 g) coarsely chopped walnuts or pecans

Makes 24 (2 ½-inch-square) blondies

The yin to brownies' yang, blondies are sold at many stores for a pretty penny, but they are not the same as fresh ones out of your oven.

1 Preheat the oven to 350°F. Line a 13 x 9 x 2-inch baking pan with foil. Lightly grease and flour the foil.
2 In a large bowl with an electric mixer on medium speed, cream the butter for 2 minutes. Add the sugar and beat for 2 minutes longer. Add the eggs and beat well; beat in the vanilla.
3 Using a wooden spoon, gradually add the flour, baking powder and salt to the creamed mixture and stir until all the ingredients are well blended. Stir in the nuts. Pour the batter into the prepared pan. Bake the blondies until a toothpick inserted in the center comes out clean, about 35 minutes. Remove the baking pan to a wire rack and let the blondies cool before cutting.

Shortbread

1 cup (250 g) butter, softened
⅔ cup (145 g) superfine sugar, plus extra for sprinkling
2½ cups (375 g) plain flour

Makes 12 shortbreads

This crisp, rich, buttery treat, which originated in Scotland, will keep in an airtight container for about 4 weeks. It is pretty cut into shapes to serve or give as gifts at Christmas or other festive occasions.

1 Preheat the oven to 325°F. Grease a large baking sheet and line with parchment paper.
2 In a large bowl, cream the butter and sugar using electric beaters until pale and fluffy. Using a large metal spoon, fold in the flour in two to three batches and mix to a soft dough.
3 Turn the dough out onto a floured work surface and knead lightly and briefly until smooth. Flatten with floured hands into a 6-inch circle and place on the baking sheet.
4 Using a rolling pin, roll the dough out into a neat 7-inch circle. With floured fingers, pinch the edges decoratively. Sprinkle with the extra sugar. With a sharp knife, mark the surface of the shortbread into 12 even wedges.
5 Bake until pale and firm, about 40 minutes. While still warm, cut the wedges along the score marks all the way through. Let the shortbreads cool completely on the baking sheet.

Sugar Cookies

1½ cups (330 g) sugar
1½ cups (375 g) butter, softened
2 eggs
2 tablespoons vanilla extract
4 cups (600 g) plain flour
1 teaspoon salt
1 teaspoon baking soda
1 teaspoon cream of tartar

Makes 7 dozen cookies

You can frost them, but these sugar cookies are also tasty on their own. These are the cookies you bake in holiday shapes with the children, and there is no store-bought equivalent to that.

1 In a large bowl, combine the sugar and butter, and beat until the mixture is well creamed. Add the eggs and vanilla, and beat until the mixture is smooth.
2 In a small bowl, combine the flour, salt, baking soda and cream of tartar. Add the flour mixture to the cream mixture, and beat until all the ingredients are well blended. Cover the bowl with plastic wrap and place in the refrigerator until the dough is chilled, about 30 minutes.
3 Preheat the oven to 350°F, set out two or more baking sheets, and ightly flour a work surface.
4 Turn out the dough onto the prepared work surface. Using a rolling pin, roll the dough out to a 1/4-inch thickness. Using cookie cutters dipped in flour, cut out as many cookies as possible. Carefully transfer the cookies to the ungreased baking sheets. Collect the dough scraps, reroll, and cut out additional cookies until there is no more dough left.
5 Bake until the cookies are just lightly browned on the edges, 10 to 12 minutes.Transfer the cookies to wire racks to cool completely.

Brownies

1 cup (150 g) chopped dark chocolate
1½ cups (225 g) plain flour
1 teaspoon baking powder
½ teaspoon salt
¾ cup (185 g) butter, softened
1½ cups (330 g) sugar
4 eggs
2 teaspoons vanilla extract
2 cups (250 g) chopped walnuts or pecans

Makes about 24 brownies

This recipe is studded with nuts, but you can substitute chocolate chips or just make a plain brownie. Bought ones are no match for warm brownies out of your oven, filling the air with the smell of chocolate and costing you much less.

1 Preheat the oven to 350°F. Line a 13 x 9 x 2-inch slab pan or baking sheet with foil. Lightly grease and flour the foil.
2 In a small, heavy saucepan over the lowest heat, melt the chocolate, stirring occasionally. Remove from the heat and let the chocolate cool. Alternatively, melt the chocolate on low power in the microwave.
3 In a small bowl or on a sheet of parchment paper, combine the flour, baking powder and salt.
4 In a large bowl, cream the butter for 2 minutes using electric beaters on medium speed. Add the sugar and beat for 2 minutes longer. Add the eggs, one at a time, beating well after each addition. Beat in the vanilla and cooled chocolate.
5 Using a wooden spoon, add the flour mixture to the chocolate mixture and stir until well blended. Stir in the nuts. Pour the batter into the slab pan.
6 Bake until a toothpick inserted in the center comes out clean, about 35 minutes. Transfer the pan to a wire rack and let the brownies cool before cutting.

If you run out of dark chocolate

If a recipe calls for 1 oz (30 g) dark chocolate and you don't have any, combine 3 tablespoons cocoa powder with 1 tablespoon softened butter, margarine or vegetable shortening. Add 1 tablespoon sugar, if you like, to make a sweeter mixture.

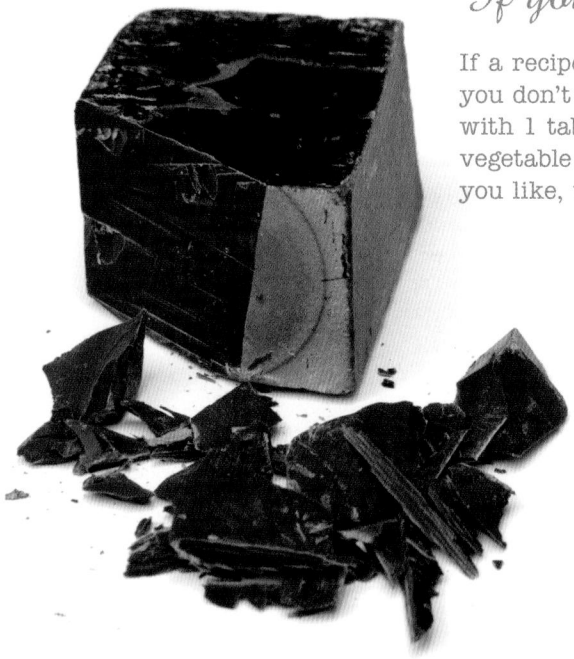

Graham Crackers

1 cup (150 g) plain flour
1¼ cups (185 g) whole wheat flour plus additional
5 tablespoons sugar
1 teaspoon baking powder
½ teaspoon salt
½ teaspoon baking soda
½ teaspoon ground cinnamon
3 tablespoons chilled butter or margarine, cut into small pieces
¼ cup (60 g) vegetable shortening
2 tablespoons honey
1 tablespoon molasses
¼ cup (60 ml) water
1 teaspoon vanilla extract

Makes 24 to 28 crackers

Store-bought just won't taste the same after you enjoy your homemade graham crackers.

1 In a medium bowl, combine the flours, sugar, baking powder, salt, baking soda and cinnamon. Using a pastry blender or two knives, cut in the butter and shortening until the mixture resembles coarse crumbs.
2 In a small bowl, combine the honey, molasses, water, and vanilla, and stir until well blended. Using a fork, gradually add the honey mixture to the flour mixture, tossing the ingredients together until they are well blended. Form the dough into a ball; the mixture may be crumbly, but do not add water. Cover the dough with plastic wrap and place in the refrigerator until the dough is chilled, for several hours.
3 Place the oven rack in the center of the oven and preheat to 350°F; set out two large baking sheets. Divide the dough in half and let it stand at room temperature for 15 minutes.
4 Spread wax paper over a work surface. Lightly sprinkle whole wheat flour over the wax paper. Place one dough half on the paper, and flatten the dough with a rolling pin. Sprinkle the dough with more whole wheat flour, and cover it with a second piece of wax paper. Using the rolling pin, roll out the dough to form a 7 x 15-inch rectangle; if the dough breaks, pinch the pieces together before continuing to roll.
5 Peel off the top piece of wax paper. Using a fork, mark dotted lines at ½- to 1-inch intervals, breaking the dough into 2 ½-inch squares. Using a spatula, transfer the dough to a baking sheet, placing the squares close together. Repeat with the remaining dough and second baking sheet. Gather the scraps and reroll until all the dough is made into squares.
6 Bake until the crackers are lightly browned on the edges, about 15 minutes.Transfer the crackers to wire racks to cool. Store the graham crackers in an airtight container at room temperature for 1 month, or freeze the crackers in a freezer-safe container for up to 6 months.

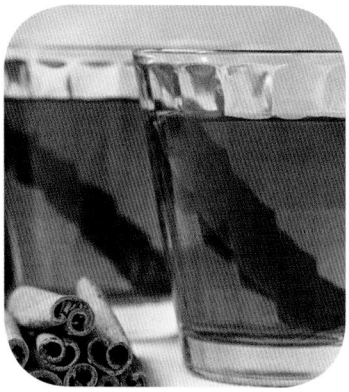

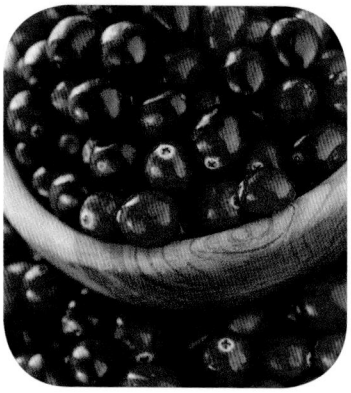

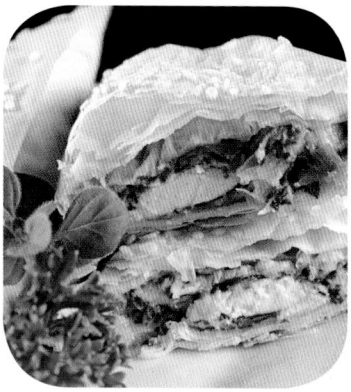

Fast Foods and Snacks

Potato Chips ❖ Spicy Nut Mix ❖ Pretzels ❖ Oven-Baked French Fries ❖ Pizza ❖ Chicken Nuggets

Breakfast Treats

Traditional French Toast ❖ Baked French Toast ❖ Granola Bar ❖ Apricot Oat Bars ❖ Scones ❖ Pancakes ❖ Waffles

Appetizing Nibbles

Antipasto Platter ❖ Chicken Liver Pâté ❖ Ham, Pork and Veal Terrine ❖ Country Pork Sausages ❖ Deviled Eggs ❖ Globe Artichokes in Olive Oil ❖ Marinated Goat's Cheese ❖ Spinach and Feta Phyllo Triangles ❖ Quesadillas ❖ Curry Puffs

Dips

Baba Ghanoush ❖ Hummus ❖ Guacamole ❖ Beet Dip ❖ Taramasalata ❖ Tapenade ❖ Tzatziki

Cold Drinks

Classic Iced Tea ❖ Cranberry Iced Tea ❖ Frosty Caramel Cappuccino ❖ Iced Coffee Slush ❖ Lemonade Syrup ❖ Ginger Beer ❖ Traditional Lemonade ❖ Lemon Squash ❖ Orange Blossom ❖ Sparkling Fruit Bowl ❖ Lemon Barley Water ❖ Bloody Mary Mix ❖ Bloody Mary ❖ Fruit Juice Spritzer ❖ Sangria

Hot Drinks

Caffe Latte ❖ Cappuccino Mix ❖ Cocoa ❖ Hot Chocolate Viennese ❖ Chai ❖ Hot Spiced Tea ❖ Hot Mulled Cider ❖ Hot Nonalcoholic Punch

Snacks, Nibbles and Drinks

When it comes to satisfying those afternoon munchies, the recipes in this chapter provide healthy alternatives to greasy fast food and bags of salty snacks from the vending machine.

You'll find real honest-to-goodness homemade potato chips, chicken nuggets and even pizza. And when you taste them, you'll finally realize why these foods became so popular in the first place. You may even spoil yourself and never be able to settle for the commercial versions again. Your own pizza dough, you'll discover, is yeasty and delicious, inviting new and interesting toppings.

You'll also find recipes for those breakfast treats that we often go out for—or buy frozen and pay far too much for. In addition, there are recipes here that can be real money savers when you entertain. You'll discover how easy it is to make your own finger foods and dips instead of hiring a caterer or buying them from the local deli. The savory treats in this chapter include an antipasto platter, pâté and rich cheesy nibbles as well as several delicious easy-to-make dips.

For an insatiable thirst or caffeine craving, the recipes here provide not only some pleasing summer quenchers but also some delightful and economical alternatives to the pricey products at your local cafe.

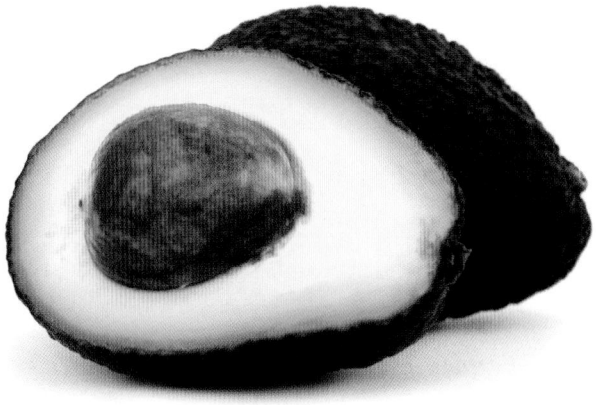

Fast Foods and Snacks

Potato Chips

vegetable oil for deep-frying (about 8 cups/2 liters)
1 lb (500 g) roasting (floury) potatoes, peeled
salt, to taste

Makes 4 servings

We are a nation of snackers, so we might as well make our own and ensure they are as healthy as they can be.

1 Pour the oil in a deep-fryer or large, heavy saucepan to a depth of about 3 inches. Insert a deep-fat thermometer and heat the oil to 375°F.
2 Meanwhile, slice the potatoes into rounds about ⅛-inch thick. As you work, drop the rounds into iced water. When ready to fry, lift the rounds from the water and pat dry on paper towels.
3 Place the potato slices in the fryer in small batches to avoid lowering the temperature of the oil; fry until crisp and golden, 3 to 5 minutes per batch. Using a slotted spoon or fryer basket, transfer the chips to paper towels to drain. Let the oil reheat to the correct temperature before frying the next batch.
4 Lightly sprinkle the chips with salt and serve.

Spicy Nut Mix

3 teaspoons vegetable oil
½ cup (80 g) almonds
½ cup (80 g) Brazil nuts
½ cup (80 g) cashew nuts
½ cup (70 g) hazelnuts
½ cup (80 g) macadamia nuts
½ cup (80 g) peanuts
½ cup (50 g) pecans
½ cup (50 g) walnut halves
2 tablespoons sugar
½ teaspoon ground cayenne pepper, or to taste
salt, to taste

Makes 4 cups

This lightly spiced mixture of nuts is perfect for lunch box snacks or party nibbles.

1 Heat the oil in a large, heavy, nonstick frying pan or skillet over medium heat. Add the nuts, tossing to coat.
2 Add the sugar, cayenne pepper and a pinch of salt and cook, stirring constantly, for 8 minutes, until the sugar has caramelized and the nuts are well coated. Serve the nuts hot or at room temperature.

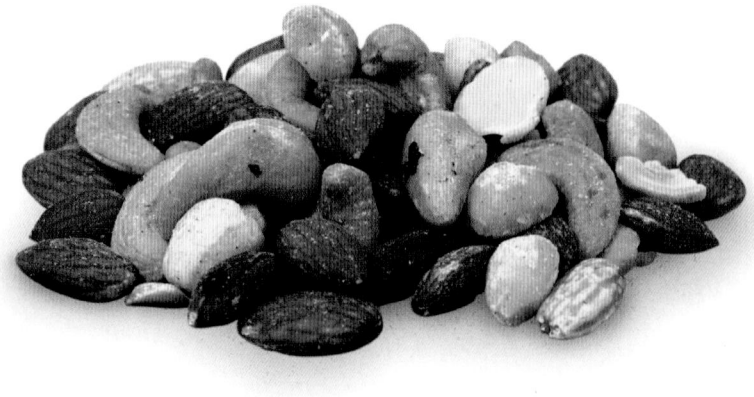

Pretzels

1½ teaspoons active dry yeast
¾ cup (200 ml) warm (110°F–115°F) water
1½ teaspoons sugar
¾ teaspoon salt
1½ cups (225 g) plain flour
2 tablespoons butter, melted
Coarse or kosher salte

Makes 6 pretzels

Big, chewy, and oh, so satisfying! You may never get to taste these pretzels—if your family gets to them first!

1 In a large mixing bowl, combine the yeast and warm water, and stir to dissolve the yeast. Stir in the sugar and the salt. Add the flour, ½ cup at a time, to form a soft dough.
2 On a lightly floured surface, turn out the dough and knead until the dough is soft and elastic, about 5 minutes (the dough will be slightly sticky). Place the dough in a lightly oiled bowl, turning once to coat the top of the dough ball with oil. Cover the bowl and let the dough rise in a warm (70°F to 80°F) place until it is doubled in size, about 1 hour.
3 Preheat the oven to 425°F. Punch down the dough and divide it into six equal portions. On a lightly floured surface, roll one dough portion into a 14-inch-long rope; twist the rope into a pretzel shape—an oval with overlapping ends in the middle. Place the pretzel on a lightly greased baking sheet. Repeat with the remaining dough portions. Brush each pretzel with the melted butter and sprinkle with salt.
4 Bake the pretzels until they are golden brown, 15 to 20 minutes. Transfer the pretzels to wire racks to cool slightly.

Oven-Baked French Fries

2 tablespoons cornstarch
2 tablespoons low-sodium soy sauce
4 potatoes, peeled and cut into strips
1 tablespoon olive oil
¼ teaspoon salt

Makes 4 servings

A healthier alternative to the perennial favorite, these fries are loaded with flavor but are low in fat.

1 In a large bowl, combine the cornstarch, soy sauce and 4 cups (1 liter) water, then whisk until well blended and smooth. Add the potatoes, toss gently, then cover and refrigerate for 1 hour.
2 Preheat the oven to 375°F. Drain the potatoes and place on paper towels to drain; pat dry. In a large bowl, toss the potatoes with the olive oil and sprinkle with the salt. Coat a baking sheet with cooking spray. Arrange the potato strips in a single layer over the baking sheet. Bake for 15 minutes, then turn the fries over and bake for 15 to 20 minutes longer, until tender and golden brown. Serve hot.

Pizza

¼ cup (60 ml) warm water (about 110°F–115°F)
¼ oz (7 g) package dry yeast
1½ cups (225 g) unsifted plain flour
¼ cup (60 ml) olive oil
½ teaspoon salt

TOPPING
cornmeal, for dusting
½ cup (125 ml) tomato sauce or paste (or use a mixture of each)
toppings as desired: grated mozzarella, sliced pepperoni, sliced mushrooms, bell pepper strips, sautéed Italian sausage, sliced olives, thinly sliced onions, bacon, pineapple, anchovies, etc

Makes a 12-inch (30 cm) pizza

Making your own pizza is not only thrifty but an easy way to please everyone—let each family member choose the topping for their part of the finished pizza. It will be easier if you have a baking stone or baking tiles for the bottom of the oven and a baker's paddle to transfer the pizza into and out of the oven. This recipe makes enough dough for a single family-sized pizza, or you can divide it into four pieces to make individual pizzas so everyone can top their own.

1 In a small bowl, combine the warm water, yeast and ¼ cup (35 g) of the flour. Stir to combine, then cover and let rise for 30 minutes.
2 Stir down the yeast mixture; add ¼ cup (60 ml) room-temperature water, the remaining flour, the olive oil and salt. On a lightly floured surface, turn out the dough and knead for 10 minutes (or use the dough hook of an electric mixer and knead for 5 minutes).
3 For use within 1 day, wrap the dough tightly in plastic wrap and store in the refrigerator; let it sit at room temperature for 1 to 2 hours before using. (To freeze the dough for later use, wrap it tightly in plastic wrap, place in a self-sealing freezer-safe plastic bag, squeeze out all the air and seal. Freeze for up to 3 months. Thaw in the plastic wrap in the refrigerator for several hours, then bring the dough to room temperature before using.)
4 Remove the racks from your oven and place a baking stone on the bottom of the oven. Preheat the oven to 450°F for about 20 minutes; it should be very hot. Dust a heavy upside-down baking sheet or a wooden baker's paddle with cornmeal. On a lightly floured surface using a lightly floured rolling pin, roll the dough into a 12-inch circle. Flop the dough over the rolling pin and unroll onto the cornmeal-covered baking sheet or paddle. (You can also sprinkle cornmeal on a regular baking sheet and cook the pizza on an oven rack, but the crust may be soggier.)
5 Spread the tomato sauce or paste over the pizza dough, leaving a 1-inch margin. Scatter the toppings as desired.
6 Gently shake the pizza off the baking sheet or paddle onto the baking stone. Bake until the crust is golden brown, about 20 minutes. Serve immediately.

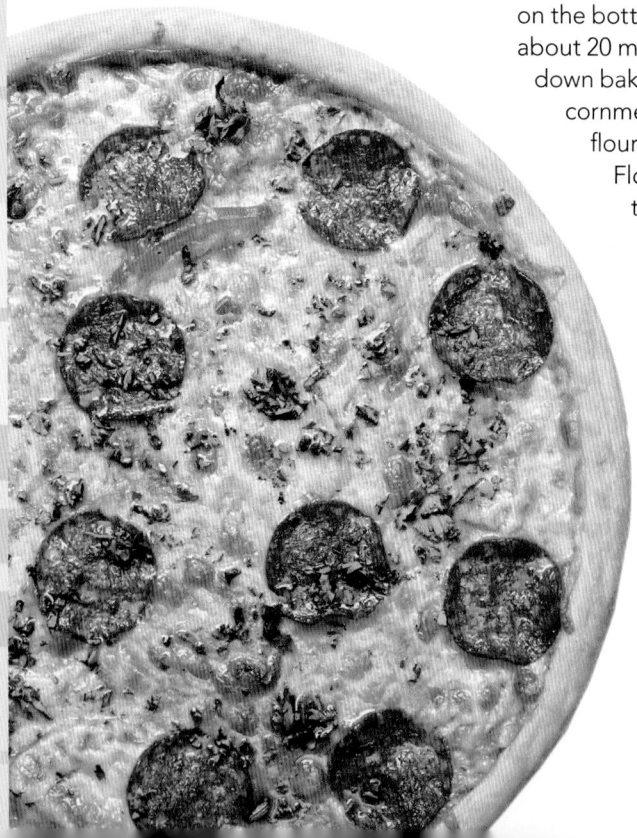

Chicken Nuggets

1½ lb (750 g) skinless chicken breasts
½ cup (75 g) Chicken Seasoning Mix (page 42)
2 cups (200 g) dry bread crumbs
2 large eggs

Makes 6 servings

For many parents, these morsels are a life- and time-saver, but the cost of regularly buying them can really eat away at your budget.

1 Cut each chicken breast into 1-inch cubes. Place the seasoning mix in a self-sealing bag. Place the bread crumbs in a large, shallow dish. In another shallow dish, whisk together the eggs and 2 tablespoons water until frothy.
2 Drop the chicken cubes, a few pieces at a time, into the bag of seasoning; seal and shake until they are well coated. Shake off any excess seasoning. Dip each cube into the beaten egg, then into the bread crumbs, gently pressing the crumbs onto the chicken until they stick. Arrange on a large, nonstick baking sheet and place in the refrigerator to chill for 30 minutes.
3 Preheat the oven to 400°F. Bake the chicken nuggets until they are golden brown and crisp, about 15 minutes, turning them once or twice during cooking. Serve hot or at room temperature.

Breakfast Treats

Traditional French Toast

4 eggs
1 cup (250 ml) milk
1 teaspoon vanilla extract
pinch of ground nutmeg
pinch of ground cinnamon
8 slices bread

Makes 4 servings

There are two methods for making French toast—this recipe is a quick fix in the morning; the recipe on the following page can be prepared the night before, then baked in the morning while the coffee brews.

1 In a bowl, lightly beat the eggs and the milk. Stir in the vanilla, nutmeg and cinnamon. Pour the mixture into a large, shallow dish with a flat base.
2 Coat a large frying pan or skillet with cooking spray. Heat the pan to hot but not smoking. Working one at a time, dip each piece of bread into the egg mixture, completely soaking it, then place the slice in the pan. Cook until the bread is brown on one side, flip it over, then cook the other side. Serve immediately, or keep warm briefly in a 200°F oven while cooking the remaining toasts.

Baked French Toast

3 eggs
1½ cups (375 ml) milk
2 tablespoons unsalted butter or margarine, melted
3 tablespoons light or dark brown sugar
½ teaspoon finely grated lemon zest
pinch of ground nutmeg
pinch of ground cinnamon
14 slices French bread (about ¾-inch/2 cm thick)
1 tablespoon confectioners' sugar

Makes 4 servings

You can make this luscious toast the night before, then pop it into the oven in the morning.

1 In a bowl, beat the eggs, milk, butter, sugar, lemon zest, nutmeg and cinnamon. Pour half the mixture into a large greased baking dish or tray. Lay the bread slices on top in a single layer, pressing them as close together as possible. Pour the remaining mixture over the bread slices and cover the pan with foil. Refrigerate overnight, or for at least 2 hours.
2 Preheat the oven to 350°F. Bake, uncovered, until the toast is puffy and golden brown, 50 to 60 minutes. Sprinkle with the confectioners' sugar. Serve hot with maple or blueberry syrup, honey, or fresh fruit, nuts and yogurt.

Granola Bar

½ cup (20 g) barley flakes
¼ cup (60 ml) cloudy apple juice, heated
⅓ cup (60 g) dried apricots
⅓ cup (40 g) golden seedless raisins
¼ cup (20 g) dried apples
¼ cup (30 g) sweetened dried cranberries
⅓ cup (60 g) dates
½ cup (50 g) toasted pecans
1 cup (100 g) rolled oats
¼ cup (35 g) whole wheat self-rising flour
2 tablespoons superfine sugar (optional)
¼ cup (30 g) sunflower seeds
¼ cup (60 g) butter or margarine
¼ cup (90 g) honey
½ teaspoon vanilla extract
1 egg

Makes 20 slices

Try this muesli bar and you'll never have a packaged one again. Full of nutritious foods, this is a great snack to take to work or pack in the lunch box. Substitute your favorite mix of dried fruit or nuts.

1 Preheat the oven to 350°F and grease a 12 x 8-inch cake pan. Line the base and two long sides with parchment paper, extending the paper an inch above the pan to help with removal later.
2 Place the barley flakes in a large heatproof bowl and pour the warm apple juice over them. Leave to stand while you chop up the dried fruit and pecans.
3 To the barley flakes, add the oats, flour, sugar (if using), dried fruit, pecans and sunflower seeds.
4 In a small saucepan, melt the butter with the honey over low heat. Cool a little, then add the vanilla extract and egg and stir to combine.
5 Pour the butter mixture over the oat mixture and mix thoroughly. Press the mixture into the cake pan and cook for 25 to 30 minutes, until lightly golden. Leave in the pan to cool, then cut into fingers or squares.

Apricot Oat Bars

1⅓ cups (240 g) dried apricots, cut into quarters
1½ cups (375 ml) orange juice
grated zest of ½ orange
⅓ cup (75 g) crystallized ginger, roughly chopped
2 cups (200 g) rolled oats
2 tablespoons soft brown sugar
1 tablespoon sunflower seeds

Makes 8 bars

These soft, chewy bars, packed with sweet fruit and ginger, make an ideal midmorning or afternoon snack.

1 Place the apricots in a saucepan with the orange juice and zest and bring to a boil. Reduce the heat and simmer, uncovered and stirring occasionally, for 25 to 30 minutes, until the liquid is absorbed. Puree in a food processor or using a hand-held mixer.
2 Meanwhile, heat the oven to 350°F. Line the base of a 9-inch round cake pan with nonstick parchment paper.
3 Stir the ginger, rolled oats, sugar and sunflower seeds into the apricot puree and mix well, then tip into the pan and spread out evenly.
4 Bake for 30 to 35 minutes, until firm and golden brown. Cool slightly, cut into wedges, then leave to cool completely in the pan. Peel off the paper before serving.

Scones

3 cups (450 g) self-rising flour
1 teaspoon salt
2 teaspoons sugar
¼ cup (60 g) butter
1 cup (250 ml) milk

Makes about 12 scones

You can add all sorts of things to scones, including currants, chopped dried apricots, or mini chocolate chips—experiment with gusto!

1 Preheat the oven to 425°F. Line two baking sheets with parchment paper.
2 In a large bowl, stir together the flour, salt and sugar. Rub in the butter using your fingertips. Make a well in the center of the flour and pour in the milk in a steady stream, stirring in the flour until a soft dough forms.
3 Turn the dough out onto a lightly floured surface and gently knead five to six times. Using a lightly floured rolling pin, roll out the dough to a ½-inch thickness and, using a floured 3-inch cutter, cut out scone rounds. Reroll the scraps as necessary (do not knead again) and cut more scones.
4 Place the scones 2 inches apart on the baking sheets and bake until golden brown, 10 to 15 minutes. Eat hot or just warm.

VARIATION

Scone Wedges: Follow steps 1–2 of the above recipe. Turn the dough out onto a lightly greased baking sheet and pat into a large round. If desired, brush the top with milk and sprinkle with sugar or a combination of sugar and cinnamon. Using a floured knife, cut the dough round into 8 wedges, but don't separate the pieces. Bake in the preheated oven for 12 minutes, or until golden brown. Carefully separate the scone wedges and serve immediately.

Pancakes

2 cups (300 g) Pancake and Waffle Mix (page 61)
2 large eggs, lightly beaten
1 cup (250 ml) milk

Makes 10 to 12 pancakes

Sliced bananas and strawberries, whole blueberries or even chocolate chips can be added to the pancake batter for a luscious breakfast treat.

1 In a large bowl, combine all the ingredients and stir until just blended. Don't overmix—the batter should be slightly lumpy.
2 Coat a large frying pan or skillet with cooking spray. Heat the pan to hot but not smoking. Spoon the batter into the pan, using about ¼ cup (60 ml) per pancake, and cook over medium heat until bubbles form across the top, about 2 minutes. Flip the pancakes and cook the other side for about 2 minutes more. Serve immediately, or keep warm briefly in a 200°F oven while cooking the remaining pancakes.

Waffles

2 large eggs, separated
1¾ cups (260 g) Pancake and Waffle Mix (page 61)
1 cup (250 ml) milk
3 tablespoons butter or margarine, melted
1 teaspoon vanilla extract (optional)

Makes about 5 waffles

A classic breakfast or brunch dish for special occasions, waffles go perfectly with maple syrup and also with fresh fruit toppings.

1 Following the manufacturer's directions, preheat a waffle iron.
2 In a large bowl, lightly beat the egg yolks. Add the remaining ingredients and stir until the mixture is just moistened.
3 In a bowl, beat the egg whites using electric beaters until soft peaks form. Using a rubber spatula, gently fold the egg whites into the batter until no white streaks remain.
4 Cook the waffles following the manufacturer's directions.

The origin of waffles

Perhaps surprisingly, waffles have been enjoyed for centuries. From the time of the ancient Greeks and throughout the Middle Ages, flat cakes were baked between two metal plates called wafer irons. These were popular into the 13th century. At that time, an enterprising craftsman forged decorative plates to resemble honeycombs. The name "waffle" is derived from the Dutch word wafel, meaning "wafer." In the 20th century, an electric waffle iron made these breakfast treats even easier to make.

Appetizing Nibbles

Antipasto Platter

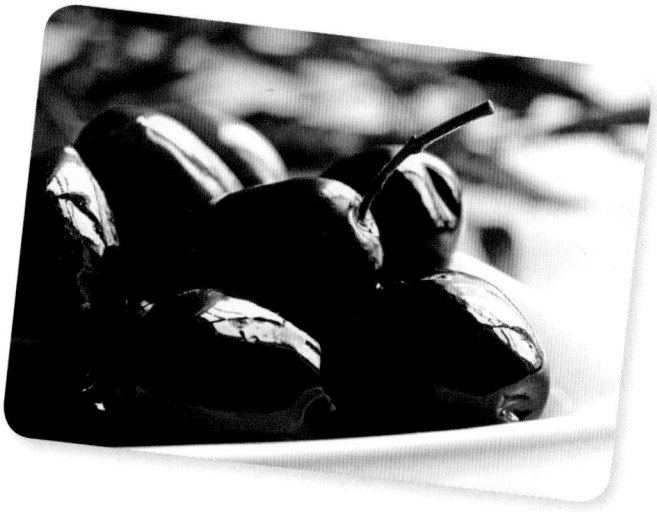

1 lb (500 g) small new potatoes, quartered
¼ cup (60 ml) olive oil
1 teaspoon dried rosemary
1 teaspoon salt
1 large red bell pepper, cut into 1-inch (2 cm) strips
1 large green bell pepper, cut into 1-inch (2 cm) strips
2 zucchini, cut into 1-inch (2 cm) slices
2 small red onions, cut into thin wedges
8 oz (250 g) button mushrooms
2 cloves garlic, crushed
8 oz (250 g) fresh mozzarella, sliced
½ lb (250 g) prosciutto, sliced
1 cup (185 g) oil-cured Greek black or green olives
sprigs of fresh rosemary or thyme

MARINADE
¼ cup (60 ml) balsamic vinegar
1 tablespoon extra virgin olive oil
1 tablespoon chopped fresh parsley
¼ teaspoon dried thyme
2 teaspoons Dijon mustard
1 small clove garlic, finely chopped
1 teaspoon lemon zest
½ teaspoon salt
¼ teaspoon freshly ground black pepper

Makes 6 to 8 servings

The star of any buffet is an antipasto ("before the meal") platter. This classic appetizer has colorful marinated vegetables, cheese and cold meats in an eye-catching arrangement. Accentuate the drama of the plate by placing contrasting colors or shapes next to each other—straight or diagonal patterns on a rectangular plate or concentric circles on a round or oval platter.

1 Preheat the oven to 450°F. In a large, shallow baking pan, combine the potatoes, olive oil, rosemary and salt. Toss to coat the potatoes well, then bake, uncovered, for 15 minutes.
2 Add the bell peppers, zucchini, onions and mushrooms to the baking pan. Sprinkle the garlic over all the vegetables. Bake, uncovered, until the vegetables are lightly browned and tender, 35 to 45 minutes.
3 Meanwhile, combine the marinade ingredients in a small bowl. Whisk until well blended and smooth.
4 Pour the marinade over the cooked vegetables in the baking pan, and stir gently until they are thoroughly coated. Let the vegetables cool to room temperature.
5 Arrange the marinated vegetables, mozzarella, prosciutto and olives in an attractive pattern on a large serving platter. Garnish with rosemary or thyme.

Chicken Liver Pâté

2 tablespoons butter
½ lb (250 g) chicken livers, cleaned, trimmed and halved
⅓ cup (90 g) cream cheese, at room temperature
1–2 tablespoons brandy
1 teaspoon salt
pinch of freshly ground black pepper
½ teaspoon dried thyme
pinch of ground nutmeg

Makes 4 servings

This smooth, rich paste is easy to make at home for your fanciest occasions. Serve it with toast wedges, water crackers or slices of baguette.

1 In a heavy frying pan or skillet, melt the butter over medium-high heat. Add the chicken livers and cook until lightly browned, 4 to 5 minutes.
2 Transfer the livers to a food processor or blender. Pour in the pan drippings, scraping up the browned bits in the pan and adding them also. Add the cream cheese, brandy, salt, pepper, thyme and nutmeg. Process until the mixture forms a smooth paste, 20 to 30 seconds. Taste and adjust the seasonings as desired.
3 Using a spatula, scrape the paste into a ramekin or serving bowl, smoothing the top. Cover and refrigerate overnight.

Ham, Pork and Veal Terrine

1 lb (500 g) diced cooked ham
1 lb (500 g) pork mince
1 lb (500 g) veal mince
1 clove garlic, crushed
1 teaspoon dried thyme
½ teaspoon dried marjoram
¼ teaspoon ground nutmeg or mace
1 teaspoon salt
pinch of freshly ground black pepper
½ cup (125 ml) dry white wine
4 small bay leaves
6–8 slices bacon
¼ lb (250 g) chicken livers, cleaned, trimmed and halved

Makes about 10 servings

A simple, classic baked terrine is perfect for a picnic in summer or sampling by a roaring fire in winter with pumpernickel or crusty French bread.

1 Preheat the oven to 300°F. In a large glass or ceramic bowl, combine the ham, pork and veal. Add the garlic, thyme, marjoram, nutmeg or mace, salt and pepper. Using clean, damp hands, mix the ingredients until they are well blended. Mix in the wine, cover and refrigerate for 1 hour.
2 Arrange the bay leaves in the bottom of a 9 x 5-inch loaf pan. Line the sides of the pan crosswise with half the bacon slices, allowing the ends to hang over the edges of the pan. Pack half the meat mixture into the loaf pan. Arrange the chicken livers along the center of the meat, then add the remaining meat mixture. Cover the terrine with the remaining bacon slices, tucking in the ends and folding the ends of the bottom slices over the top of the loaf.
3 Set the pan in a baking dish. Pour enough warm water into the baking dish to come halfway up the sides of the pan. Bake for 2 to 2½ hours, until the terrine pulls away from the sides of the pan and the juices run clear when it is pierced with a clean skewer or toothpick.
4 Set the pan on a wire rack and let the terrine cool. Pour off any liquid. When the terrine is completely cool, turn it out onto a plate, cover with plastic wrap and refrigerate overnight.

Country Pork Sausages

2 lb (1 kg) lean pork, trimmed
¼ lb (250 g) uncooked pork fat
1½ teaspoons sea salt
1½ teaspoons dried sage, crumbled
½ teaspoon dried thyme, crumbled
¼ teaspoon crushed black peppercorns
1 small onion, finely chopped

Makes 10 to 12 sausages

Needing no casings, these hearty and delicious homemade sausages are ready to star at your next brunch. Because you make them, you know what's in them and you can adjust the seasonings to suit your own tastes.

1 Cut the pork and pork fat into ½-inch cubes. Place in a large bowl, cover and refrigerate until the meat is chilled.
2 In a small bowl, combine the salt, sage, thyme and the peppercorns. Sprinkle the seasoning mixture over the meat, add the onion, then thoroughly mix all the ingredients together using your hands.
3 Place half the sausage mixture in a food processor or blender and process to a medium-coarse consistency. Scrape the pureed mixture into another large bowl and repeat with the remaining sausage mixture. Cover and refrigerate for 12 hours or overnight to let the texture firm up and allow the flavors to develop fully.
4 Using damp hands, divide the sausage mixture into 10 or 12 equal portions and roll each portion into a ball. Form each ball into a small sausage patty. Either cook immediately or place the sausages on parchment paper or freezer paper, with pieces of paper between any layers. Wrap the entire package of sausages in foil or a self-sealing plastic bag. Refrigerate the uncooked sausages for up to 2 days or store in the freezer for up to 3 weeks.
5 To cook the sausages, heat a large, heavy frying pan over medium heat. Add the sausages and cook, turning them often, until browned on all sides and cooked through, 13 to 15 minutes. Drain off any fat as it accumulates, and transfer the cooked sausages to paper towels to drain completely before serving.

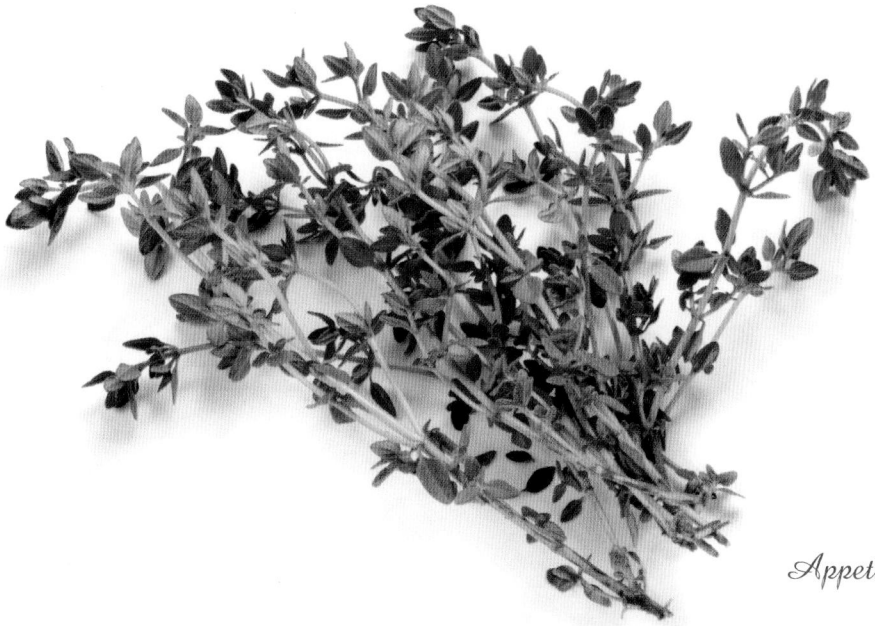

Deviled Eggs

12 eggs
½ cup (125 g) Classic Mayonnaise (page 29)
1 tablespoon mustard
1 tablespoon white wine vinegar
1 teaspoon salt
1 teaspoon sugar
1 teaspoon ground white pepper
½ cup (70 g) finely chopped celery
paprika (optional)

Makes 12 servings

Contrary to popular terminology, eggs should never actually be boiled or they will turn gray. You can cook the eggs up to 1 day ahead, but to avoid contamination they should not be stuffed until just before serving.

1 Place the eggs in a single layer in a large saucepan. Add enough cold water to cover the eggs by 1 inch. Set the saucepan over high heat and bring to a full boil; immediately remove the pan from the heat, cover and let stand for 15 minutes.
2 Drain the eggs and crack the wide end of each, then plunge into a large bowl of iced water. To peel, crack each shell all over by tapping it on a work surface. Hold each egg under cold running water while removing the shell. Set each shelled egg on a paper towel to drain as you peel them.
3 Using a small, sharp knife, cut each egg in half lengthwise. Using a small spoon, scoop out the yolks and put them in a sieve set over a bowl. Arrange the egg white halves on a plate and refrigerate. Using the back of a spoon, press the egg yolks through the sieve into the bowl.
4 Add the mayonnaise, mustard, vinegar, salt, sugar, pepper and celery to the sieved yolks. Using a fork, stir gently to combine all the ingredients well.
5 Using a small spoon or a piping bag fitted with a number 6 star tip, fill each egg white half with about 1 tablespoon of the egg-yolk mixture. If desired, sprinkle the eggs with a little paprika before serving.

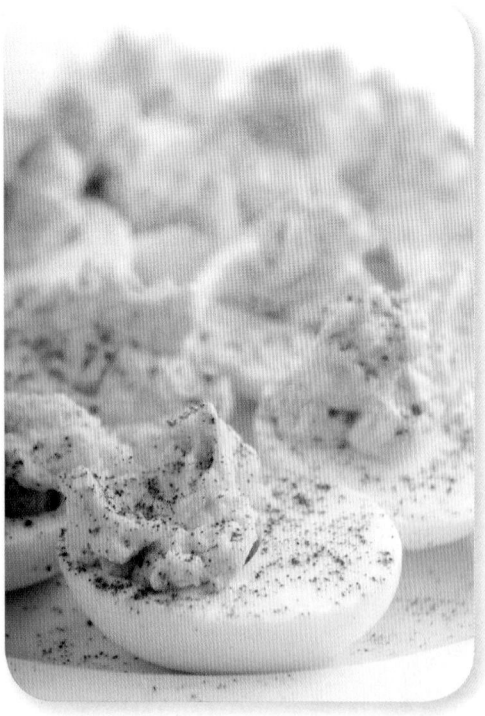

VARIATIONS

Caper-Dill Eggs: To the mayonnaise, add 3 tablespoons drained and chopped capers, 3 tablespoons finely chopped fresh dill and ½ teaspoon ground white pepper.
Chili Eggs: To the mayonnaise, add ½ teaspoon chili powder, or to taste, and 1 teaspoon ground cumin.
Curried Eggs: To the mayonnaise, add 1 tablespoon curry powder, or to taste, and 3 tablespoons chopped tomato chutney.
Spicy Eggs: To the mayonnaise, add 3 tablespoons bottled horseradish, or to taste, and 2 tablespoons finely chopped fresh parsley.

Globe Artichokes in Olive Oil

2 lb (1 kg/about 6 small) fresh young globe artichokes
1 large lemon, halved
4 cups (1 liter) white wine vinegar
1 tablespoon sea salt
1 tablespoon dill seeds
1 tablespoon black peppercorns
2 bay leaves
2 sprigs fresh herbs such as rosemary, dill or marjoram
2 cloves garlic, sliced
2 small fresh red chile peppers
3–4 cups (750 ml–1 liter) extra virgin olive oil

Makes 6 servings

The end of winter is the time to find small, tender baby artichokes at the markets. Use these seasoned artichokes in salads or as part of an antipasto platter, serve them with strong-flavored cheeses or just enjoy them on their own.

1 Using scissors, cut off the outer, tough leaves of each artichoke; trim off the pointed tip of each remaining leaf. Using a sharp knife, cut each artichoke in half lengthwise and rub the cut halves with the lemon halves to prevent browning. Fill a bowl with cold water and place the artichoke halves in the bowl with any remaining juice in the lemons. Let stand for 1 hour.
2 In a large, nonreactive saucepan, combine the vinegar, salt, dill seeds, peppercorns and bay leaves. Bring the mixture to a boil over medium-high heat.
3 Drain the artichokes and add them to the saucepan; reduce the heat to medium-low and simmer for 10 minutes.
4 Drain the artichokes again and let them dry; discard the cooking liquid. Transfer the artichokes to two large, warmed, sterilized, widemouthed jars, dividing them equally (see Safe Bottling and Preserving, page 72). Add 1 herb sprig, half the garlic slices and 1 chile pepper to each jar. Pour the olive oil over the artichokes, leaving a ¼-inch space between the top of the oil and the rim of the jar. Wipe the rims, cover and store in the refrigerator for up to 1 month. The artichokes will be ready for eating in a few days.

Marinated Goat's Cheese

1 goat's cheese (3–4 oz/100–125 g)
¼ teaspoon mixed peppercorns (black, white, green)
⅛ teaspoon coriander seeds, crushed
fresh thyme sprigs
fresh rosemary sprigs
fresh fennel sprigs
1 bay leaf
1 small red chile pepper
1 clove garlic
½ cup (125 ml) olive oil

Makes 1 round

How do you make a good thing even better? In the case of goat's cheese, you marinate it yourself in herb-infused olive oil. You can buy marinated goat's cheese, but this is easy and made to your own taste.

1 Center the goat's cheese in a warmed, sterilized, widemouthed jar. Tuck the peppercorns, coriander seeds, herb sprigs, bay leaf, chile pepper and garlic around the cheese.
2 Pour in the olive oil until the top of the oil is ¼-inch from the rim of the jar. Wipe the rim, cover the jar, then label and date it. Store in the refrigerator for up to 1 month; the cheese will be ready for eating in 1 week.

Spinach and Feta Phyllo Triangles

4 tablespoons (80 g) butter or margarine, plus an extra 2 teaspoons, melted
1 small onion, finely chopped
10 oz (300 g) frozen chopped spinach, thawed and squeezed dry
1 tablespoon finely chopped fresh dill or ¼ teaspoon dried dill, crumbled
½ cup (75 g) crumbled feta
1 egg, lightly beaten
6 sheets frozen phyllo pastry, thawed

Makes 12 triangles

It's true that phyllo, the multilayered Greek dough, is difficult and time-consuming to make. Purchased phyllo dough, however, is a wonderful base for appetizers, desserts or other dishes that can be expensive to buy finished. Follow the package directions to thaw the frozen dough; once opened, the dough will keep in the refrigerator for about 1 week.

1 Preheat the oven to 350°F. Melt the butter in a large frying pan or skillet over medium heat. Add the onion and sauté until translucent, 3 to 5 minutes. Add the spinach and cook for 2 minutes longer. Stir in the dill, then transfer to a large bowl. Add the feta and egg and stir until the mixture is well blended.
2 Lay one sheet of the phyllo pastry on a work surface and brush lightly with 1 teaspoon of the melted butter. Top the pastry with a second sheet of phyllo, brush with butter, and repeat with a third sheet of phyllo.
3 Using a sharp knife or pizza cutter and a ruler if you like, cut the stack of buttered phyllo sheets lengthwise into six strips about 1¾-inch wide. Cut the strips in half to make 12 in total. Place 1 tablespoon of the spinach–feta mixture at the end of each strip. Fold the end of each strip diagonally over the filling to form a triangle. Continue folding diagonally along the entire strip, alternating directions and ending with a triangular package. When each triangle is complete, brush the top with some of the butter. Repeat to make 12 triangles in total.
4 Line a baking sheet with parchment paper. Arrange the phyllo triangles on the sheet and bake until golden brown, about 25 minutes.

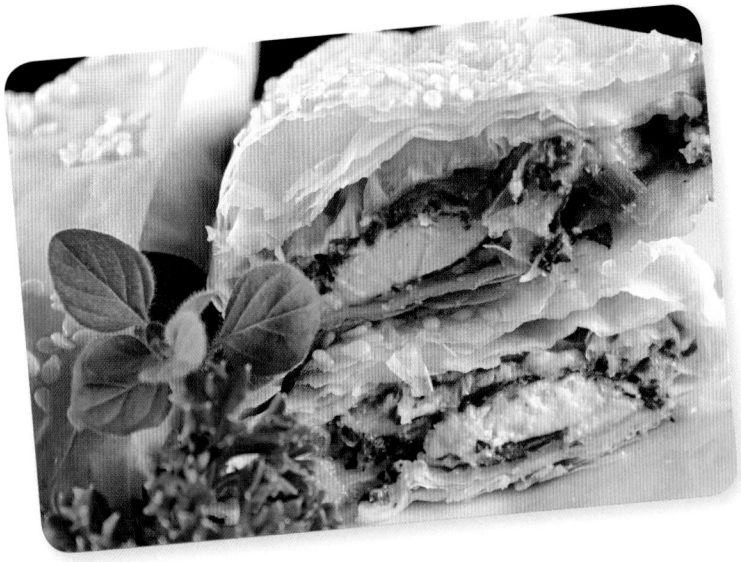

Quesadillas

four 8-inch (20 cm) flour tortillas
1 cup (4 oz/125 g) grated cheddar or other tasty cheese
1 large red bell pepper, cut into ¼-inch (5 mm) slices
¼ cup (50 g) cooked fresh or thawed frozen corn kernels
3 spring onions with tops, thinly sliced
3 tablespoons chopped fresh coriander
¼ cup (60 g) homemade or prepackaged salsa
Guacamole (page 151), sour cream or natural yogurt (optional)

Makes 4 servings

You can serve a quesadilla as a lunch dish or use a pizza cutter to cut it into small triangles and arrange on a plate with sour cream and guacamole as an appetizer.

1 Preheat the oven to 425°F. Place each tortilla on a 12-inch square of foil. Sprinkle each tortilla with the cheese, bell pepper, corn, spring onion, coriander and salsa, dividing the toppings equally. Moisten the edges of one tortilla and fold in half, encasing the toppings; press the edges together. Repeat with the remaining tortillas.
2 Move a folded tortilla so it is centered on the top half of the foil square. Fold each side edge of the foil over the quesadilla. Fold the bottom half of the foil up and over the quesadilla until the top and bottom foil edges are even; fold the edges over twice to make a package. Repeat with the remaining quesadillas and arrange on a baking sheet.
3 Bake the quesadillas until the cheese melts, about 7 minutes. Remove the baking sheet from the oven, unwrap the quesadillas and arrange them on a plate or serving platter. If desired, serve with a dollop of guacamole, sour cream or yogurt.

Curry Puffs

1¾ lb (800 g) potatoes, peeled and diced
1¼ cups (160 g) frozen baby peas
1½ tablespoons curry powder
½ teaspoon salt
6 sheets frozen butter puff pastry, just thawed
1 egg, beaten

Makes 24

These traditional Malaysian snacks are usually deep-fried, but using puff pastry and baking them in the oven gives a much lighter, puffier result.

1 Preheat the oven to 400°F. Put the potatoes in a saucepan of cold water, bring to a boil and cook, covered, until they are just tender. Add the peas and cook for a further 2 minutes. Remove from the heat and drain well. Add the curry powder and salt, then roughly mash.
2 Using a 4-inch cookie cutter, cut four circles from each sheet of pastry. Put 1 tablespoon of the potato mixture on each pastry circle. Fold in half and press the edges together. Starting at one end, fold a little of the pinched edge back over itself and continue to the other end, forming a neatly braided edge.
3 Arrange the curry puffs on baking sheets, brush with beaten egg and bake for 20 to 25 minutes, until puffed and golden.

Dips

Baba Ghanoush

1 large eggplant, about 1¼ lb (1.2 kg)
¼ cup (60 ml) lemon juice
1 tablespoon extra virgin olive oil
2 cloves garlic, quartered
¼ cup (65 g) tahini (sesame paste)
salt and freshly ground black pepper, to taste

Makes about 2 cups (440 g)

Much loved in the Middle East, this smoky favorite, available in supermarkets and delis, gets its flavor from charring the eggplant first. You can make this delicious dip yourself and serve it with pita triangles.

1 Preheat the broiler. Using a sharp fork or skewer, prick the eggplant all over. Place the eggplant in the broiler 6 inches from the heat source. Broil, turning every 5 minutes, until the skin is blackened and the eggplant is soft, about 20 minutes. Remove the eggplant and leave until cool to the touch.
2 Using a sharp knife, peel the eggplant. Roughly chop the flesh and place in a food processor or blender. Add the lemon juice, olive oil, garlic and tahini. Pulse until the mixture is well blended and of a spreadable consistency. Taste and season as desired with salt and pepper.
3 Scrape the dip into a bowl, then cover and refrigerate for at least 2 hours before serving to let the flavors develop.

Hummus

2 cups (480 g) cooked or drained, rinsed, canned chickpeas
1 tablespoon extra virgin olive oil
2 cloves garlic, quartered
½ teaspoon ground cumin
¼ cup (65 g) tahini (sesame paste)
¼–½ cup (60–125 ml) lemon juice
salt and freshly ground pepper, to taste
finely chopped fresh parsley or paprika, for sprinkling

Makes 1½ cups (330 g)

Another staple of Middle Eastern cooking, hummus is excellent with pita triangles, crudités or bagel chips, but it can be used as a spread in sandwiches too.

1 In a food processor or blender, combine the chickpeas, olive oil, garlic, cumin and tahini. Process until the mixture is of a rough consistency.
2 With the motor running, slowly pour in the lemon juice a little at a time until the desired consistency is reached. Taste the hummus and season with salt and pepper. Before serving, sprinkle with parsley or paprika.

Guacamole

2 ripe avocados, halved
1 tomato, cored, seeded and finely chopped
½ cup (80 g) finely chopped red onion
4 tablespoons chopped fresh coriander
2 tablespoons lime juice
¾ teaspoon salt
¾ teaspoon ground cumin (optional)
hot pepper sauce (optional)

Makes 2½ cups (550 g)

This creamy blend of avocados, tomato, red onion and coriander is a divine dip for chips, crudités, pretzels and more. It can also be a memorable addition to taco salads, grilled poultry or fish and is a must for wraps.

1 Using a spoon, scoop out the avocado flesh into a glass or ceramic bowl. Using a fork, mash the avocado, but not until completely smooth—there should be small chunks of flesh.
2 Add the tomato, onion, coriander and lime juice, and stir with the fork until the ingredients are well blended but the consistency is still slightly rough. If desired, stir in the cumin and hot pepper sauce to add more heat to the guacamole.
3 Spoon the dip into a serving bowl. Serve immediately, or cover and refrigerate until ready to serve.

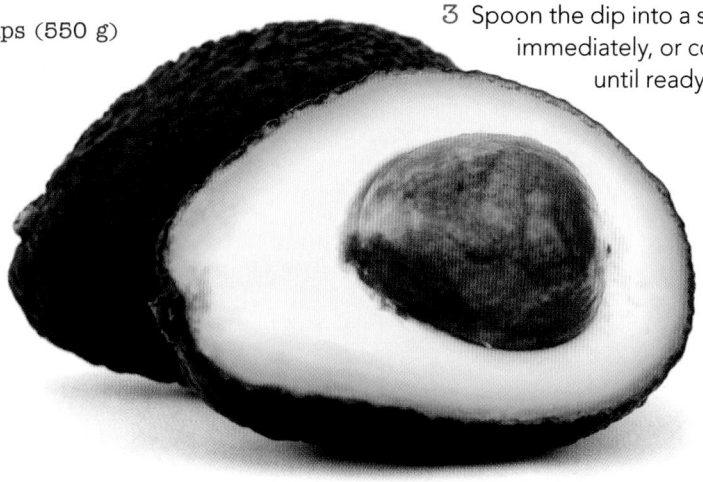

Beet Dip

5 red beets (about 2 lb/1 kg)
1¼ cups (310 g) natural low-fat yogurt
2 cloves garlic, crushed
¼ cup (60 ml) lemon juice
2 tablespoons extra virgin olive oil
½ teaspoon ground cumin
½ teaspoon ground coriander
½ teaspoon ground cinnamon
½ teaspoon paprika
freshly ground black pepper, to taste

Makes 4 servings

Serve this beautifully vibrant dip with chargrilled pita toasts for a casual start to a barbecue, or use it as a scrumptious sandwich filler.

1 Cut off the beet stems ½ inch from the roots (no closer). Scrub the roots very gently but thoroughly, being careful not to nick the skin.
2 Cook the beets in a large pot of simmering, salted water for 40 to 60 minutes, until tender. Drain and allow to cool slightly. When cool enough to handle, rub off the skins. It is a good idea to wear rubber gloves when doing this so your hands don't become stained.
3 Finely chop, grate or process the beets in a food processor, then transfer to a serving bowl.
4 Add the yogurt, garlic, lemon juice, oil, cumin, coriander, cinnamon and paprika and mix well. Season to taste with pepper, cover and refrigerate until required. Serve with warm crusty bread.

Taramasalata

7 oz (200 g) smoked cod's roe
1½ oz (40 g) (1 thick slice) stale white bread, crusts removed
2 tablespoons milk
⅓ cup (80 ml) vegetable oil
¼ cup (60 ml) olive oil
¼ cup (60 ml) lemon juice
1 clove garlic, crushed
freshly ground black pepper, to taste
wedge of lemon
sprigs of fresh flat-leaf parsley

Makes 4 servings

Quick and easy to make, this classic smoked cod's roe dip can be served as a snack with drinks or as a more formal starter with strips of pita bread.

1 Soak the cod's roe in a bowl of cold water for about 1 hour to remove some of the saltiness.
2 When you're ready to prepare the dip, soak the bread in the milk for 5 minutes. Rinse and drain the roe thoroughly, cut in half lengthwise, then, with the skin side down on a board, scrape the roe off the skin with a knife. Put the roe in a blender or food processor.
3 Squeeze the bread dry and add it to the roe. Blend together, trickling in first the vegetable oil, then the olive oil, while the motor is running.
4 Now add the lemon juice, a little at a time, adding a little extra, if desired, for a sharper taste. If the mixture is slightly thick, you can loosen it with a little boiling water rather than adding more oil or lemon juice. Add the garlic and season to taste with pepper.
5 Spoon the taramasalata into a bowl, cover and refrigerate until ready to serve. Garnish with a lemon wedge and parsley sprigs.

Dips are not just for dipping

So much more than something to plunge crackers, chips or crudités into, dips are a versatile culinary performer. Many can be used as condiments, toppings for various dishes, fillings for omelettes or spreads for sandwiches. Experiment!

Tapenade

1 cup (185 g) oil-cured Mediterranean or Greek black olives, pitted
6–8 anchovy fillets
¼ cup (40 g) capers, rinsed and squeezed dry
2 cloves garlic, halved
2 teaspoons lemon juice
3–4 tablespoons extra virgin olive oil
freshly ground black pepper, to taste

Makes about 1 cup (250 g)

Not for the timid palate, this rich spread combines the heady taste of olives, anchovies, capers and garlic. When bought from a deli, it's a pricey treat. Make your own and enjoy it on toasted slices of Italian bread, drizzled with extra virgin olive oil.

1 In a food processor or blender, puree the olives, anchovy fillets, capers, garlic and lemon juice until the mixture is finely chopped.
2 Add 3 tablespoons of the olive oil, pulsing on and off, until the mixture is a spreadable, grainy paste; add more olive oil as needed to reach the desired consistency. Taste the tapenade and season with pepper.

Tzatziki

1 cucumber, peeled, sliced lengthwise and seeded
2 cups (500 g) natural yogurt
1 clove garlic, crushed
1 tablespoon finely chopped fresh mint
2 tablespoons olive oil, plus extra for drizzling
sea salt and freshly ground black pepper, to taste

Makes about 2½ cups (625 g)

A creamy cucumber concoction to cool the fires of the spiciest dish, this quintessential Greek dip is a logical choice in summer, when cucumbers are plentiful. You can buy it in supermarkets, but it is easy to make your own. Serve it with crudités, chips or pita triangles, as a dressing for Greek salad or as an accompaniment for grilled kabobs or fish.

1 Cut the cucumber into small dice and spread between layers of paper towel to dry well.
2 In a bowl, combine the yogurt, cucumber, garlic, mint and olive oil and stir until well blended. Taste the tzatziki and season with salt and pepper.
3 Spoon into a serving bowl, cover and refrigerate until required. Serve drizzled with olive oil.

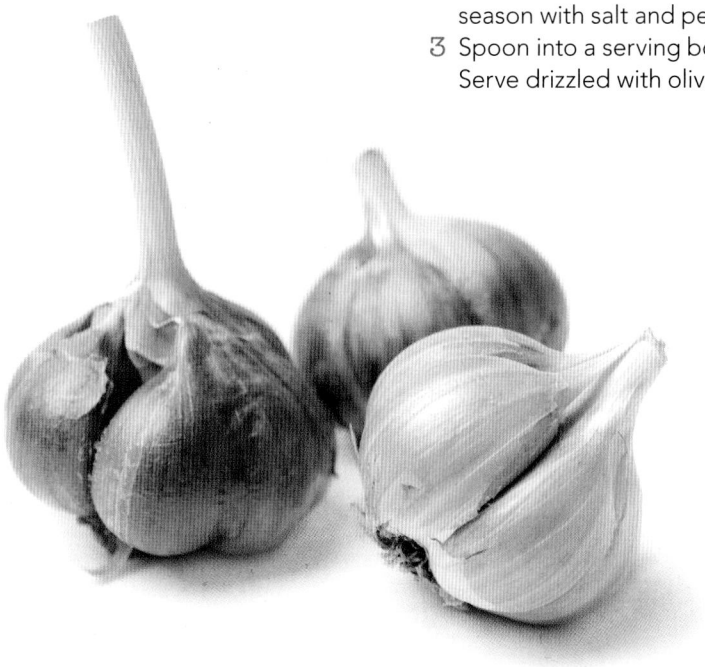

Cold Drinks

Classic Iced Tea

2 tablespoons tea leaves, or 6 tea bags
Sugar Syrup (opposite), to taste
ice cubes
lemon wedges or small fresh mint sprigs (optional)

Makes 4 servings

Always best when it is freshly made, iced tea is an economical thirst quencher.

1 In a kettle, bring 2 cups (500 ml) cold water to a full, rolling boil.
2 Rinse a teapot with boiling water and discard the water. Place the tea in the pot and slowly pour the boiling water over the tea. Cover the teapot and let the tea steep for 3 to 5 minutes.
3 Stir the tea once. Strain the tea into a large jug, add another 2 cups (500 ml) cold water and sweeten to taste with sugar syrup.
4 To serve, fill glasses with ice cubes and pour the cold tea over the ice; if desired, garnish each serving with a lemon wedge or mint sprig.

Cranberry Iced Tea

4 tablespoons tea leaves, or 6 tea bags
2 cups (500 ml) cranberry juice
Sugar Syrup (opposite), to taste
ice cubes
fresh or frozen whole cranberries or lime slices (optional)

Makes 4 servings

This fruity red tea is perfect for a special occasion.

1 In a kettle, bring 2 cups (500 ml) cold water to a full, rolling boil.
2 Rinse a teapot with boiling water and discard the water. Place the tea in the pot and slowly pour the boiling water over the tea. Cover the teapot and let the tea steep for 3 to 5 minutes.
3 Stir the tea once. Strain the tea into a large jug, add the cranberry juice and sweeten to taste with sugar syrup.
4 To serve, fill glasses with ice cubes and pour the cold tea over the ice; if desired, garnish each serving with a few whole cranberries or a lime wedge.

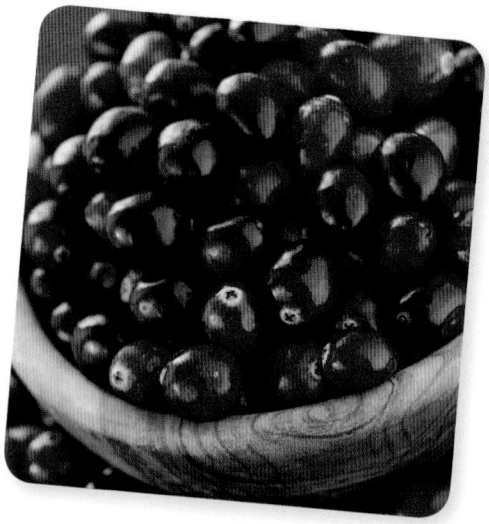

Sugar syrup: the perfect sweetener

Keep a jar of this sugar syrup in your refrigerator to sweeten iced teas and coffees. Because the sugar is already dissolved, you'll get the ideal sweetness without any graininess added. Here's how to make it:

In a small saucepan, combine 2 cups (440 g) sugar and 2½ cups (625 ml) water over medium heat. Cook, stirring frequently, until the mixture boils and the sugar has dissolved completely. Remove the saucepan from the heat, cover and let stand for 1 to 2 minutes to allow the steam to dissolve any unmelted crystals on the side of the saucepan. Pour the cooled syrup into a 1-quart (750 ml) jar, seal tightly and store in the refrigerator. Makes 3 cups (750 ml)

Frosty Caramel Cappuccino

2 cups (500 ml) milk
3 tablespoons Caramel Sauce (page 60), plus 2 teaspoons extra (optional)
2 teaspoons instant espresso coffee granules
8–10 ice cubes
4 tablespoons whipped cream

Makes 2 servings

Whip up this gourmet-style coffee concoction for almost nothing without leaving home or standing in line.

1. In a food processor or blender, combine the milk, 3 tablespoons of the caramel sauce, if using, the coffee granules and ice cubes. Process until the mixture is smooth.
2. Pour the mixture into two chilled glasses. Top with whipped cream and drizzle with the remaining caramel sauce if desired. Serve immediately.

Iced Coffee Slush

3 cups (750 ml) hot strong brewed coffee
½–1 cup (110–220 g) sugar
6 cups (1.5 liters) milk
1½ teaspoons vanilla extract

Makes 12 servings

This chilly delight will take the heat out of summer without making a hole in your purse or requiring a trip to a coffee shop.

1. In a freezer-safe bowl, combine the coffee and the amount of sugar desired. Stir until the sugar has completely dissolved, then cover and refrigerate until thoroughly chilled. Stir in the milk and vanilla. Re-cover the bowl and place in the freezer until the mixture is solid.
2. Several hours before serving, transfer the bowl to the refrigerator. Using a mallet, break up the coffee mixture, then place in a food processor or blender and process until slushy. Serve immediately.

Lemonade Syrup

3 cups (660 g) sugar
3 cups (750 ml) lemon juice (about 16 lemons)
2 tablespoons grated lemon zest

Makes about 5½ cups (1.4 liters) syrup

Whip up a batch of this syrup whenever you see lemons on sale, then keep it on hand to make the best homemade lemonade you've ever tasted—in a flash! This makes a much less expensive and better-tasting lemonade than anything you can buy.

1 Place the sugar in a 6-cup (1.5-liter) heatproof container. Add 1 cup (250 ml) boiling water, stirring constantly until the sugar has completely dissolved. Leave to cool.
2 Stir in the lemon juice and zest until well blended. Cover and store in the refrigerator for up to 1 week.

VARIATION
Limeade Syrup: Substitute 3 cups (750 ml) fresh lime juice and 2 tablespoons grated lime zest and proceed as above.

Ginger Beer

GINGER BEER "MOTHER"
½ teaspoon dried yeast
2 tablespoons sugar
2 tablespoons ground ginger

SUGAR SYRUP
4 cups (900 g) sugar
½ cup (125 ml) strained lemon juice

Makes 6 quarts (6 liters)

This fizzy and refreshing treat is made by fermenting sugar syrup with a yeast mixture called the "ginger beer mother" or "ginger beer plant."

1 For the ginger beer "mother," place the yeast and ½ teaspoon of the sugar in a large jar. Add 1 cup (250 ml) warm water and ½ teaspoon of the ginger. Mix well, cover the jar with a cloth and leave at room temperature for 8 days, mixing in ½ teaspoon each of the remaining sugar and ginger every day.
2 For the sugar syrup, put the sugar in a large saucepan with 6 cups (1.5 liters) cold water. Heat, stirring, just until the sugar has dissolved. Remove from the heat and add 4¾ quarts (4.5 liters) warm water and the lemon juice. Stand, if necessary, until lukewarm.
3 Strain the yeast mixture into the syrup through a sieve lined with a double thickness of cheesecloth, and stir well. Keep the sediment on the cheesecloth for making further batches of ginger beer. Stir the syrup mixture well and pour into clean, sturdy bottles, preferably fitted with clip-on seals or else with screw tops. Fill the bottles only to the base of the necks, and seal. Leave in a cool place for about 5 days—in hot weather, the ginger beer will be ready in 3 to 4 days.
4 To make further batches of ginger beer, return half the ginger beer "mother" left on the cheesecloth to the jar (discard the rest), and add 1 teaspoon each of ground ginger and sugar and 1 cup (250 ml) water (no more yeast is needed).
5 Repeat the process as before, feeding the "mother" with ½ teaspoon each of ginger and sugar daily. After 8 days, mix with the sugar syrup and bottle as before.

Traditional Lemonade

¼–⅓ cup (60–80 ml) Lemonade Syrup (opposite)
ice cubes
lemon wedge or fresh mint sprig (optional)

Makes 1 serving

Tart, sweet and very refreshing, this old-fashioned syrup-based lemonade is quick, delicious and cheap.

In a tall glass, combine the desired amount of syrup with ¾ cup (185 ml) water and stir until well blended. Add some ice cubes and, if desired, garnish with a lemon wedge or mint sprig.

Lemon Squash

4 strips (about 3 inches/8 cm each) lemon zest, cut into thin slices
1 cup (250 ml) Lemonade Syrup (opposite)
3 cups (750 ml) chilled club soda or sparkling mineral water
ice cubes
lemon slices or small fresh mint sprigs (optional)

Makes 4 servings

This is the fizzy version of economical lemonade, loaded with bright lemon taste and bubbles.

1. In a 2-quart (2 liter) jug, combine the lemon zest and syrup to taste. Stir until well blended.
2. Just before serving, pour in the club soda or sparkling mineral water; stir gently to blend the ingredients. Fill glasses with ice cubes, pour the lemon squash over the ice and, if desired, garnish with a lemon wedge or small mint sprig.

VARIATION

Lime Squash: Prepare as directed, substituting lime zest and Limeade Syrup (opposite) for the lemon zest and Lemonade Syrup or to taste. Garnish with lime wedges or strawberries.

Orange Blossom

1 large strip orange zest
1 teaspoon superfine sugar, plus a saucer of extra sugar for dipping
¼ cup (60 ml) gin
1 oz (30 ml) orange juice
1 slice orange

Makes 1 serving

For a nonalcoholic version of this festive drink, you can substitute sparkling water for the gin and add it after shaking the orange juice and sugar. This is a popular cocktail that is easy and inexpensive to make at home.

1. Rub the orange zest around the rim of a chilled martini glass. Dip the rim into the saucer of sugar.
2. In a cocktail shaker, combine the 1 teaspoon of sugar, gin and orange juice. Cover and shake until well blended. Place a strainer over the glass and pour the mixture through. Garnish with the orange slice.

Sparkling Fruit Bowl

1 package (10 oz/300 g) frozen raspberries
1 package (10 oz/300 g) frozen strawberries
1½ cups (330 g) sugar
10 whole cloves
½ teaspoon ground cardamom
6 strips (about 3 x ½ inch/8 x 1 cm each) orange zest
1 vanilla bean, split
2 cups (500 ml) orange juice
2 cups (500 ml) club soda or sparkling mineral water
ice cubes

Makes 10 servings

Beautifully colored and with the tang of raspberries, strawberries and oranges, this is a spicy, fizzy fruit punch for parties.

1 In a large, nonreactive saucepan, combine the berries, sugar, cloves, cardamom, orange zest, vanilla bean and 6 cups (1.5 liters) water. Bring to a boil over medium-high heat. Reduce the heat to medium-low and simmer, uncovered, for about 10 minutes, stirring occasionally.
2 Place a large sieve over a large jug. Pour the berry mixture through, straining out the solids; do not press the solids. Let cool to room temperature, then stir in the orange juice.
3 Just before serving, stir in the club soda or sparkling mineral water. Serve the punch over ice.

Lemon Barley Water

⅔ cup (140 g) pearl barley
2 oz (60 g) sugar cubes
2 lemons, washed
ice cubes and lemon slices, to serve

Makes 4 servings

Less sweet and heavy than most bought varieties, homemade lemon barley water is free from artificial colorings and flavorings.

1 Rinse the barley in a sieve under cold running water and drain well. Place in a saucepan, cover with cold water and bring to a boil, then reduce the heat and cook gently for 5 minutes. Pour the barley back into the sieve and rinse again.
2 Put the barley in a large jug or bowl. Rub each sugar cube over the skins of the lemons to extract the oils, then add the cubes to the jug or bowl.
3 Pour in 6 cups (1.5 liters) boiling water and stir until the sugar has dissolved. Cover the jug or bowl with a clean dish towel and leave to infuse for 3 hours, or until cold.
4 Squeeze the juice from both lemons and add it to the barley water. Strain through a nylon sieve into a serving jug. Cover and chill for 1 hour. Put several ice cubes and a few lemon slices in each of four tall glasses, pour in the lemon barley water and serve.

Bloody Mary Mix

2¼ cups (560 ml) tomato juice
¼ cup (60 ml) lemon juice
½ teaspoon black pepper
½ teaspoon salt
½ teaspoon celery seeds
1 teaspoon Worcestershire sauce
½ teaspoon hot red pepper sauce, such as Tabasco

Makes 2½ cups (625 ml)

Keep this mix ready to go in the refrigerator and you can whip up fantastic Bloody Marys in a flash—or just serve it over ice as a spicy tomato juice treat. You can buy Bloody Mary mixes, but the homemade version is livelier and much, much cheaper.

Combine all the ingredients in a 1-quart (1-liter) jar with a tight-fitting lid. Seal tightly and shake to blend well. Refrigerate for up to 1 week; shake well before using.

Bloody Mary

½ cup cracked ice
⅓ cup (80 ml) vodka
5 oz (150 ml) Bloody Mary Mix (above)
1 celery stalk

Makes 1 serving

This spicy drink stands up to even the most flavorful foods. Homemade with your own mix, it's a treat without being a threat to your budget.

Place the cracked ice in a tall glass. Pour the vodka and Bloody Mary mix over the ice. Garnish with the celery stalk.

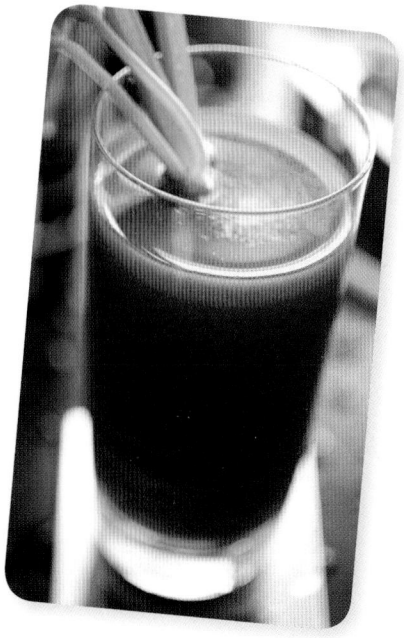

Fruit Juice Spritzer

3 cups (750 ml) chilled dry white wine or fruit juice of choice
1½ cups (375 ml) chilled fruit juice of choice, or a complementary juice
1½ cups (375 ml) chilled carbonated beverage (soda water, lemonade or ginger ale)
ice cubes
fresh mint leaves or citrus wedges (optional)

Makes 8 servings

Here is a lovely, light, fizzy cooler that you can customize to suit your taste and your menu—try cranberry-raspberry juice, pineapple juice, grape juice, pink grapefruit juice, tangerine juice or anything else that takes your fancy. If you don't use wine, you can blend two juices instead. A wonderful start to a summer party that won't break the bank.

1 Combine all the liquids in a 2-quart (2-liter) jug.
2 Serve straight or over ice cubes. If desired, garnish individual glasses with mint leaves or citrus wedges.

Sangria

2 oranges, sliced
2 lemons, sliced
2 cinnamon sticks
¾ cup (185 ml) brandy
1 bottle (750 ml) red wine
1 bottle (750 ml) sparkling cider, chilled
ice cubes

Makes about 7 cups (1.75 liters)

The color of garnets, full of fruit and always welcome whatever the season, sangria is an easy-to-make, delightful wine punch from Spain. Homemade is fresher tasting and a lot less pricey.

1 In a large punch bowl or glass jug, combine the oranges, lemons, cinnamon and brandy.
2 Pour the wine and cider over the fruit mixture, gently stirring until the punch is well blended. Just before serving, add ice cubes as desired.

Hot Drinks

Caffe Latte

1½ cups (375 ml) milk
⅔ cup (170 ml) freshly brewed espresso
sweetened cocoa powder (optional)

Makes 2 servings

Why buy a cup of special coffee when you can so easily make it yourself at a fraction of the price and without having to leave home?

1 In a small saucepan over low heat, cook the milk just until tiny bubbles begin to form around the edges of the saucepan, 10 to 15 minutes; do not let the milk come to a boil. If a skin forms on the milk's surface, remove it with a spoon.
2 Divide the espresso between two 8-ounce cups or mugs. Add ⅓ cup (80 ml) of the hot milk to each cup.
3 Using an electric mixer or wire whisk, beat the remaining hot milk until it is frothy. Spoon the milk froth into the cups, dividing it equally. If desired, sprinkle a little sweetened cocoa powder over the foam before serving.

VARIATIONS

Chocolate Mint Latte: Prepare as directed above, adding a finely chopped ½-ounce (15 g) chocolate-covered peppermint patty to each cup along with the espresso.

Caffe Latte à l'Orange: Prepare as directed above, adding 1 tablespoon Grand Marnier or other orange-flavored liqueur to each cup along with the espresso.

Cappuccino Mix

1 cup (100 g) skim powdered milk
1 cup (100 g) instant chocolate milk powder
⅔ cup (30 g) instant coffee granules or espresso powder
½ cup (110 g) sugar
½ teaspoon ground cinnamon
¼ teaspoon ground nutmeg

Makes about 3 cups (350 g) dry mix

Love the convenience of instant special coffees to keep at the office or to brew a fast cup for an afternoon pick-me-up? Make your own and you'll save a bundle.

Combine the ingredients in an airtight container. Cover and shake until well blended. For 1 cup (250 ml) of instant cappuccino, place 3 tablespoons in a mug or coffee cup. Add ¾ cup (185 ml) boiling water and stir until the mix has completely dissolved.

Cocoa

2 tablespoons sugar
1 tablespoon cocoa powder
¾ cup (185 ml) milk
miniature marshmallows (optional)
1 stick cinnamon (optional)

Makes 1 serving

On a cold, blustery day, there's nothing quite like hot cocoa made the good old-fashioned way.

1. In a small saucepan, combine the sugar, cocoa and ¼ cup (60 ml) water. Over medium heat, bring the mixture to a boil, stirring constantly until the sugar has dissolved. Lower the heat and simmer for 2 minutes, whisking constantly.
2. Stir in the milk. Increase the heat to medium and cook until the cocoa is heated through; do not allow the mixture to boil.
3. To serve, pour the cocoa into a mug or cup. If desired, top with several marshmallows and use the cinnamon stick as a stirrer.

Hot Chocolate Viennese

⅓ cup (40 g) cocoa powder
⅓ cup (75 g) sugar
2½ cups (625 ml) milk
1½ cups (375 ml) freshly brewed strong coffee or espresso

Makes 4 servings

Chocolate, coffee and hot milk—triple yum! This is a cafe treat that you can enjoy much more cheaply at home.

1. In a saucepan, combine the cocoa powder and sugar, pressing out any lumps. Stirring constantly, pour in enough of the milk to moisten the dry mixture, about ½ cup (125 ml); whisk in the coffee and the remaining 2 cups (500 ml) milk.
2. Cook over medium-low heat, stirring occasionally, until the mixture steams but does not boil, 8 to 10 minutes. Pour the hot chocolate into mugs or coffee cups and serve.

Chai

2 tea bags
1 stick cinnamon
6 cardamom pods, crushed
1 whole clove
¼ teaspoon ground ginger
2½ cups (625 ml) milk
⅓ cup (75 g) sugar
cinnamon sticks (optional)

Makes 4 servings

The spicy, creamy tea drink that is ever-more popular, chai is a lovely afternoon soother or stimulator. It is convenient and economical to make your own.

1. In a small saucepan, combine the tea bags, cinnamon stick, cardamom, clove, ginger and 2 cups (500 ml) water; bring the mixture to a boil over medium-high heat. Reduce the heat, cover and simmer for 5 minutes.
2. Stir in the milk. Increase the heat, return the mixture to a boil, then boil for 1 minute. Remove the saucepan from the heat, place a sieve over a warmed teapot and pour the mixture through; discard the solids. Add the sugar and stir until it has dissolved.
3. Divide among four mugs or cups and, if desired, serve with a cinnamon stick as a stirrer.

Hot Spiced Tea

2 sticks cinnamon
6–12 whole allspice
1 teaspoon whole cloves
12 tea bags
1 cup (230 g) packed brown sugar
1 cup (250 ml) cranberry juice
½ cup (125 ml) orange juice
¼ cup (60 ml) lemon juice

Makes 3 quarts (3 liters)

Give extra zest to hot tea with this inviting spice mixture—it will make your kitchen smell fabulous while it warms you to your toes. No mix can match this hot spiced tea at any price. It's the perfect drink for a winter afternoon.

1. Cut a 4-inch square of double-thickness cheesecloth. Put the cinnamon sticks, allspice and cloves in the center. Bring together the corners of the fabric to form a bag; secure with a piece of kitchen string.
2. Place the spice bag in a large, nonreactive saucepan and add 12 cups (3 liters) water. Bring to a boil over high heat, then remove from the heat and add the tea bags. Cover the pan and let the tea steep for 5 minutes. Remove and discard the tea bags and spice bag.
3. Stir in the sugar until dissolved. Add the juices, stirring until the ingredients are well blended. Return the saucepan to low heat, and gently heat the spiced tea through before serving.

Hot Mulled Cider

4 cups (1 liter) apple cider
10 whole cloves
10 black peppercorns
4 strips (about 3 x ½ inch/8 x 1 cm each) orange zest
1 stick cinnamon, cracked
1 vanilla bean, split

Makes 4 servings

One of the best warm-me-ups, this cider has some surprises in its spice. You don't have to go to a ski lodge to enjoy it.

1. In a saucepan, combine all the ingredients and bring to a boil over medium heat. Remove the saucepan from the heat and let the mixture steep for 30 minutes. Remove and discard the spices.
2. Return the saucepan to low heat and slowly cook until the cider begins to steam. Ladle the cider into warm mugs, wait 3 to 5 minutes and serve.

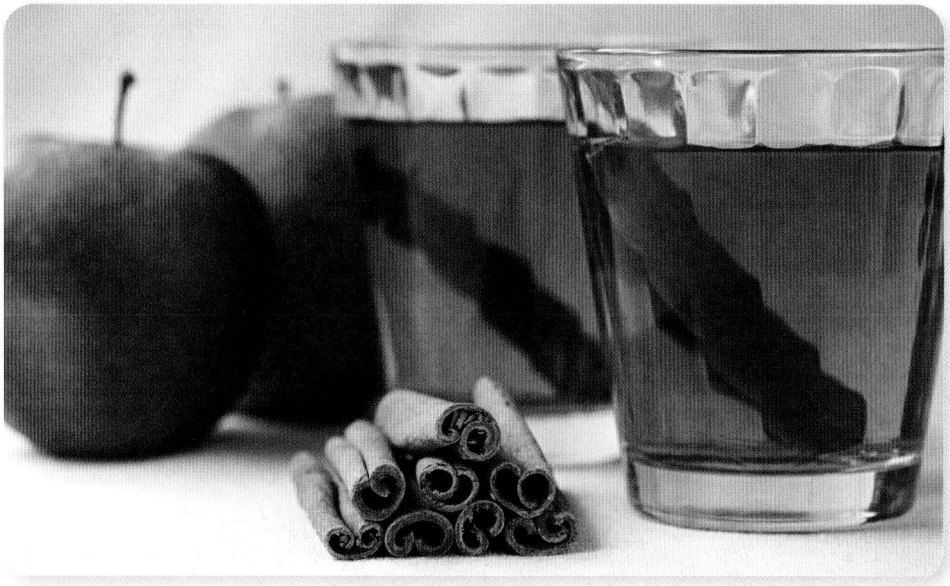

Hot Nonalcoholic Punch

4 cups (1 liter) hot brewed tea
1 cup (220 g) sugar
4 cups (1 liter) cranberry juice
4 cups (1 liter) apple juice
2 cups (500 ml) orange juice
¾ cup (185 ml) lemon juice
24 whole cloves
2 sticks cinnamon
1 orange, sliced

Makes 12 to 16 servings

A traditional holiday punch served warm or cool, this recipe is festive for parties and quite economical when you make it up fresh.

1. In a large, nonreactive saucepan over medium-high heat, combine the hot tea and sugar, stirring until the sugar has dissolved. Add the juices, 12 cloves and the cinnamon sticks. Bring the mixture to a boil and boil for 2 minutes.
2. Remove the saucepan from the heat. Pour the mixture into a heatproof punch bowl. Insert the remaining cloves into the orange slices and float them on the punch as garnish. Serve the punch warm or cooled to room temperature.

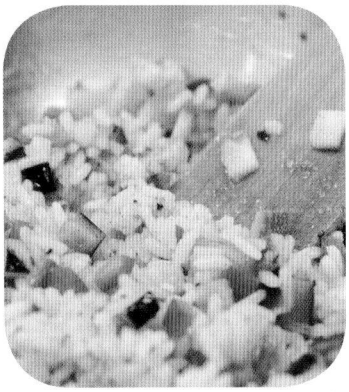

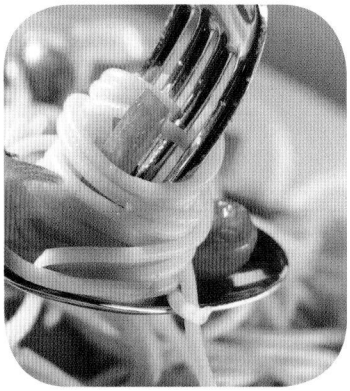

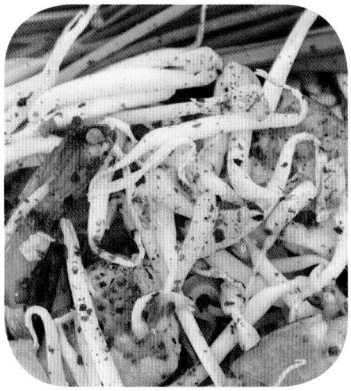

Deli-Style Dishes

Savory Meat Mix ❖ Chili Con Carne ❖ Tomato Herb Tarts ❖ Barbecue Sauce ❖ Barbecued Spareribs ❖ Baked Beans ❖ Stir-Fried Vegetables ❖ Chinese Crispy Beef Stir-Fry ❖ Refried Beans ❖ Curry with Rice ❖ Pork Korma with Potatoes and Spinach ❖ Thai Green Chicken Curry ❖ Pad Thai Noodles with Shrimp ❖ Singapore Noodles ❖ Chinese Fried Rice ❖ Basic Rice Pilaf ❖ Tandoori Chicken

Main-Dish Pies

Chicken Pot Pie ❖ Shepherd's Pie ❖ Spicy Beef Pie ❖ Quiche Lorraine

Pasta Dishes

Spaghetti Bolognese ❖ Spaghetti with Speedy Tomato Sauce ❖ Pasta with Fresh Tomato Sauce ❖ Pasta Puttanesca ❖ Fettuccine Alfredo ❖ Penne with Four-Cheese Sauce ❖ Pasta with Seafood ❖ Penne All'amatriciana ❖ Pasta with Classic Basil Pesto ❖ Pasta with Mushroom Pesto ❖ Pasta with Sun-Dried Tomato Pesto ❖ Ravioli ❖ Lasagna

Soups

Beef Barley Soup ❖ Black Bean Soup ❖ Chicken Noodle Soup ❖ New England Clam Chowder ❖ Cream of Tomato Soup ❖ Quick Shrimp Laksa ❖ Minestrone ❖ Lentil Soup ❖ Gumbo ❖ French Onion Soup ❖ Vegetable Soup ❖ Split Pea Soup ❖ Gazpacho

Salads

Classic Coleslaw ❖ Greek Salad ❖ Potato Salad ❖ Thai Beef Salad ❖ Egg Salad ❖ Pasta Salad ❖ Caesar Salad ❖ Creamy Chicken Salad ❖ Curried Chicken Salad ❖ Turkey Salad ❖ Tuna Salad ❖ Cobb Salad ❖ Shrimp Salad ❖ Tuscan-Style Three-Bean Salad ❖ Salade Niçoise

Take-Out and Prepared Food

Have you noticed how the prepared-food aisles are taking up more and more space in your supermarket? We are increasingly reliant on ready-made meals, and supermarkets are simply responding to this demand.

The only problem is that these eat-as-they-are or pop-in-the-microwave dishes carry an enormous price premium for the little extra convenience that they provide.

This chapter is devoted to the true convenience foods you can make fresh in your own kitchen. Most make minimal demands on your time. And many are foods that you can make ahead—or leave simmering in a slow cooker—for a meal later.

On the following pages, you'll find tasty meat and bean dishes and satisfying savory pies similar to those that you might find at the deli counter or in the supermarket freezer section. You'll also find a tempting selection of delicious, easy-to-make pasta dishes. (For a special treat, try them with the fresh pastas from Chapter 1.) There are hearty soups that will fill your kitchen with wonderful aromas, delight your family, and use up leftovers—and unlike the canned versions, homemade soups can provide more flavor with a lot less salt. You'll also find a wide selection of deli-style salads that you can make with minimal fuss, ranging from versatile sides such as Coleslaw to main dishes like Caesar Salad and Creamy Chicken Salad—and unlike some deli salads, they will never have too much mayonnaise!

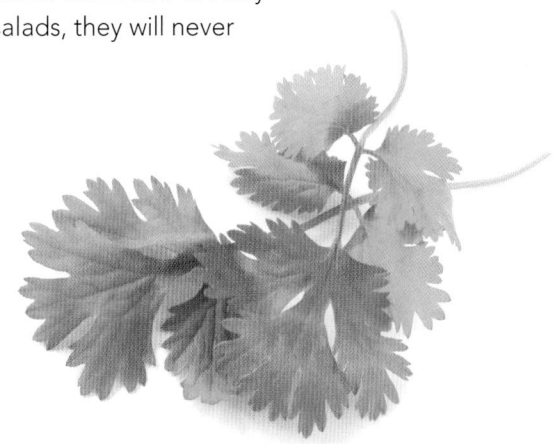

Deli-Style Dishes

Savory Meat Mix

2 tablespoons olive or canola oil
2 onions, chopped
2 cloves garlic, finely chopped
1 celery stalk, chopped
2 carrots, chopped
2½ lb (1 kg) lean ground beef or pork
2 teaspoons dried basil
1 teaspoon dried oregano
1 teaspoon salt
½ teaspoon freshly ground black pepper
large pinch of sugar
1 tablespoon Worcestershire sauce
14½ oz (410 g) can chopped tomatoes

Makes about 6 cups (1.5 kg)

This versatile base recipe can be made with either beef or pork. You can use it in the following recipe and in the Spaghetti Bolognese on page 179.

1. In a large, heavy saucepan, heat the oil over medium heat. Add the onions, garlic, celery and carrots and sauté until softened, about 5 minutes, stirring occasionally. Crumble the beef or pork into the pan, breaking it up with a large spoon; cook, stirring occasionally, until the meat is no longer pink. Drain off as much fat as possible.
2. Add the remaining ingredients and stir until well mixed. Reduce the heat, cover and simmer for 20 to 25 minutes.
3. Remove from the heat and allow to cool completely. Spoon off any visible fat, then divide the mixture among three or four 2-cup (500 ml) self-sealing, freezer-safe plastic bags. Seal, label, date and freeze. The mixture will keep for up to 3 months in the freezer.

Chili Con Carne

2 cups (350 g) Savory Meat Mix (above), thawed
1 tablespoon chili powder, or to taste
1 teaspoon ground cumin
2 cans (15½ oz/420 g each) red kidney beans, drained and rinsed
hot pepper sauce, to taste
hot cooked rice, tortilla chips, grated cheddar, sour cream or natural yogurt (optional)

Makes 6 servings

This will be the fastest chili you've ever put together using fresh meat.

1. In a saucepan, combine the meat mix, chili powder, cumin and kidney beans. Mix well, then cover and cook over medium-high heat until heated through, about 10 minutes. Add some hot pepper sauce to your desired level of spiciness.
2. Serve over rice or with tortilla chips, if desired. Sprinkle a little cheese over each serving or top with a dollop of sour cream or yogurt, if desired.

Tomato Herb Tarts

1 sheet frozen puff pastry
½ cup (60 g) finely grated cheddar
2 tablespoons grated Parmesan cheese
1 lb (450 g) ripe tomatoes, peeled and sliced
2 tablespoons finely chopped fresh parsley
2 tablespoons finely chopped fresh basil
2 tablespoons finely chopped fresh thyme
1 tablespoon virgin olive oil
freshly ground black pepper, to taste

Makes 4 to 6 tarts

Using frozen puff pastry means you can rustle up these individual tarts in a jiffy.

1 Preheat the oven to 400°F.
2 Place the puff pastry on a work surface. Using a large, round cutter, cut out 4 to 6 circles and place on a baking sheet. Bake until puffed and golden brown, 10 to 12 minutes.
3 Remove from the oven and sprinkle some of the cheddar and Parmesan cheese over each pastry circle, leaving a small border around the edges. Layer the tomato slices over the cheese, then sprinkle with the herbs. Drizzle with the olive oil and sprinkle with pepper.
4 Return to the oven and bake until the cheese is completely melted, about 5 minutes. Turn the oven off and let the tarts stand for a few minutes before removing them from the oven. Serve immediately or at room temperature.

Barbecue Sauce

1½ cups (375 ml) tomato sauce
1 cup (250 ml) cider vinegar
⅔ cup (170 ml) peanut or safflower oil
⅓ cup (80 ml) Worcestershire sauce
½ cup (115 g) firmly packed dark brown sugar
3 tablespoons mild yellow mustard
½ teaspoon freshly ground black pepper
juice of 1 large lemon
1–2 fresh red chile peppers, finely chopped (optional)

Makes about 3 cups (750 ml)

Meant for spareribs (see Barbecued Spareribs, page 168), this tangy homemade sauce also goes well with chicken. As well as saving you money, it's a satisfying condiment to make as you can adjust the ingredients to suit your own tastes.

Put all the ingredients in a saucepan and mix to combine. Bring to a boil over medium heat; immediately reduce the heat to low, then cover and simmer until the sugar has completely dissolved and the sauce has thickened slightly, about 20 minutes.

If you run out of brown sugar

If a recipe calls for ½ cup (115 g) firmly packed brown sugar and you don't have any on hand, stir 1 tablespoon molasses into ½ cup (110 g) regular granulated sugar.

Barbecued Spareribs

5 lb (2.25 kg) pork spareribs, in 6–8 rib portions
3 cups (750 ml) Barbecue Sauce (page 167)

Makes 6 servings

You get the most succulent results when you prepare your own ribs at home; a side benefit is that it's also very economical.

1 Place the ribs in a large self-sealing bag, glass baking dish or nonreactive bowl. Pour 2 cups (500 ml) of the barbecue sauce over the ribs and toss to coat. Cover and refrigerate overnight.
2 On a covered kettle-style barbecue, follow the manufacturer's directions to prepare the coals for the indirect method of cooking. Add the ribs and cook for 1 to 1½ hours, basting frequently with the marinating sauce.
3 In a small saucepan, warm the remaining barbecue sauce over low heat and serve on the side with the ribs.

Baked Beans

1 lb (450 g) dried beans, picked through and rinsed
⅓ cup (115 g) maple syrup
1 teaspoon mustard powder
1 teaspoon salt
½ teaspoon freshly ground black pepper
¼ lb (125 g) salt pork
1 onion, peeled

Makes 6 servings

Why buy a can when you can make your own baked beans? Use borlotti, cannellini or haricot (navy) beans, or use a mixture of all three. The beans can be baked slowly one day, then reheated or served cold for breakfast or lunch the next.

1 Place the beans in a large saucepan and add enough water to cover by 2 inches. Bring to a boil and boil for 2 minutes. Remove the saucepan from the heat, cover and leave to soak for 1 hour.
2 Add more water to cover the beans and return the pan to the heat. Bring to a boil, reduce the heat and simmer until the beans are tender, about 1 hour, adding more water as necessary to keep the beans covered. Drain the beans, reserving the cooking liquid.
3 Preheat the oven to 250°F. Transfer the beans to a casserole dish. In a bowl, combine the maple syrup, mustard, salt and pepper and pour the mixture over the beans. Cut the pork into ½-inch slices, up to but not through the rind. Add the pork and onion to the bean mixture, pressing them down to immerse them. If needed, add the reserved cooking liquid until the beans are completely covered.
4 Cover and bake for 4 hours, adding more reserved cooking liquid or water as needed so the beans don't dry out. Remove the lid and bake for 1 hour more, or until the beans are tender.

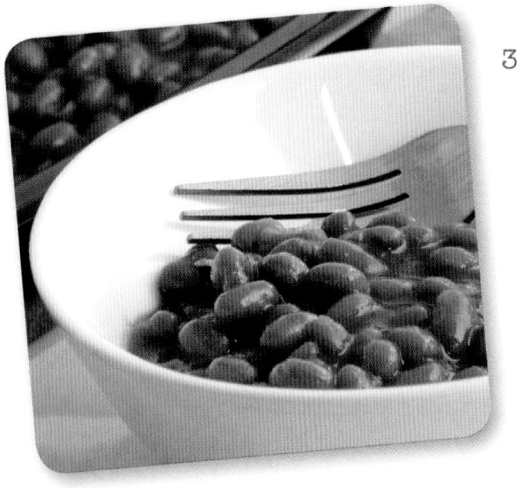

Stir-Fried Vegetables

1½ tablespoons soy sauce
1½ tablespoons mirin or dry sherry
1 tablespoon honey
2 tablespoons Vegetable Stock (page 51)
2 tablespoons vegetable oil
1½ lb (750 g) mixed fresh vegetables, prepared and cut into even-sized pieces
1 clove garlic, crushed
1-inch (2–3 cm) piece fresh ginger, peeled and grated
2 teaspoons sesame oil

Makes 4 servings

Stir-frying really makes the most of vegetables, retaining their color, crunch, flavor and texture.

1 In a small jug, combine the soy sauce, mirin or sherry, honey and stock. Mix well, then set aside.
2 In a wok or large deep frying pan or skillet, heat the oil. Add any of the tougher, slower-cooking vegetables (such as carrots, broccoli, celery, green beans and baby corn) and stir-fry over high heat for 30 seconds. Pour in 1 to 1½ tablespoons of water, cover with a lid and cook over high heat for 2 minutes.
3 Next add the more tender, quicker-cooking vegetables (such as bell peppers, snow peas, bean sprouts and spring onions), along with the garlic and ginger. Stir-fry until they are almost tender, about 2 minutes.
4 Finally, stir in any delicate leafy vegetables (such as shredded greens or bok choy) and cook for 1 more minute, until all are cooked but still retain some bite and their bright color.
5 Pour in the reserved sauce and stir-fry for 1 minute, until all the vegetables are coated in the sauce. Transfer to a serving platter, drizzle with the sesame oil and serve.

Chinese Crispy Beef Stir-Fry

7 oz (200 g) lean beef steak
2 teaspoons cornstarch
1 teaspoon five-spice
1 carrot, peeled
1 small leek, white part only, trimmed
6 spring onions, sliced diagonally
½ red bell pepper, cut into strips
3½ oz (100 g) dried rice noodles
1½ tablespoons soy sauce
1½ tablespoons rice wine
1½ tablespoons vegetable oil
1 large clove garlic, finely chopped
1-inch (2–3 cm) piece fresh ginger, peeled and finely chopped
1 red chile pepper, seeded and finely chopped
soy sauce, for drizzling

Makes 2 servings

Make the most of prime lean beef by stir-frying it with healthy vegetables, wholesome noodles and aromatic Asian-style flavorings.

1 Cut the meat across the grain into 2-inch-wide pieces, then cut each piece into very thin strips. Place in a small bowl with the cornstarch and five-spice and mix together until meat is coated.
2 Cut the carrot and leek into 2-inch lengths, then cut each piece into thin matchsticks. Combine in a bowl with the spring onions and bell pepper.
3 Put the noodles in a heatproof bowl, pour some lightly salted boiling water over them and soak for 3 minutes. Drain and refresh in cold water, then drain again. Mix the soy sauce, rice wine and 1½ tablespoons of water in a small jug or bowl.
4 Place a wok or a large frying pan or skillet over high heat. When hot, add 1 tablespoon of the oil. When the oil begins to smoke, toss in the meat and stir-fry until cooked through, 2 to 3 minutes; remove with a slotted spoon. Add the remaining oil with the garlic, ginger and chile pepper. Stir-fry for 30 seconds, then add the vegetables and toss for another 30 seconds.
5 Stir in the soy sauce mixture. As soon as the liquid is bubbling, mix in the drained noodles, then the meat. Serve immediately, with soy sauce to drizzle over the top.

Refried Beans

2 tablespoons vegetable oil
1 large onion, chopped
2 cans (15 oz/420 g each) pinto, black or red kidney beans, drained and rinsed
1 teaspoon ground cumin
salt, to taste
chili powder, to taste (optional)

Makes 4 to 6 servings

Craving homemade refried beans but crunched for time? That's not a problem with this recipe.

1 In a large, heavy saucepan, heat the oil over medium heat. Add the onion and sauté until just softened. Add the beans, cumin, salt and chili powder, if using. Cook, stirring, until heated through, 5 to 10 minutes. Remove the pan from the heat.
2 Using a potato masher, mash the bean mixture to the desired consistency. Place back over medium heat and cook until the mixture is thick and creamy in texture, about 15 minutes.

Curry with Rice

¼ cup (35 g) plain flour
½ teaspoon salt
¼ teaspoon freshly ground black pepper
1½ lb (650 g) boneless, skinless chicken or turkey breasts or thighs (or lamb), cut into 1-inch (2–3 cm) cubes
¼ cup (60 ml) vegetable oil
1 large yellow onion, chopped
2 cloves garlic, finely chopped
2 small celery stalks, chopped
1–2 tablespoons Curry Powder (page 45)
1¾ cups (440 ml) Chicken Stock (page 50)
4 carrots, cut crosswise into ½-inch (1 cm) slices
½ cauliflower, cut into florets
1¼ cups (250 g) basmati rice

Makes 4 servings

Flavorful, economical and easy to prepare, curry is deliciously adaptable and a tasty way to use up leftovers. Meat, poultry, seafood, vegetables—just about anything goes when it comes to making a curry.

1 In a large, self-sealing bag, combine the flour, salt and pepper. Working in small batches, add the meat to the bag, seal well, then shake to coat the meat with the flour mixture.
2 In a large, heavy saucepan with a tight-fitting lid, heat the oil over medium-high heat. Add half the meat to the pan and sauté until lightly brown, about 5 minutes. Remove and drain on paper towels. Repeat with the remaining meat.
3 In the oil and juices left in the pan, sauté the onion, garlic and celery until soft, about 5 minutes. Add the curry powder, stock, carrots, cauliflower and reserved meat. Reduce the heat to low, then cover and simmer until the cauliflower is just tender, 20 to 30 minutes.
4 Meanwhile, in a large saucepan, cook the rice according to the package directions. Transfer to a large warm serving bowl, spoon the curry over the rice and serve immediately.

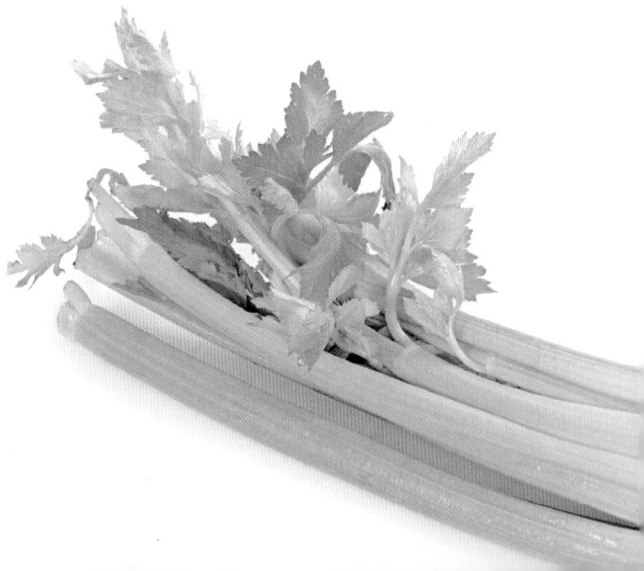

Pork Korma with Potatoes and Spinach

1 tablespoon vegetable oil
2 large onions, sliced
1 lb (500 g) lean ground pork
2 cloves garlic, crushed
8 green cardamom pods, crushed and pods discarded
1 tablespoon cumin seeds
2½ cups (600 ml) Chicken Stock (page 50), hot
1½ lb (750 g) small new potatoes, scrubbed and halved
2 teaspoons cornstarch
1 cup (250 g) natural yogurt
¾ cup (80 g) ground almonds
salt and freshly ground black pepper, to taste
9 oz (250 g) baby English spinach leaves
¼ cup (25 g) flaked almonds, lightly toasted

Makes 4 servings

Thickened with ground almonds and yogurt, this dish is rich and creamy, yet not as indulgent as traditional kormas. Serve with warm chappati or naan breads.

1 In a large, heavy saucepan or flameproof casserole dish, heat the oil. Add the onions and cook over medium heat for 10 minutes. Transfer to a bowl.
2 Add the pork, garlic, cardamom and cumin seeds to the pan or dish. Cook, stirring often and breaking up the meat with a large spoon, until the meat has changed color, about 5 minutes. Return about half the onions to the pan, pour in the stock and bring back to a boil. Reduce the heat, cover and simmer for 15 minutes.
3 Stir in the potatoes and bring back to the simmering point, then cover and cook until the potatoes are tender, about 20 minutes.
4 Meanwhile, blend the cornstarch with about ½ cup (125 g) of the yogurt and the ground almonds to make a paste. Stir this mixture into the curry and bring just to a boil, stirring. Reduce the heat and simmer until slightly thickened, about 1 minute. Season to taste with salt and pepper.
5 Reserve a few small spinach leaves for garnishing, then fold the rest through the korma until they are just wilted and bright green. Mix the flaked almonds with the remaining onions.
6 Serve the curry drizzled with the remaining yogurt and topped with the almond and onion mixture and spinach leaves.

Thai Green Chicken Curry

4 boneless, skinless chicken breasts (21 oz/600 g total)
12 oz (350 g) new potatoes, scrubbed
6 spring onions
8 grape or cherry tomatoes
14 oz (400 ml) can light coconut milk
2½ cups (600 ml) Chicken Stock (page 50), hot
2 tablespoons Green Curry Paste (page 46)
2 tablespoons lime juice
¾ cup (115 g) shelled fresh or thawed frozen peas
4 tablespoons chopped fresh coriander
salt and freshly ground black pepper, to taste

Makes 4 servings

Keep the fat content low in a tangy Thai curry by not prefrying the ingredients; simply simmer them in light coconut milk and stock with potatoes, peas and tomatoes.

1 Cut the chicken breasts into thin strips across the grain and cut the potatoes into chunks. Slice the spring onions diagonally and halve the cherry or grape tomatoes.
2 Pour the coconut milk and stock into a wok or large frying pan or skillet. Stir in the curry paste and heat until boiling. Stir in the chicken strips and potatoes, then bring back to a boil.
3 Reduce the heat and simmer, uncovered, until the chicken and potatoes are just tender, about 15 minutes.
4 Stir in the spring onions, lime juice, peas and tomatoes and simmer for a further 3 to 4 minutes. Stir in the coriander and season to taste with salt and pepper.

Pad Thai Noodles with Shrimp

1 tablespoon lime juice
2 tablespoons low-sodium soy sauce
1 tablespoon fish sauce
24 small peeled raw shrimp, about 9 oz (250 g) in total
9 oz (250 g) package dried rice noodles (medium thickness)
¼ cup (60 ml) vegetable oil
1 teaspoon sesame oil
2 small red chile peppers, deseeded and finely chopped
5 oz (150 g) fresh baby corn, halved lengthwise
2¼ cups (200 g) bean sprouts
7 oz (200 g) bok choy, finely shredded
8 oz (220 g) can water chestnuts, drained and sliced
1 cup (250 ml) canned reduced-fat coconut milk
1 lime, cut into wedges

Makes 4 servings

Typical Thai flavors, including chile peppers, lime and coconut, combine in this aromatic stir-fry of shrimp, noodles and Asian vegetables.

1 In a bowl, mix together the lime juice, soy sauce and fish sauce. Add the shrimp and toss together, then set aside to marinate for a few minutes.
2 Meanwhile, put the noodles in a large heatproof bowl. Pour boiling water over to cover, add 1 teaspoon of the vegetable oil and stir gently. Soak for 4 minutes, then drain thoroughly.
3 Lift the shrimp out of the marinade and pat dry with a paper towel. Heat a wok or heavy frying pan or skillet until very hot, then add 1 teaspoon of the vegetable oil and all of the sesame oil and swirl to coat the wok. Add the shrimp and chile peppers and stir-fry until the shrimp turn pink, about 2 minutes. Remove with a slotted spoon, leaving any remaining oil in the wok.
4 Add the rest of the oil to the pan. Toss in the corn and stir-fry for 30 seconds. Add the bean sprouts and bok choy and stir-fry for 1 minute, then add the reserved marinade. Cook for a few seconds, stirring all the time, then add the water chestnuts and drained noodles. Stir-fry for a further 1 minute.
5 Return the shrimp to the wok and pour in the coconut milk. Toss everything together over high heat until bubbling. Serve immediately, with lime wedges to squeeze over.

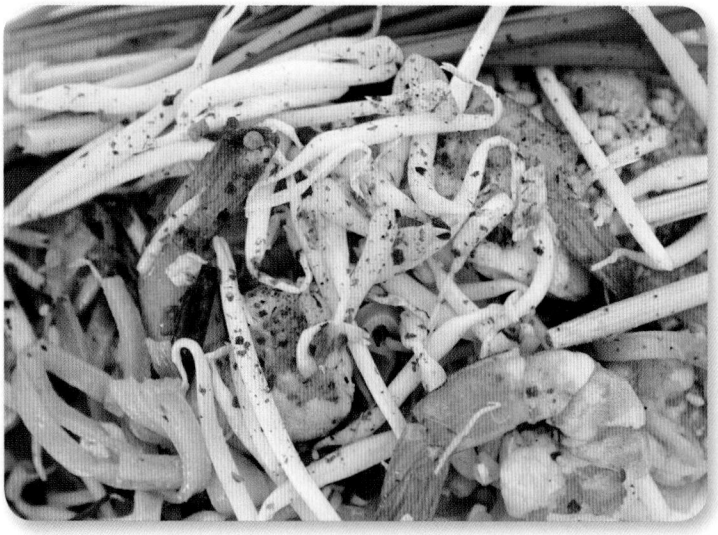

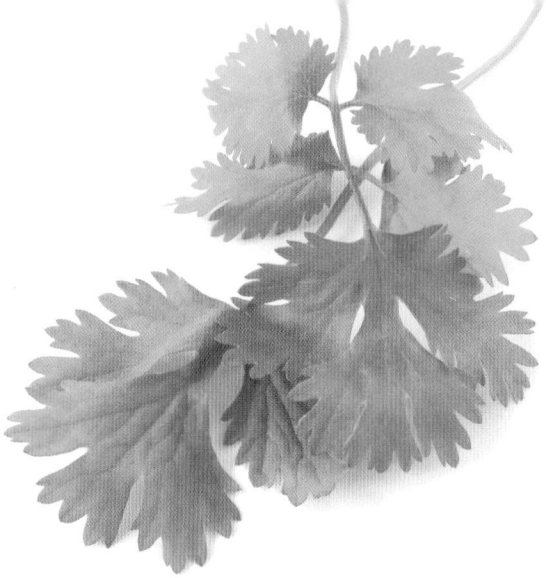

Singapore Noodles

6 oz (170 g) dried rice vermicelli noodles
2 tablespoons peanut oil
7 oz (200 g) peeled small raw shrimp
7 oz (200 g) boneless, skinless chicken breasts, thinly sliced
6 spring onions, thinly sliced diagonally
3 teaspoons grated fresh ginger
1 small red bell pepper, thinly sliced
2 teaspoons curry powder
1 teaspoon ground turmeric
3 teaspoons Chinese rice wine
2 tablespoons light soy sauce
2 tablespoons Chicken Stock (page 50)
¾ cup (115 g) frozen peas, thawed
3 eggs, beaten
fresh coriander sprigs, to garnish
lime quarters, to serve

Makes 4 servings

A perennial favorite at Singaporean food stalls and a popular take-out dish all over the world, this tasty, home-cooked version will feed the family for much less than purchased noodles—and they'll taste much fresher and less oily, too.

1 Soak the noodles according to the package directions, then drain and set aside.
2 In a wok, heat 1 tablespoon of the oil. Fry the shrimp and chicken, in batches, until just cooked, then remove to a plate.
3 Heat the remaining oil and stir-fry the spring onions, ginger and bell pepper until just beginning to soften, then stir in the curry powder and turmeric and cook for 1 minute.
4 Stir in the rice wine, soy sauce and stock until combined, then add the peas and drained noodles and toss until the peas are tender.
5 Push the noodles to one side of the wok and pour in the beaten eggs. Cook stirring, for 1 minute, then mix the egg through the noodles.
6 Return the shrimp and chicken to the wok and toss until warmed through and well combined.
7 Serve the noodles in bowls, garnished with coriander sprigs and a wedge of lime.

Chinese Fried Rice

1½ cups (300 g) long-grain white rice
2 tablespoons vegetable oil
2 eggs, lightly beaten
2 cloves garlic, chopped
1 red bell pepper, diced
1 carrot, diced
3 Chinese sausages, sliced, or 3½ oz (100 g) diced ham
½ cup (80 g) frozen peas, thawed and drained
2 spring onions, sliced
2 tablespoons soy sauce
2 teaspoons sugar
2 teaspoons shrimp paste (optional)

Makes 4 servings

Once you have made fried rice the first time, you'll realize how versatile it is. Use whatever leftover or seasonal vegetables you like. Fried rice is so easy to make at home that you'll never need to go out and buy it again! The secret is to cook the rice the night before to obtain the right texture—or use up any leftover rice that happens to be in the fridge.

1 Wash the rice under cold running water until the water almost runs clear. Drain, then place in a saucepan with 2¼ cups (560 ml) cold water. Cover with a tight-fitting lid and place over medium heat until the water comes to a boil, then reduce the heat to a simmer and cook until the rice has absorbed all the liquid, about 15 minutes. Remove from the heat and stand, covered, for 10 minutes.
2 Spread the rice out on a tray, allow to cool, then cover lightly with plastic wrap. Refrigerate overnight.
3 In a wok or large frying pan or skillet, heat 1 tablespoon of the oil over medium heat. Add the eggs and cook for 1 minute, stirring until lightly scrambled, then remove from the wok. Add the remaining oil to the wok and briefly cook the garlic until fragrant, then add the bell pepper and carrot and toss until softened, 1 to 2 minutes.
4 Add the Chinese sausage or ham, toss for another minute, then add the cooked rice. Keep tossing until the rice is reheated, breaking up any large clumps as you go. At the last minute, add the peas, spring onions, soy sauce, sugar, egg and shrimp paste, if using. Mix together well and serve.

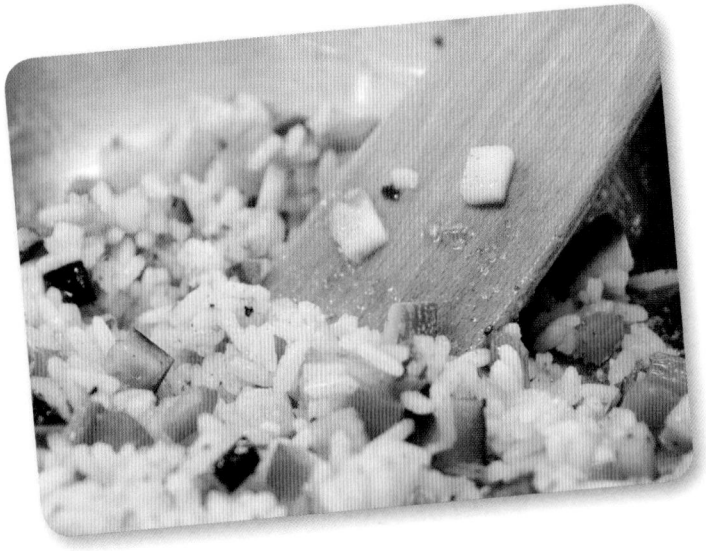

Basic Rice Pilaf

1 tablespoon olive oil or vegetable oil
1 cup (200 g) long-grain white rice
2 cups (500 ml) Chicken Stock (page 50)

Makes 4 to 6 servings

Once you know how to make pilaf (seasoned rice or other grains), you have the base for an almost infinite variety of dishes. Try using brown rice, wild rice, bulgur or barley instead of white rice; stir in cooked meats, seafood or vegetables, add a handful of toasted pine nuts, pistachios or pecans—and suddenly you have a gourmet meal in minutes.

1. In a heavy saucepan, heat the oil over medium-high heat until very hot. Add the rice and stir constantly until the oil is absorbed and the rice is translucent, about 5 minutes.
2. Add the stock, increase the heat to high and bring the mixture to a boil. Stir once, lower the heat and cover the pan tightly. Simmer until the liquid is absorbed and the rice is tender, 15 to 20 minutes.

Tandoori Chicken

3 cloves garlic, crushed
1 teaspoon paprika
¾ teaspoon ground cumin
¾ teaspoon ground coriander
½ teaspoon cinnamon
½ teaspoon chili powder
½ teaspoon freshly ground black pepper
2 cups (500 g) natural yogurt
4 skinless, bone-in chicken breast halves (about 2 lb/ 1 kg in total)
1 small red onion, finely chopped
1 cucumber, seeded and diced
½ cup (25 g) chopped fresh coriander

Makes 4 servings

A favorite at many Indian restaurants around the world, Tandoori Chicken isn't difficult to make at home. Marinating the chicken overnight in the yogurt ensures a great result as the enzymes in the yogurt tenderize the flesh and make it creamy and moist.

1. In a shallow glass or ceramic baking dish, combine the garlic, spices and a dash of salt. Stir in 1 cup (250 g) of the yogurt until well blended. Make several slashes in the flesh of the chicken with a sharp knife, cutting almost to the bone. Place the chicken, cut side down, in the yogurt mixture. Cover and refrigerate for at least 2 hours or overnight, turning the chicken several times.
2. Preheat the oven to its highest setting. Lift the chicken from its marinade and place in a shallow baking dish; discard any leftover marinade. Bake the chicken for 20 minutes, then reduce the oven temperature to 250°F and bake for a few more minutes, until cooked through but still juicy.
3. Meanwhile, combine the onion, cucumber, coriander and the remaining yogurt in a bowl and mix well. Serve the chicken with the yogurt mixture on the side.

Main-Dish Pies

Chicken Pot Pie

1 large potato, peeled and chopped
1 carrot, sliced
½ cup (125 g) butter
1 small yellow onion, chopped
½ cup (75 g) plain flour
¾ teaspoon salt
½ teaspoon dried thyme, crumbled
½ teaspoon freshly ground black pepper
1½ cups (375 ml) Chicken Stock (page 50)
¾ cup (185 ml) milk
2 cups (300 g) chopped cooked chicken
½ cup (80 g) frozen peas
½ cup (75 g) frozen corn
Basic Double Crust Pie Pastry (page 123)

Makes 6 servings

Frozen chicken pies are no match for this lovely dish, which cleverly uses up the leftovers from a roast chicken. The pie can be made ahead and frozen, tightly covered with freezer-safe foil, for up to 3 months.

1 Put the potato and carrot in a large saucepan and cover with water. Bring to a boil, then reduce the heat, cover and simmer until just tender, 8 to 10 minutes. Drain the vegetables and set aside.
2 Melt the butter in a large, heavy saucepan over medium heat. Add the onion and sauté until tender. Stir in the flour, salt, thyme and pepper until well blended, then gradually add the stock and milk, stirring constantly. Bring the mixture to a boil; cook, stirring constantly, until it has thickened. Stir in the chicken, peas, corn, potato and carrot. Remove the mixture from the heat.
3 Preheat the oven to 425°F. Roll out the pastry to line a 9-inch pie plate. Ease the pastry into the dish, then trim the edge. Spoon the chicken mixture into the pastry case. Roll out the remaining pastry to make a lid, then cut some slits or decorative vents in the pastry. Carefully place the pastry lid over the filling; fold the top edge over and under the bottom crust edges, then pinch the edges together to seal. If desired, you can form a decorative edge around the rim using a fork or with your fingers.
4 Bake the pie until the crust is golden brown, 35 to 40 minutes. Remove from the oven and allow the pie to stand for 15 minutes before serving. To bake a frozen pie, cover the edge with pieces of foil, place on a baking sheet and bake in a 425°F oven for 30 minutes. Reduce the oven temperature to 350°F and bake for an additional 70 to 80 minutes, or until the crust is golden brown.

Shepherd's Pie

5 boiling (waxy) potatoes
⅔ cup (170 ml) light cream or creamy milk
3 tablespoons butter
salt and freshly ground black pepper, to taste
freshly grated nutmeg
2 tablespoons vegetable oil
1 onion, chopped
1 clove garlic, crushed
2 teaspoons Worcestershire sauce
2 tablespoons tomato sauce
2 tablespoons chopped fresh mixed herbs (such as parsley, thyme, marjoram or mint)
1 lb (500 g) cooked lamb, trimmed of fat, then ground
⅔ cup (170 ml) lamb gravy or Beef Stock (page 49)

Makes 4 servings

This is a favorite way to transform leftovers from the weekend roast into a satisfying meal for all the family.

1 Preheat the oven to 350°F. Peel and quarter the potatoes. Boil or steam until the potatoes are tender, then drain and mash well. Heat the cream or milk and half the butter in a saucepan and beat into the mashed potatoes. Season well with salt, pepper and a little nutmeg. Cover and keep warm.
2 In a saucepan, heat the oil over medium heat. Add the onion and garlic and sauté until soft and golden, about 5 minutes. Stir in the Worcestershire sauce, tomato sauce and herbs. Stir in the lamb and gravy or stock. Transfer to a baking dish and spoon the mashed potatoes over the top. Smooth the potato topping, then score the surface decoratively.
3 Dot the remaining butter over the mashed potato and bake for 45 minutes, or until the pie is golden brown and thoroughly heated through.

Spicy Beef Pie

2 potatoes
1 lb (450 g) lean ground beef
2–3 spring onions, sliced
1 large carrot, finely chopped
1 clove garlic, finely chopped
½ teaspoon dried thyme
½ teaspoon dried sage
½ teaspoon salt
½ teaspoon freshly cracked black pepper
¼ teaspoon celery salt
pinch of ground cinnamon
3 tablespoons finely chopped fresh parsley
¼ cup (60 ml) chili sauce
Basic Double Crust Pie Pastry (page 123)
1 tablespoon Dijon mustard
1 tablespoon milk

Makes 6 servings

Transform the humble meat pie into a special dish.

1 Peel and quarter the potatoes. Cook in a large saucepan of boiling water until tender. Drain, mash and set aside.
2 Meanwhile, brown the beef in a large, heavy saucepan over medium heat until no pink remains. Drain the liquid from the pan and return to the heat. Stir in the spring onions, carrot, garlic, thyme, sage, salt, pepper, celery salt and cinnamon and sauté for 4 to 5 minutes. Add the mashed potatoes, parsley and chili sauce. Stir to combine, then remove from the heat.
3 Preheat the oven to 450°F. Roll out the pastry to line a 9-inch pie plate. Ease the pastry into the dish, then trim the edge. Brush the mustard over the inside of the pastry case, then spoon the beef mixture into the pastry case. Roll out the remaining pastry to make a lid, then cut some slits or decorative vents in the pastry. Carefully place the pastry over the filling; fold the top edge over and under the bottom crust edges, then pinch the edges together to seal. If desired, form a decorative edge around the rim using a fork or with your fingers. Brush the top of the pastry with the milk.
4 Bake for 10 minutes, reduce the temperature to 350°F and bake until the crust is golden brown, about 25 minutes.

Quiche Lorraine

Basic Single Crust Pie Pastry (page 124)
6 slices good-quality bacon, diced and lightly fried
1½ cups (185 g) grated Gruyère
1½ cups (375 ml) light cream
4 eggs
½ teaspoon salt
small pinch of ground cayenne pepper
small pinch of ground nutmeg

Makes 6 main course or 12 appetizer servings

Deliciously creamy, this much-loved quiche takes its name from the Lorraine region in France. The filling was originally made with just eggs, cream and bacon, but now includes cheese—a good Gruyère or other Swiss cheese. A store-bought quiche, while convenient, will never taste as good as your own, fresh from the oven.

1 Preheat the oven to 400°F. Line a 9-inch pie plate with the pastry and flute the edges. Place in the refrigerator and rest for 15 to 20 minutes.
2 Fill the pastry case with pie weights or beans and bake for 10 minutes. Remove from the oven and remove the weights or beans.
3 Sprinkle the cooked bacon around the pastry case, then sprinkle with the cheese. In a large bowl, beat the cream, eggs, salt, cayenne pepper and nutmeg until well blended. Carefully pour the cream mixture into the pastry case.
4 Bake for 15 minutes, then reduce the oven temperature to 350°F. Bake for another 15 to 20 minutes, or until the filling is set in the center. Remove from the oven and allow the quiche to stand for 10 minutes before serving to allow the custard to set.

If you run out of cream

Heavy cream: If a recipe calls for 1 cup (250 ml) heavy cream (not for whipping) and you don't have any on hand, whisk together ¾ cup (185 ml) milk with ⅓ cup (80 ml) melted butter until well blended.

Light cream: If a recipe calls for 1 cup (250 ml) light cream and you don't have any on hand, whisk together ¾ cup (185 ml) milk with ¼ cup (60 ml) melted butter until well blended.

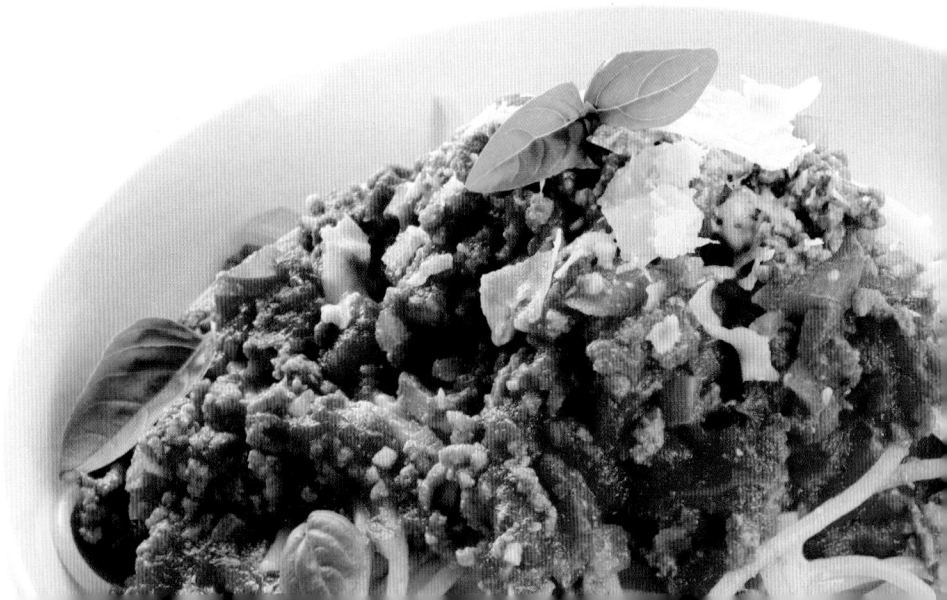

Pasta Dishes

Spaghetti Bolognese

2 cups (350 g) Savory Meat Mix (page 166), thawed
14½ oz (410 g) can chopped tomatoes
¾ cup (185 g) tomato paste
½ cup (125 ml) dry red wine
2 teaspoons dried basil, crumbled
1 teaspoon dried oregano, crumbled
16 oz (500 g) spaghetti
grated Parmesan cheese, for sprinkling

Makes 6 to 8 servings

Please a hungry crowd in just 30 minutes with this classic spaghetti recipe.

1. In a large, heavy saucepan over medium heat, combine the meat mix, tomatoes, tomato paste, wine, basil and oregano. Stir until well combined. Bring to a boil over high heat, then reduce the heat to low and simmer, stirring occasionally, for about 30 minutes.
2. Meanwhile, cook the spaghetti according to the package directions, then drain.
3. Serve the spaghetti topped with the meat sauce and sprinkled with Parmesan cheese.

Spaghetti with Speedy Tomato Sauce

16 oz (410 g) can Italian plum tomatoes
¾ cup (185 g) tomato paste
1 teaspoon dried oregano, crumbled
1 teaspoon dried basil, crumbled
1 teaspoon sugar
½ teaspoon salt
¼ teaspoon freshly ground black pepper
1 lb (500 g) spaghetti
grated Parmesan cheese, for sprinkling

Makes about 6 servings

You'll never need to buy bottled sauce again with this super recipe. Using the most basic pantry ingredients, this entire meal is ready in no time at all. In summer, when fresh tomatoes are plentiful and cheap, substitute fresh, chopped tomatoes for the canned variety.

1. In a large saucepan over medium heat, combine the tomatoes, tomato paste, oregano, basil, sugar, salt and pepper. Bring to a boil, then reduce the heat and simmer for 15 to 20 minutes.
2. Meanwhile, cook the spaghetti according to the package directions, then drain.
3. Serve the sauce over the spaghetti and sprinkle with Parmesan cheese.

Pasta with Fresh Tomato Sauce

3 lb (1.25 kg) ripe fresh tomatoes, or a 35 oz (800 g) can Italian plum tomatoes, chopped
2 tablespoons olive oil
3 cloves garlic
2 tablespoons tomato paste
2–3 tablespoons chopped fresh basil leaves, or 2 teaspoons dried basil, crumbled
1 teaspoon sugar
1 teaspoon salt
¼ teaspoon freshly ground black pepper
1 lb (500 g) pasta, such as spaghetti, vermicelli or linguine, cooked and drained
grated Parmesan cheese, for sprinkling

Makes about 6 servings or 3 cups (750 ml) sauce

Bursting with rich, juicy, vine-ripened tomatoes, this classic sauce forms the base for many other pasta sauces. This is a great way to use up overripe tomatoes as they impart an especially intense flavor. If tomatoes are not in season, you can use canned, but the flavor won't be nearly as good.

1 If using fresh tomatoes, score a cross in the base of each tomato and place in a heatproof bowl. Cover with boiling water, leave for 30 seconds, then plunge in cold water and peel the skin away from the cross. Cut the tomatoes in half and scoop out the seeds, then chop the flesh.
2 In a large, heavy saucepan, heat the olive oil over medium heat. Add the garlic and cook for 1 minute. Add the tomatoes, tomato paste, basil and sugar and bring to a boil, stirring constantly. Reduce the heat to low and simmer until the sauce thickens, 12 to 15 minutes.
3 Stir in the salt and pepper. Serve over hot cooked pasta sprinkled with a little Parmesan cheese.

Pasta Puttanesca

2 tablespoons olive oil
2 cloves garlic, finely chopped
1 cup (135 g) halved, pitted, large black Greek olives
¼ cup (35 g) drained capers
8 chopped anchovies
3 cups (750 ml) Fresh Tomato Sauce (above)
¼ teaspoon crushed red pepper flakes, or to taste
1 lb (500 g) pasta, cooked and drained

Makes 6 servings

For a true taste of the Mediterranean without leaving home, try this rich tomato sauce—salty, piquant and just a little spicy!

1 In a large, heavy saucepan, heat the olive oil over medium-low heat. Add the garlic and sauté until soft, about 2 minutes. Add the olives, capers, anchovies, tomato sauce and pepper flakes to taste.
2 Increase the heat to medium-high. Simmer the sauce for 15 minutes, stirring often. Serve over hot cooked pasta.

If you run out of tomato sauce

If a recipe calls for 2 cups (500 ml) tomato sauce and you don't have any on hand, combine ¾ cup (185 g) tomato paste and 1 cup (250 ml) water and whisk until well blended.

Fettuccine Alfredo

3 tablespoons butter
4 tablespoons finely chopped shallots
1¼ cups (300 ml) heavy cream
1 cup (250 ml) light cream
½ teaspoon salt
pinch of ground nutmeg
¾ cup (75 g) grated Parmesan cheese
1 lb (500 g) fettuccine, cooked and drained

Makes 4 servings

The king of cream sauces, Alfredo has a rich flavor that is entirely dependent on the quality of the cheese, so indulge in the best. You will still pay less than restaurant prices—and you'll find that store-bought Alfredo sauces just don't compare.

1 In a saucepan over medium heat, melt the butter. Add the shallots and sauté until they are soft, 3 to 4 minutes. Stir in all the cream, with the salt and nutmeg. Increase the heat to high and bring the mixture to a boil, stirring constantly. Reduce the heat to low and simmer until the sauce thickens, 4 to 5 minutes. Stir in the Parmesan cheese.
2 Place the hot cooked fettuccine in a large, warm serving bowl. Pour the sauce over, toss well and serve.

Penne with Four-Cheese Sauce

3 tablespoons butter
2 cloves garlic, finely chopped
2 tablespoons plain flour
1 cup (250 ml) light cream
1 cup (250 ml) milk
1 cup (125 g) grated fontina cheese
1 cup (150 g) grated provolone cheese
½ cup (75 g) grated mozzarella
½ cup (50 g) grated Parmesan cheese
½ teaspoon salt
¼ teaspoon ground white pepper
1 lb (500 g) penne or other pasta, such as farfalle or rotini, cooked and drained

Makes 4 servings

If you love cheese, this dish is for you—not one, but four intriguing cheeses combine to make a superb pasta sauce. It's so simple to make and much, much better than anything you'll find in a bottle!

1 In a large, nonstick saucepan over medium heat, melt the butter. Add the garlic and sauté until soft, about 2 minutes. Stir in the flour and cook until bubbly, about 1 minute. Remove the pan from the heat and gradually whisk in the cream and milk. Place back over medium heat and cook, stirring often, until the sauce just boils and thickens, 3 to 5 minutes.
2 Add the cheeses, salt and pepper and cook, stirring constantly, until the cheeses melt and the sauce is smooth, 1 to 2 minutes.
3 Place the hot cooked pasta in a warm serving bowl. Pour the sauce over, toss well and serve.

Pasta with Seafood

2 tablespoons extra virgin olive oil
1 onion, chopped
2–3 cloves garlic, chopped
2 tablespoons chopped fresh parsley
1 cup (250 ml) dry white wine
14½ oz (410 g) can chopped tomatoes
pinch of crushed red pepper flakes
¼ teaspoon sugar
pinch of saffron threads
freshly ground black pepper, to taste
8 mussels, scrubbed and beards removed
2 cleaned squid, tentacles cut into bite-sized pieces and the bodies cut into rings
10 oz (300 g) raw tiger or king shrimp, peeled and deveined
14 oz (400 g) spaghetti
fresh oregano or marjoram sprigs, to garnish

Makes 4 servings

Turn your kitchen into a cheery Italian trattoria with this delightful old classic. You could pay a small fortune for this dish in a restaurant—or make it at home and have it just the way you like it.

1 In a large saucepan, heat the olive oil. Add the onion and sauté until softened but not browned, 5 to 7 minutes. Add the garlic and parsley and cook for 1 minute more.
2 Pour in the wine and bring to a boil. Adjust the heat so that the wine boils steadily, and cook until the wine has almost all evaporated, about 15 minutes.
3 Stir in the tomatoes, pepper flakes, sugar and saffron. Reduce the heat and cook gently for 15 minutes. Season to taste with pepper.
4 Add the mussels. Cover and cook over medium heat until the mussels start to open, about 5 minutes. Add the squid and shrimp and cook until the shrimp turn pink, a further 3 to 4 minutes. Remove the pan from the heat. Discard any mussels that have not opened, then cover the pan to retain the heat.
5 Meanwhile, cook the spaghetti according to the package directions, then drain. Return the pasta to the empty pan, add some of the tomato sauce and toss until the pasta is coated.
6 Serve the pasta with the remaining tomato sauce and seafood piled on top, garnished with small herb sprigs.

Penne All'amatriciana

⅓ cup (80 ml) olive oil, plus extra, for drizzling
1 onion, finely chopped
2 cloves garlic, crushed
7 oz (200 g) bacon slices or pancetta, chopped
2 cans (14½ oz/410 g each) chopped tomatoes
½ teaspoon crushed red pepper flakes, or to taste
salt and freshly ground black pepper, to taste
14 oz (400 g) penne
⅓ cup (35 g) grated Parmesan cheese, plus extra, to serve
2 tablespoons finely chopped fresh parsley

Makes 4 servings

This is a great stand-by for a super-quick pasta dish as all the ingredients are usually in the fridge or pantry. Vary the red pepper flakes to suit your family's tastes.

1 In a heavy saucepan, heat the olive oil over medium heat. Add the onion and garlic and sauté until soft but not brown, about 5 minutes. Add the bacon and fry lightly. Stir in the tomatoes and pepper flakes and cook, stirring from time to time, for about 20 minutes. Season to taste with salt and pepper.
2 Meanwhile, cook the penne according to the package directions, then drain.
3 Transfer the tomato sauce mixture to a large serving bowl. Add the hot pasta and Parmesan cheese and toss until well combined. Sprinkle with chopped parsley and serve immediately, with a little extra olive oil for drizzling and grated cheese.

Pasta with Classic Basil Pesto

6½ cups (250 g/about 2 bunches) fresh basil, leaves picked
2 cloves garlic
¼ cup (60 ml) extra virgin olive oil
2 tablespoons butter, softened
½ cup (50 g) grated Parmesan cheese
¾ cup (115 g) pine nuts
½ teaspoon grated lemon zest
1 teaspoon salt
¼ teaspoon freshly ground black pepper
1 lb (500 g) pasta, cooked and drained

Makes 1½ cups (375 g) or 4 servings

It pays to use extra virgin olive oil when making pesto, because the sauce is not cooked and the flavor of the oil shines through, marrying beautifully with the basil, garlic and Parmesan cheese. Homemade pesto tastes so much fresher than any bottled pesto sauce—and is almost as quick and simple as opening a jar.

1 Pack the basil leaves and garlic cloves into a food processor or blender. Process at high speed until all the leaves are pureed, about 2 minutes, scraping down the side of the bowl as needed. With the motor still running, pour in the olive oil in a slow, steady stream.
2 Add the butter, Parmesan cheese, pine nuts, lemon zest, salt and pepper. Scraping down the sides of the bowl several times, puree until the mixture forms a paste, about 3 minutes. Add 1 to 2 tablespoons of water if the mixture seems too stiff.
3 While the pasta is still very hot, add the pesto, about ½ cup (125 g) at a time, tossing thoroughly after each addition to evenly distribute it through the pasta; if the pesto is too sticky, add 1 tablespoon hot water to thin it slightly. Serve hot.

Pesto: more than green basil sauce

In Italian, "pestare" means "to pound"—and that is the technique used to make the simple, classic sauce known as pesto. Most people are familiar with the green sauce made from pulverized basil leaves, but not all pestos are made from basil—they're not even all green. The technique used is what makes a sauce a pesto.

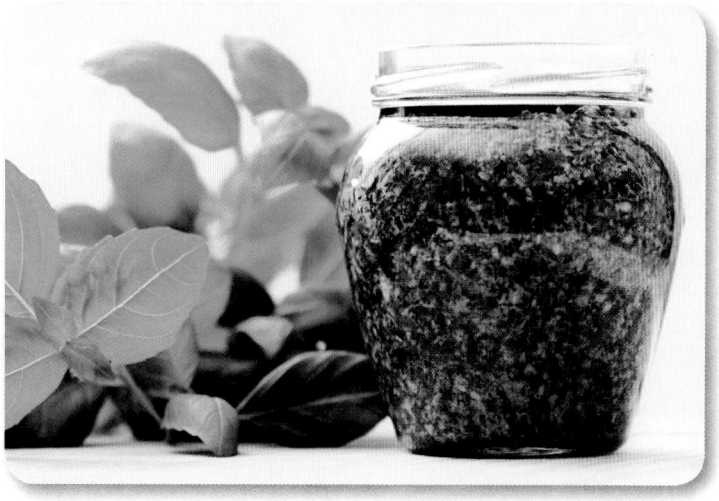

Pasta with Mushroom Pesto

2 tablespoons butter
1 clove garlic, finely chopped
10 oz (300 g) fresh mushrooms, thinly sliced
2 tablespoons butter, softened
2 tablespoons snipped fresh chives or spring onion tops
½ cup (50 g) grated Parmesan cheese
¾ teaspoon salt
¼ teaspoon freshly ground black pepper
1 lb (500 g) pasta, cooked and drained

Makes about ¾ cup (185 g) or 4 servings

When mushrooms are on sale, try this delightfully earthy variation on the pesto theme. Experiment with different-flavored varieties or even use a mixture.

1 In a large frying pan or skillet over medium-high heat, melt the butter. Add the garlic and mushrooms and sauté until golden, 2 to 3 minutes.
2 Transfer the mushroom mixture to a food processor or blender. Add the softened butter, chives, Parmesan cheese, salt and pepper and process to a smooth puree.
3 While the pasta is still very hot, add the mushroom pesto, a few good dollops at a time, tossing thoroughly after each addition to evenly distribute it through the pasta; if the pesto is too sticky, add 1 tablespoon hot water to thin it slightly. Serve hot.

Pasta with Sun-Dried Tomato Pesto

1 cup (50 g) tightly packed fresh basil leaves
½ cup (75 g) sun-dried tomatoes in oil, undrained
¼ cup (30 g) chopped walnuts, raw or lightly toasted
1 small red chile pepper, seeded and chopped (optional)
½ cup (125 ml) extra virgin olive oil
⅓ cup (35 g) grated Parmesan cheese
1 lb (500 g) pasta, cooked and drained

Makes about 1 cup (250 g) or 4 servings

Intense tomato flavors are enhanced by walnuts in yet another version of pesto—and again, you'll find it always tastes far better when it is freshly made.

1 Put the basil in a food processor or blender. Process at high speed until all the leaves are pureed, about 2 minutes, scraping down the side of the bowl as needed. Add the tomatoes with their liquid, walnuts and chile pepper, if using, and process to a puree. With the motor still running, pour in the olive oil in a slow, steady stream.
2 Scrape the pesto mixture into a large bowl. Fold in the Parmesan cheese until it is incorporated.
3 While the pasta is still very hot, add the pesto, a few good dollops at a time, tossing thoroughly after each addition to evenly distribute it through the pasta; if the pesto is too sticky, add 1 tablespoon hot water to thin it slightly. Serve hot.

Ravioli

1 batch Simple Fresh Pasta (page 62)

PROSCIUTTO-RICOTTA FILLING
2 teaspoons olive oil
1 oz (30 g) prosciutto, roughly chopped
3 cloves garlic, finely chopped
1 cup (250 g) ricotta
½ cup (50 g) grated Parmesan cheese
1 egg yolk
½ cup (30 g) finely chopped fresh basil
½ teaspoon salt
¼ teaspoon freshly ground black pepper

TOMATO SAUCE
2 teaspoons olive oil
1 small yellow onion, chopped
2 cloves garlic, finely chopped
28 oz (800 g) can chopped Italian plum tomatoes
½ teaspoon salt
grated or shaved Parmesan cheese, for sprinkling

Makes 12 ravioli, about 4 servings

You can fill these mouthwatering morsels with just about anything you like—plus a soft cheese of some kind, such as the ricotta used below.

1 Prepare the pasta dough. Cover dough and let sit for 1 hour.
2 Meanwhile, prepare the prosciutto-ricotta filling. In a large nonstick frying pan or skillet, heat the olive oil over medium heat. Add the prosciutto and garlic and cook until the garlic is soft, about 2 minutes. Transfer the mixture to a bowl and allow to cool to room temperature. Add the ricotta, Parmesan cheese, egg yolk, basil, salt and pepper and stir gently to blend; set aside.
3 Divide the dough into two equal portions. Cover one portion. On a lightly floured surface, roll out the second portion into a 9 x 12-inch rectangle, about 1/16-inch thick. Using a sharp knife or pastry wheel, cut the rectangle into four strips about 3 inches wide and 9 inches long.
4 On two of the dough strips, drop three equal mounds of the filling, spacing the mounds about 1 inch apart and leaving a ½-inch margin all around the edges. Using a pastry brush, brush the dough margins with water. Carefully place the remaining dough strips on top; firmly press along the edges and around each mound to seal the dough strips together firmly. Cut each strip crosswise into three ravioli. Repeat with the remaining dough portion to make 12 ravioli.
5 Prepare the tomato sauce. In a heavy saucepan, heat the olive oil over medium heat. Add the onion and sauté until soft, about 5 minutes. Add the garlic and cook for 2 minutes more. Add the tomatoes and salt and bring to a boil over medium heat; reduce the heat to a bubbling simmer and cook, stirring often, until the sauce thickens slightly, about 10 minutes.
6 Meanwhile, in a large pot of boiling water, cook the ravioli until firm-tender, about 6 minutes. Drain well, divide among warm serving plates and top with some of the tomato sauce. Serve with Parmesan cheese for sprinkling over.

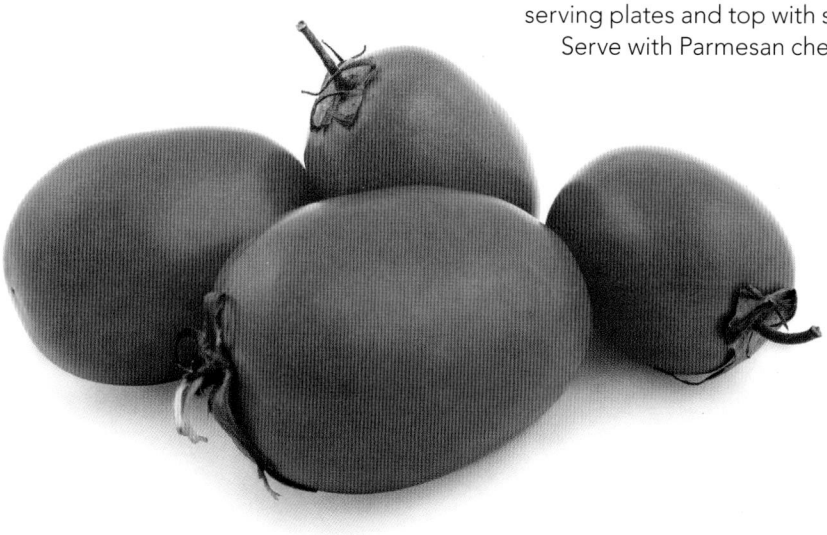

Lasagna

2 tablespoons butter or olive oil
10 oz (300 g) mushrooms, roughly chopped
1 quantity Spaghetti Bolognese sauce (page 179)
1 batch Simple Fresh Pasta (page 62), cooked until almost tender and drained, or 1 lb (500 g) no-boil lasagna sheets
½ cup (50 g) grated Parmesan cheese
1 cup (150 g) grated mozzarella

TOMATO SAUCE
2 cans (28 oz/800 g each) chopped Italian plum tomatoes
1 yellow onion, finely chopped
4 cloves garlic, finely chopped
3 tablespoons chopped fresh basil
½ teaspoon dried thyme, crumbled
½ teaspoon salt
½ teaspoon freshly ground black pepper
2 tablespoons plain flour, mixed with ¼ cup (60 ml) cold water

Makes 6 servings

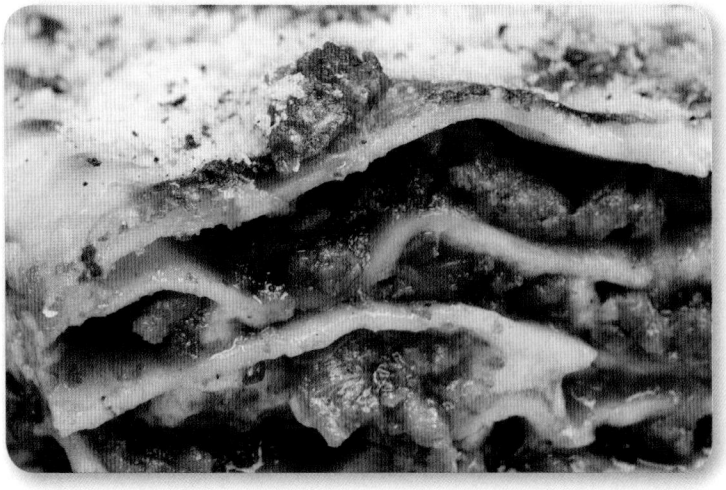

Homemade lasagna is a wonderfully welcoming dish. When you make it yourself, you know exactly what's in it—and you can use the ingredients that you happen to like best. A winner all around.

1 Prepare the tomato sauce. In a large, heavy saucepan, combine the tomatoes, onion, garlic, basil, thyme, salt and pepper. Mix well and bring to a boil over medium-high heat. Reduce the heat to medium-low and simmer for 15 minutes, stirring occasionally to break up the tomatoes. Slowly whisk in the flour paste and simmer, stirring constantly, until the sauce thickens, about 2 minutes.
2 In a large frying pan or skillet, melt the butter or heat the olive oil over high heat. Add the mushrooms and cook until light brown, about 5 minutes. Transfer to a large bowl and add the bolognese sauce and 4 cups (1 liter) of the tomato sauce. Mix well.
3 Spread the remaining tomato sauce over the bottom of an ungreased 9 x 13-inch baking dish. Top with a single layer of slightly overlapping lasagna sheets, half the bolognese sauce and half the Parmesan cheese. Repeat the layers, beginning with the lasagna sheets. Scatter the mozzarella over the top of the lasagna.
4 Cover the dish with foil and bake until the sauce is bubbly, 45 to 55 minutes. Remove from the oven and stand for 10 minutes before serving.

Beef Barley Soup

1 tablespoon butter
1 carrot, chopped
1 celery stalk, chopped
1 onion, chopped
4 cups (1 liter) Beef Stock (page 49)
2 cups (350 g) chopped cooked roast beef
14½ oz (410 g) can chopped tomatoes
1 cup (220 g) quick-cooking barley
1½ teaspoons salt
½ teaspoon dried basil, crumbled
½ teaspoon dried oregano, crumbled
½ teaspoon freshly ground black pepper
½ cup (80 g) frozen peas

Makes 8 servings

The culinary use of barley can be traced back to the Stone Age. Pearl barley is the type most often used for soups—it is polished and the bran has been removed. Homemade beef barley soup is filling and delicious, a bargain all around.

1 In a large, heavy saucepan, melt the butter over medium heat. Add the carrot, celery and onion and sauté until the vegetables are tender, about 5 minutes.
2 Pour in the stock and 4 cups (1 liter) water. Add the roast beef, tomatoes, barley, salt, basil, oregano and pepper and bring to a boil. Reduce the heat, cover and simmer for 20 minutes, stirring occasionally.
3 Remove the lid and stir in the peas. Simmer, uncovered, for 5 minutes longer. Ladle into bowls and serve.

Make the most of soup

One of the all-time, soul-satisfying comfort foods, homemade soup is simple to prepare, highly nutritious and usually extremely economical. It is a wonderful way to use up all kinds of leftovers, from vegetable peelings to pot roast. Best of all, it is a filling meal you can make in a single pot. Add a tossed green salad and crusty bread or rolls and you've got all the bases covered.

Black Bean Soup

- 2 cups (440 g) dried black beans, sorted and rinsed
- 8 thick slices bacon, rind removed, cut crosswise into ½ inch (1 cm) strips
- 2 large yellow onions, chopped
- 2 celery stalks, chopped
- 2 carrots, chopped
- 2 cloves garlic, finely chopped
- 2 bay leaves
- 1 teaspoon dried thyme, crumbled
- ½ teaspoon hot red pepper sauce
- 3 tablespoons chopped fresh coriander
- 2 tablespoons lemon juice
- sour cream or natural yogurt (optional)
- 8 fresh coriander sprigs (optional)

Makes 8 servings

Southwestern flavor fills every bowl of this stick-to-your-ribs favorite. Black beans are loaded with fiber, are a good source of iron and contain plenty of B vitamins. Homemade black bean soup can feed a crowd for practically nothing. You just can't buy anything this good in a can!

1. Place the beans in a large, heavy saucepan and add enough cold water to cover. Over high heat, bring the mixture to a boil, then cook for 2 minutes. Remove the saucepan from the heat, cover and let the beans stand for 1 hour. Drain the beans and discard the cooking liquid; set the beans aside.
2. Return the saucepan to medium-high heat and add the bacon strips. Sauté until the bacon is crisp, 5 to 8 minutes. Using a slotted spoon, transfer the bacon to paper towels to drain.
3. In the bacon drippings in the saucepan, sauté the onions, celery, carrots, garlic, bay leaves and thyme over medium heat until the vegetables are tender, 8 to 10 minutes.
4. Add 8 cups (2 liters) water and the reserved beans and return to a boil. Reduce the heat to medium-low, cover and simmer for 45 minutes. Remove and discard the bay leaves.
5. Place 1 cup (250 ml) of the bean mixture in a food processor or blender. Process to a smooth puree, then pour back into the saucepan. Add the reserved bacon, hot pepper sauce, coriander and lemon juice and stir until well combined.
6. Ladle into soup bowls. Serve garnished with a dollop of sour cream or yogurt and a coriander sprig, if desired.

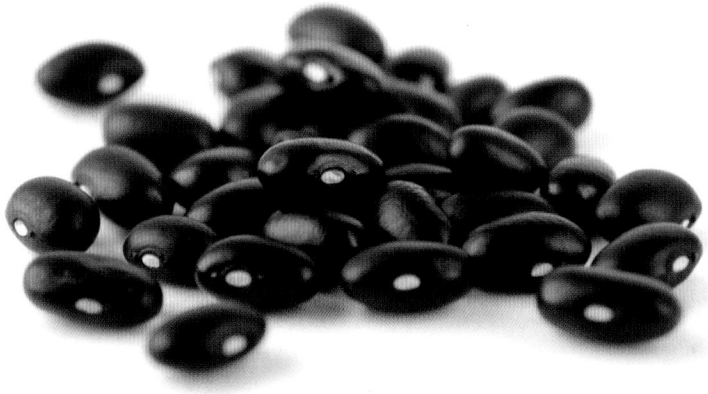

Chicken Noodle Soup

1 teaspoon butter
1 carrot, chopped
1 celery stalk, chopped
1 onion, chopped
6 cups (1.5 liters) Chicken Stock (page 50)
1½ cups (225 g) chopped cooked chicken
1 teaspoon salt
½ teaspoon dried marjoram
½ teaspoon dried thyme
pinch of freshly ground pepper
1½ cups (200 g package) egg noodles
1 tablespoon finely chopped fresh parsley

Makes 6 servings

There is nothing quite as comforting as a steaming bowl of homemade chicken noodle soup. Our version is so quick and easy that you may never bother with commercially produced varieties again. This soup is also very versatile. For a more exotic version, borrow from the kitchens of South East Asia: Leave out the marjoram, thyme and parsley and instead flavor the soup with herbs and spices such as fresh ginger, chile pepper and coriander—you could also add some sliced shiitake mushrooms and bean sprouts at the end for some slippery, crunchy texture.

1 In a large saucepan, melt the butter over medium heat. Add the carrot, celery and onion and sauté until the vegetables are tender, 8 to 10 minutes.
2 Add the stock, chicken, salt, marjoram, thyme and pepper. Bring to a boil, then reduce the heat and stir in the noodles. Cook until the noodles are tender, about 10 minutes. Stir in the parsley, ladle into bowls and serve.

New England Clam Chowder

2 lb (1 kg/about 24) clams in shells, scrubbed
4 slices bacon, rind removed, chopped
1 large onion, chopped
2 tablespoons plain flour
1 lb (500 g) all-purpose potatoes, peeled and cubed
2 cups (500 ml) milk
2 teaspoons fresh thyme leaves
1 bay leaf
pinch of ground cayenne pepper
3 tablespoons chopped fresh flat-leaf parsley

Makes 4 servings

This creamy, rich soup is how New Englanders like their clam chowder. If clams aren't available, substitute vongole (baby clams), mussels or a 7 oz (200 g) can of clams.

1 In a large saucepan over high heat, bring the clams and 2 cups (500 ml) water to a boil. Reduce the heat, cover and simmer for 5 minutes, then remove the lid. Using tongs or a slotted spoon, transfer the clams to a large bowl as they open. Strain the clam broth, then add enough water to make up 1½ cups (375 ml); set aside.
2 Wipe out the saucepan and place over medium heat. Sauté the bacon and onion until the onion is golden, about 7 minutes. Sprinkle with the flour and cook, stirring constantly, just until bubbling but not browned, about 1 minute.
3 Add the potatoes, milk, reserved clam broth, thyme, bay leaf and cayenne pepper. Bring to a simmer over medium heat. Simmer, stirring occasionally, until the potatoes are tender, about 10 minutes.
4 Meanwhile, remove the clams from their shells and cut into bite-sized pieces if necessary. Stir the clams into the chowder and cook until heated through, about 2 minutes. Discard the bay leaf. Ladle the chowder into individual bowls and serve sprinkled with parsley.

Cream of Tomato Soup

2½ cups (500 g) chopped peeled tomatoes, fresh or canned
1 small celery stalk, diced
1 small onion, diced
1 tablespoon vegetable oil
2 tablespoons plain flour
1 cup (250 ml) light cream
1 teaspoon salt (optional)
pinch of freshly ground black pepper
3 tablespoons sour cream (optional)
3 teaspoons finely chopped fresh parsley (optional)

Makes 3 servings

Pair this with a grilled cheese sandwich and you've got the ultimate comfort meal. If you have eaten canned tomato soup all your life, you're in for a big treat!

1. In a saucepan over medium-high heat, combine the tomatoes, celery and onion. Bring to a boil, reduce the heat to low, cover and simmer for 15 minutes, stirring often. Remove from the heat and let the mixture cool for 10 minutes.
2. Transfer the tomato mixture to a food processor or blender. Process to a smooth puree.
3. Heat the oil in a large saucepan over medium heat. Add the flour and stir until the mixture is smooth. Gradually add the cream, stirring constantly. Bring to a boil and cook for 2 minutes.
4. Gradually add the tomato mixture, stirring constantly. Add the salt, if using, and the pepper. Continue to cook until the soup is heated through.
5. Ladle into bowls and garnish each with a dollop of the sour cream and a sprinkle of the parsley, if desired.

Quick Shrimp Laksa

9 oz (250 g) package rice vermicelli
1 tablespoon peanut oil
3 tablespoons Laksa Paste (page 44)
3 cups (750 ml) Fish, Chicken or Vegetable Stock (pages 50 and 51)
14 oz (400 ml) can coconut milk
2 lb (1 kg) raw shrimp, peeled and deveined, tails left on
1 teaspoon salt
1 heaped cup (100 g) bean sprouts
3 tablespoons roughly chopped fresh Vietnamese mint
⅔ cup (20 g) fresh coriander leaves
1 small red chile pepper, seeded and sliced
lime wedges, to serve

Makes 4 servings

Vary the ingredients in this traditional South East Asian noodle soup to suit the ingredients you have on hand. You can use cooked chicken, tofu, mixed seafood or a combination of all three, if you desire.

1. Put the noodles in a heatproof bowl and pour in boiling water to cover. Leave to soak for 10 minutes, then drain and set aside.
2. In a wok, heat the oil over medium heat. Add the laksa paste and fry until fragrant, about 1 minute. Stir in the stock and bring to a boil. Add the coconut milk and simmer for 2 to 3 minutes. Add the shrimp and cook until they turn pink, about 4 minutes. Stir in the salt.
3. Divide the noodles among four bowls and top each with some bean sprouts and fresh herbs. Pour the soup over the noodles, dividing the shrimp evenly. Serve garnished with chile pepper slices and lime wedges on the side.

Minestrone

1 tablespoon olive oil
1 large yellow onion, chopped
2 cloves garlic, finely chopped
3½ cups (875 ml) Beef Stock (page 49)
15 oz (420 g) can white beans, drained
14½ oz (410 g) can chopped Italian plum tomatoes
2 cups (150 g) roughly shredded cabbage
2 large carrots, thinly sliced
1 teaspoon dried oregano
1 teaspoon dried basil
½ teaspoon salt
½ teaspoon freshly ground black pepper
2 oz (50 g) pasta shells
1 small zucchini, sliced
grated Parmesan cheese, for sprinkling

Makes 8 servings

Italian cooks have no definite rules for what goes into minestrone—so long as there's a hearty mix of vegetables, white beans and pasta or rice. Humble and inexpensive, a homemade minestrone trumps the canned variety every time. To make it vegetarian, use vegetable stock instead of beef stock.

1 In a large, nonstick saucepan, heat the olive oil over medium-high heat. Add the onion and garlic and sauté until the onion is soft, about 5 minutes. Stir in the stock, beans, tomatoes, cabbage, carrots, oregano, basil, salt and pepper.
2 Bring to a boil and stir in the pasta. Reduce the heat, cover and simmer for 15 minutes, or until the vegetables and pasta are tender. Stir in the zucchini and cook, uncovered, for 3 minutes.
3 Ladle into bowls and serve sprinkled with Parmesan cheese.

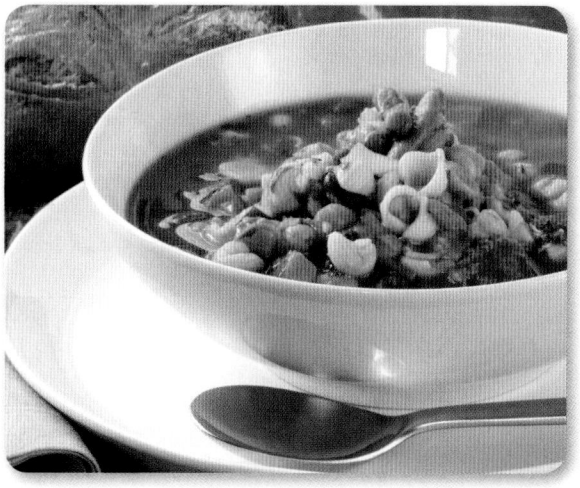

Lentil Soup

1 cup (185 g) dried brown or green lentils, sorted and rinsed
6 cups (1.5 liters) Chicken Stock (page 50)
1 tablespoon vegetable oil
1 large onion, chopped
1 clove garlic, finely chopped
2½ cups (500 ml) chopped fresh tomatoes
2 small carrots, sliced
½ teaspoon dried thyme
¼ teaspoon dried marjoram

Makes 8 servings

Long a staple of Indian and Middle Eastern cooking, lentils are an excellent source of fiber, protein, folate and iron, which makes this soup very good for you—the perfect low-cost, one-dish dinner.

1 In a large saucepan over medium-high heat, combine the lentils and the stock. Bring to a boil, reduce the heat to low and simmer for 30 minutes.
2 Meanwhile, heat the oil in a large frying pan or skillet over medium-high heat. Add the onion and garlic and sauté until tender, about 5 minutes.
3 Add the onion mixture to the lentils. Stir in the tomatoes, carrots, thyme and marjoram and cook until the lentils and vegetables are tender, about 30 minutes.

Gumbo

¼ cup (60 ml) olive oil
1 pound (500 g) beef brisket or chuck steak, cut into ½-inch (1 cm) chunks
6 ounces (175 g) baked ham, cut into ½-inch (1 cm) chunks
1 large yellow onion, chopped
6 scallions, including green tops, thinly sliced
1 large red bell pepper, cored, seeded and diced
3 tablespoons plain flour
1 cup (200 g) thinly sliced fresh okra or ½ package (10 ounces/200 g) frozen okra
4 cups (1 liter) Chicken Stock (page 50) or reduced-sodium canned chicken broth
8 ounces (225 g) cabbage, cored and cut into ½-inch chunks
4 cups (300g) thinly sliced mustard greens
3 cups (225 g) thinly sliced turnip greens
½ teaspoon salt
¼ teaspoon ground black pepper
1 bay leaf
½ teaspoon dried thyme, crumbled
½ teaspoon dried marjoram, crumbled
4 whole allspice
2 whole cloves
⅛ teaspoon ground cayenne pepper
6 cups (450 g) trimmed, washed and chopped spinach
1 bunch watercress, tough stems removed and leaves chopped

Makes 4 servings

Is it soup or is it stew? We just know it's delicious if you whip it up yourself from scratch. This good Cajun flavor doesn't come in a can.

1 In a large saucepan or an 8-quart Dutch oven over moderate heat, heat the olive oil about 2 minutes. Add the brisket or chuck steak and ham, and cook, stirring frequently, until the meat is lightly browned, about 5 minutes. Using a slotted spoon, transfer the meat to a bowl and set aside.
2 Add the onion and scallions to the Dutch oven and cook, stirring frequently, until the vegetables are softened, about 5 minutes. Add the red bell pepper and cook, stirring frequently, until it is crisp-tender, about 4 minutes. Stir in the flour until the vegetables are well coated. Add the okra and cook, stirring constantly, until all the ingredients are well combined. Gradually pour in the stock, stirring until well blended..
3 Add the cabbage, mustard greens, turnip greens, salt, pepper, bay leaf, thyme, marjoram, allspice, cloves, cayenne, and reserved meats. Bring the mixture to a boil, reduce the heat to moderately low and simmer, stirring occasionally, until the gumbo is thickened and the beef is tender, about 1½ hours.
4 Add the spinach and watercress. Cover the Dutch oven and cook until tender, about 15 minutes longer. Remove and discard the bay leaf.

French Onion Soup

2 tablespoons butter
5 yellow onions, thinly sliced
2 tablespoons sugar
3½ cups (875 ml) Beef Stock (page 49)
¼ cup (60 ml) brandy (optional)
½ teaspoon salt
½ teaspoon freshly ground black pepper
4 baguette slices, about ½-inch (1 cm) thick, toasted
4 tablespoons grated Gruyère

Makes 4 servings

Easier to make than you may think, this classic of French cooking is mostly a matter of slicing onions! Nothing in a can or a package compares.

1 Preheat the oven to 400°F. In a large, heavy saucepan, melt the butter over medium-high heat. Add the onions and sugar, increase the heat to high and sauté until the onions are lightly golden, about 10 minutes. Reduce the heat to medium-low and sauté for 10 minutes longer, stirring occasionally.
2 Add the stock and 5 cups (1.25 liters) water. Increase the heat to high and bring to a boil, then reduce the heat to medium-low and simmer for 20 minutes. Add the brandy, if using, and the salt and pepper. Increase the heat to high and return to a boil.
3 Place four 1-cup (250 ml) ramekins or soup bowls on a sturdy baking sheet. Ladle soup into the bowls. Place a baguette slice on top of each soup and sprinkle each slice with 1 tablespoon of the cheese.
4 Bake until the cheese has melted, about 5 minutes. Serve hot.

Vegetable Soup

3 tablespoons olive oil
1 large red onion, diced
5 cloves garlic, finely chopped
2 large carrots, thinly sliced
4 yellow summer squashes, diced
2 zucchini, diced
½ lb (250 g) green beans, sliced
2 lb (1 kg) tomatoes, peeled and chopped
1 lb (500 g) new potatoes, diced
5 cups (1.25 liters) Vegetable Stock (page 51)
¾ teaspoon salt
¾ teaspoon dried marjoram
½ teaspoon freshly ground black pepper

Makes 4 servings

The best vegetable soup is made with the freshest produce and it doesn't come from a can. You make it yourself from what's ripe in the garden or what's in season at the local farmers' market.

1 In a large saucepan, heat the olive oil over medium heat. Add the onion and garlic and cook until soft, about 5 minutes. Add the carrots and cook, stirring frequently, until the carrots are soft, about 5 minutes.
2 Add the squashes, zucchini, green beans, tomatoes, potatoes, stock, salt, marjoram and pepper. Increase the heat to high and bring to a boil, then reduce the heat to medium-low. Cover and simmer until the vegetables are tender, 40 to 50 minutes.

Split Pea Soup

16 oz (500 g) package dried green split peas
1 ham bone
1 large onion, chopped
1 teaspoon salt
½ teaspoon freshly ground black pepper
½ teaspoon dried thyme, crumbled
1 bay leaf
1 large carrot, diced
1 celery stalk, diced

Makes 10 servings

This is a great soup to make when you have a ham bone in the house. It's hearty, filling, supremely economical and will feed a whole family with plenty to spare.

1. Put the split peas in a large, heavy saucepan and pour in enough water to cover them by 2 inches. Bring to a boil over high heat, then boil for 2 minutes. Remove from the heat, cover and let stand for 1 hour. Drain and rinse the peas, discarding the soaking liquid. Return the peas to the saucepan.
2. Add 10 cups (2.5 liters) water, the ham bone, onion, salt, pepper, thyme and bay leaf. Bring the mixture to a boil over high heat, then reduce the heat to low. Cover and simmer for 1½ hours, stirring occasionally.
3. Transfer the ham bone to a cutting board and leave until cool enough to handle. Remove the meat from the bone; discard the bone. Dice the meat and return to the saucepan.
4. Add the carrots and celery and simmer over medium-low heat until the soup reaches the desired consistency and the vegetables are tender, 45 to 60 minutes. Remove and discard the bay leaf before serving.

Gazpacho

3 cups (600 g) chopped tomatoes
2 celery stalks, chopped
1 green bell pepper, chopped
1 cucumber, chopped
3 tablespoons fresh parsley, finely chopped
1 tablespoon fresh chives, finely chopped
1 spring onion, thinly sliced
1 clove garlic, finely chopped
5 cups (1.25 liters) tomato juice
⅓ cup (80 ml) red wine vinegar
¼ cup (60 ml) olive oil
1 teaspoon salt
½ teaspoon Worcestershire sauce
½ teaspoon freshly ground black pepper

Makes 10 servings

One of the great joys of summer is fresh tomatoes—and this chilled soup is the most refreshing way to use that bounty. Whip up a batch and keep it in the refrigerator for a quick, refreshing snack, lunch or start to a barbecued dinner. It's a treat you can make better than supermarkets or delis because you can adapt it to your individual taste.

In a large, nonreactive bowl, combine all the ingredients. Stir until well blended, then cover and refrigerate for several hours or overnight.

Salads

Classic Coleslaw

1 small green cabbage, shredded and immersed in iced water for 1 hour
3 carrots, grated
1 cup (250 g) Classic Mayonnaise (page 29)
⅓ cup (75 g) sugar
¼ cup (60 ml) cider vinegar

Makes 10 to 12 servings

The quintessential side salad for a perfect picnic, tangy slaw offers crunchy texture and good nutrition. No deli slaw—at any price—can compare with your own.

1 Drain the cabbage and transfer to paper towels. Blot with additional towels until it is completely dry. Place in a large bowl, add the carrots and toss until thoroughly mixed.
2 In a small bowl, combine the mayonnaise, sugar and vinegar. Stir until well blended and smooth.
3 Pour the dressing over the cabbage mixture and toss until well coated.

Greek Salad

3 ripe tomatoes
3 small Lebanese (short) cucumbers
2 large red onions
2 green bell peppers
⅔ cup (115 g) black olives
3½ oz (100 g) pickled mild or hot chile peppers
⅓ cup (80 ml) olive oil
2 tablespoons red wine vinegar
salt and freshly ground black pepper, to taste
10 oz (300 g) feta
1 teaspoon dried oregano, or 2 teaspoons fresh oregano leaves

Makes 4 servings

This popular salad has many variations and can even include rice-stuffed vine leaves and anchovies. Interestingly, it does not traditionally include lettuce.

1 Cut the tomatoes into wedges. Thickly slice the cucumbers in rounds. Slice the onions, but not too thinly. Cut the bell peppers into strips.
2 Place all the vegetables in a salad bowl. Top with the olives and pickled chile peppers.
3 To make the vinaigrette, whisk 3 tablespoons of the olive oil and all the vinegar until combined; add salt and pepper to taste. Drizzle over the salad.
4 Cut the feta into thick cubes or crumble coarsely, then add to the salad. Sprinkle with the oregano, drizzle with the remaining olive oil and serve.

Potato Salad

- 1½ lb (1 kg) potatoes, skin left on, cut into same-sized chunks
- 1 tablespoon cider vinegar
- 1 teaspoon sugar
- 1 small celery stalk, chopped
- 1 small red onion, chopped
- ¼ cup (45 g) chopped stuffed olives
- ½ teaspoon salt
- ½ teaspoon celery seeds
- ¾ cup (185 g) Classic Mayonnaise (page 29) or salad dressing
- 2 hard-boiled eggs, peeled and chopped

Makes 4 servings

What would a picnic or barbecue be without this stalwart standby adding its creamy goodness? Shun the deli version and make your own. Boiling or "waxy" potatoes, such as new potatoes, are ideal for potato salads as they hold their texture when cooked.

1. Put the potatoes in a large saucepan with enough water to cover. Bring to a boil over high heat and boil until the potatoes are tender, 20 to 30 minutes. Drain the potatoes and remove the peels. When the potatoes are cool enough to handle, cut into large dice and place in a bowl.
2. Drizzle the vinegar over the potatoes, then sprinkle with the sugar. Add the celery, onion, olives, salt and celery seed. Add the mayonnaise and eggs and fold gently until well combined. Cover and refrigerate for at least 1 hour before serving.

Thai Beef Salad

- 1 lb (500 g) rump steak
- ½ cup (125 ml) low-sodium soy sauce
- 2 cloves garlic, crushed
- 3 oz (100 ml) lime juice
- 1 lb (500 g) broccoli florets
- 4 tablespoons fresh mint leaves
- 4 tablespoons fresh basil leaves
- 3 tablespoons fresh coriander leaves
- 1 small cucumber, halved lengthwise and sliced
- 2 red chile peppers, thinly sliced
- 2 teaspoons soft brown sugar

Makes 4 servings

A salad with substance that even the men enjoy! Drenched with flavor, beautiful beef makes a meal of this fresh and zingy salad. Adjust the chile pepper heat to suit your taste.

1. In a large nonreactive bowl, combine the steak, ¼ cup (60 ml) of the soy sauce, the garlic and 2 tablespoons of the lime juice. Toss to coat, then leave to marinate for 10 minutes.
2. Preheat the broiler to high. Cook the steak for 2 minutes on each side, then set aside to rest.
3. Steam or microwave the broccoli until tender-crisp. Leave to cool for 10 minutes, then place in a large bowl with the mint, basil and coriander. Add the cucumber slices.
4. Slice the steak and add to the salad. Mix together the chile peppers, sugar, remaining soy sauce and remaining lime juice. Stir gently through the salad and serve.

Egg Salad

4 hard-boiled eggs, peeled and chopped
¼ cup (55 g) chopped green olives
¼ cup (60 g) Classic Mayonnaise (page 29) or salad dressing

Makes 4 servings

Dark pumpernickel or a flavorful rye bread sets off the creamy texture and taste of this old favorite—always infinitely better when you make it yourself with the ingredients you like best.

In a bowl, combine all the ingredients; gently fold until they are all well blended.

Pasta Salad

8 oz (250 g) pasta, such as fusilli, farfalle or penne
1 red bell pepper, cut into thin strips
1 yellow bell pepper, cut into thin strips
2 tablespoons olive oil
2 tablespoons red wine vinegar
½ teaspoon salt
¼ teaspoon freshly ground black pepper
2 tablespoons finely chopped fresh parsley
2 tablespoons finely chopped fresh basil
2 tablespoons drained capers
2 cloves garlic, finely chopped
1 small red onion, diced
1 cup (200 g) peeled, seeded and chopped tomatoes

Makes 4 servings

This salad uses bell peppers for a splash of color, but this basic pasta salad is also a good place to use whatever vegetables are in season—just blanch or sauté them before tossing them through the pasta. Again, fresh is definitely best!

1. Cook the pasta according to the package directions. Drain and place in a large serving bowl.
2. Add the remaining ingredients and toss until well combined.
3. Cover and leave to stand at room temperature for 30 minutes for the flavors to develop. Toss gently again before serving.

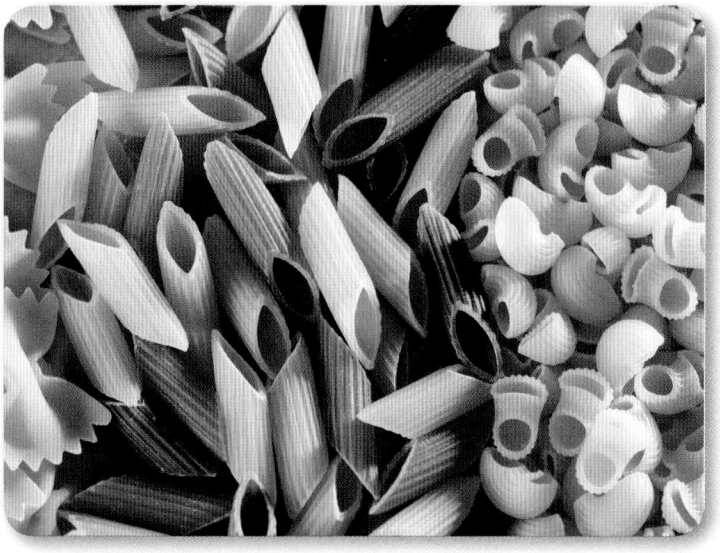

Caesar Salad

2 small romaine lettuces
4 large iceberg lettuce leaves
2 oz (50 g) block of Parmesan cheese
2 slices sourdough bread, crusts removed
2 tablespoons olive oil

ANCHOVY DRESSING
4 anchovy fillets
1 clove garlic, roughly chopped
3 oz (100 ml) olive oil
1 very fresh large egg yolk
2 tablespoons lemon juice
2 tablespoons Dijon mustard
1 tablespoon Worcestershire sauce
salt and freshly ground black pepper, to taste

Makes 4 servings

In 1924 in Tijuana, Mexico, Caesar Cardini first mixed romaine lettuce, Parmesan cheese and croutons, and dressed it with a mixture of garlic, lemon juice, egg, olive oil and Worcestershire sauce. People have been enjoying it ever since. You can pay good money for a rather ordinary caesar salad in a cafe or restaurant; naturally, it will never be as good as the one you make at home!

1 Cut the romaine and iceberg lettuce leaves into bite-sized pieces. Using a vegetable peeler or cheese grater, shave the Parmesan cheese into thin slivers.
2 To make the anchovy dressing, place the anchovy fillets and garlic in a bowl and mash to a paste. Whisk in the olive oil, egg yolk, lemon juice, mustard and Worcestershire sauce. Season with salt and pepper.
3 To make the croutons, cut the bread into small cubes. In a large nonstick frying pan or skillet, heat the olive oil over medium heat. Add the bread cubes and cook until golden brown on all sides, taking care they do not burn. Set aside and keep warm.
4 Arrange the lettuce leaves and shaved Parmesan cheese on individual serving plates. Drizzle the dressing over the salad, sprinkle with the croutons and serve.

Creamy Chicken Salad

2 cups (500 g) Classic Mayonnaise (page 29)
2 celery stalks, chopped
1 tablespoon mustard
1¼ teaspoons poppy seeds
½ teaspoon salt
4 cooked skinless, boneless chicken breasts, cubed
chopped pecans, to serve

Makes about 10 servings

Serve this old favorite on a bed of lettuce, with fruit, or as a filling for sandwiches. It's especially exquisite if you use homemade mayonnaise.

1 In a large bowl, combine the mayonnaise, celery, mustard, poppy seeds and salt. Stir until well blended.
2 Add the cooked chicken and gently fold to coat. Cover and place in the refrigerator for 3 to 4 hours, until the salad is chilled. Sprinkle with pecans before serving.

Curried Chicken Salad

½ cup (125 g) Classic Mayonnaise (page 29)
½ cup (140 g) chutney
1–3 tablespoons curry powder, to taste
2 cooked skinless, boneless chicken breasts, cubed

Makes about 6 servings

A piquant filling for pita bread, this salad is also sensational served with tropical fruit or cooked rice.

1 In a large bowl, combine the mayonnaise, chutney and curry powder. Stir until well blended.
2 Add the cooked chicken and gently fold to coat. Cover and place in the refrigerator for 3 to 4 hours, until the salad is chilled and the flavors have developed.

Turkey Salad

1 cup (150 g) chopped cooked turkey
¼ cup (60 g) Classic Mayonnaise (page 29)
1 small celery stalk, finely chopped
1 tablespoon chili sauce

Makes 4 servings

A great way to use up leftover Christmas turkey, this recipe gives you wonderful sandwiches for next to nothing. Serve the salad on whole wheat rolls with lettuce or salad leaves.

In a bowl, combine all the ingredients; gently fold until they are all well blended.

Tuna Salad

¼ cup (60 g) plus 1 tablespoon Classic Mayonnaise (page 29)
3 tablespoons finely chopped red onion
3 tablespoons sweet pickle relish
2 tablespoons chopped celery
2 tablespoons lemon juice
1 tablespoon drained capers
1 tablespoon finely chopped fresh dill
¼ teaspoon salt
2 cans (6½ oz/185 g each) tuna, drained

Makes 4 servings

Not your average tuna salad, this version is made special with capers, red onion and dill. It's much better than any you'll find at the deli.

1 In a bowl, combine the mayonnaise, onion, relish, celery, lemon juice, capers, dill and salt. Stir until the dressing is well blended and smooth.
2 Add the tuna and gently fold until well combined.

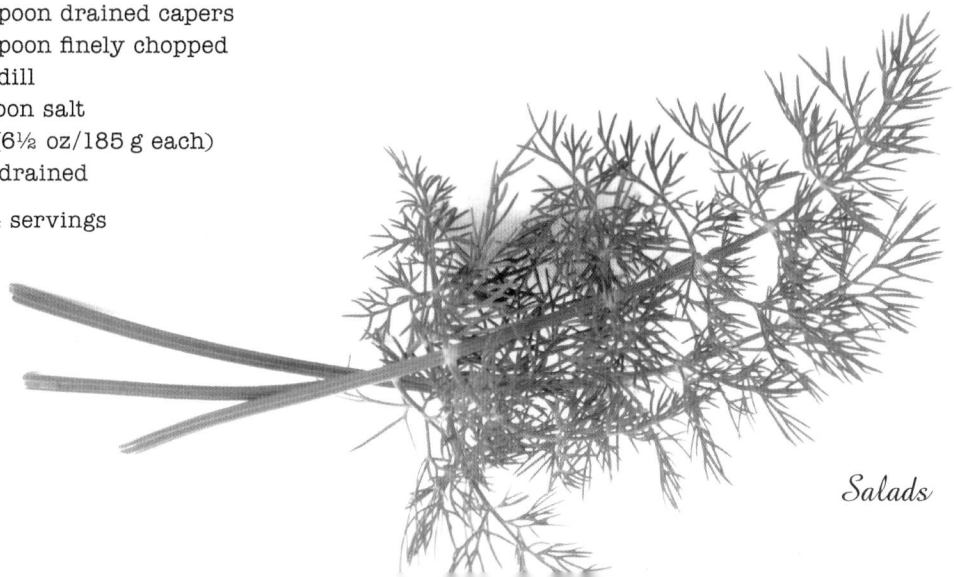

Cobb Salad

1 large shallot, minced
1 tablespoon Dijon mustard
1 tablespoon red wine vinegar
3 tablespoons olive oil
1 medium head romaine lettuce, cut into 2-inch-long (5 cm) pieces
2 hard-cooked eggs, peeled and coarsely chopped
½ cup Roasted Bell Peppers in Oil (page 73) or bottled red bell peppers, drained and cut into 2-inch-long (5 cm) strips
3 plum tomatoes, cut lengthwise into 8 wedges
1 peeled, pitted and sliced avocado
2 cups cooked chicken, cubed
24 niçoise olives
½ cup (60 g) crisp-cooked, crumbled bacon
½ cup (60 g) crumbled blue cheese

Makes 4 servings

Created at Hollywood's famed Brown Derby restaurant in 1936 by the owner, Robert Cobb, this noteworthy salad always features cooked chicken or turkey, bacon, eggs, avocado, and tomato in an eyepleasing arrangement. Your own will be less expensive than any restaurant version.

1 In a large bowl, combine the shallot, mustard, vinegar and oil. Whisk until the dressing is well blended. Pour half of the dressing into a small bowl and set aside.
2 Add the romaine lettuce to the bowl and toss to coat with the remaining dressing. Divide the lettuce equally among four individual serving plates.
3 Arrange the eggs, bell pepper strips, tomatoes, avocado slices, chicken, and olives, divided equally, on top of the lettuce on each plate. Drizzle some of the reserved dressing over each salad and sprinkle with ⅛ cup of the bacon and ⅛ cup of the blue cheese.

Shrimp Salad

¼ cup (60 g) Classic Mayonnaise (page 29)
¼ cup finely chopped celery
2 tablespoons lemon juice
2 tablespoons finely chopped fresh tarragon
¼ teaspoon salt
pinch of ground cayenne pepper
1 lb (500 g) peeled cooked shrimp

Makes 4 servings

This luscious salad is lovely served on a bed of mixed greens, as a filling for soft rolls or with flatbreads. Buy the freshest shrimp, use your own mayonnaise and you'll have restaurant quality in your own kitchen for a fraction of the price.

1 In a bowl, combine the mayonnaise, celery, lemon juice, tarragon, salt and cayenne pepper. Stir until well blended and smooth.
2 Add the shrimp and gently fold until well combined.

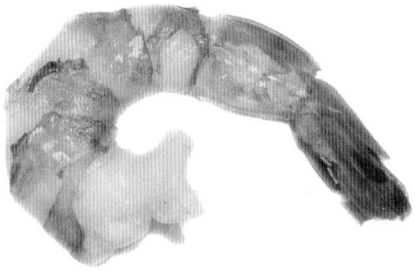

Tuscan-Style Three-Bean Salad

10 oz (300 g) green beans, trimmed and halved
14 oz (400 g) can red kidney beans, rinsed and drained
14 oz (400 g) can cannellini or butterbeans, rinsed and drained
1 small red onion, finely chopped
2 large tomatoes, seeded and chopped
3 tablespoons chopped fresh flat-leaf parsley
3 tablespoons olive oil
2 tablespoons lemon juice
1 clove garlic, crushed
salt and freshly ground black pepper

Makes 4 servings

This classic salad uses cannellini beans, red kidney beans and fresh green beans, but depending on what you have in your pantry, combinations of different beans can be used. Another great stand-by for when the cupboards run bare.

1 Half-fill a saucepan with water and bring to a boil. Add the green beans and cook until just tender, 5 to 7 minutes. Drain, rinse with cold water and drain again. Place in a serving bowl.
2 Add the canned beans, onion, tomatoes and parsley.
3 Mix together the olive oil, lemon juice and garlic, season with salt and pepper, then mix through the salad.
4 Serve immediately, or cover and refrigerate until required.

Salade Niçoise

2 carrots, peeled
½ lb (250 g) green beans, trimmed
1 lb (500 g) small red new potatoes
1 large shallot, finely chopped
1 tablespoon Dijon mustard
1 tablespoon drained capers
1 tablespoon red wine vinegar
¼ cup (60 ml) olive oil
1 romaine lettuce, washed and cut 2 inches (5 cm) thick
2 hard-boiled eggs, peeled and halved lengthwise
½ cup Roasted Red Bell Peppers in Oil (page 73) or bottled red bell peppers, drained and cut into long strips
3 Italian plum tomatoes, cut lengthwise into 8 wedges
24 niçoise olives
6½ oz (185 g) can oil-packed tuna, drained

Makes 4 servings

A gorgeous and appetizing array of tuna, eggs and vegetables, this great classic from the south of France is a picture-perfect composed salad. Delight your family and friends with your own version—fresh and custom-made. No restaurant can match that or your costs.

1 Parboil the carrots and slice thinly. Blanch the beans and cut in half, crosswise. Boil the new potatoes and slice thinly.
2 In a large bowl, combine the shallot, mustard, capers, vinegar and oil. Whisk until well blended, then pour half the dressing into a small bowl and set aside.
3 Add the lettuce to the large bowl and toss to coat with the dressing. Divide the lettuce among four serving plates.
4 Arrange the egg halves, bell pepper strips, tomatoes, carrots, beans, potatoes, olives and tuna over the lettuce on each plate. Drizzle some of the reserved dressing over each salad, or serve it on the side.

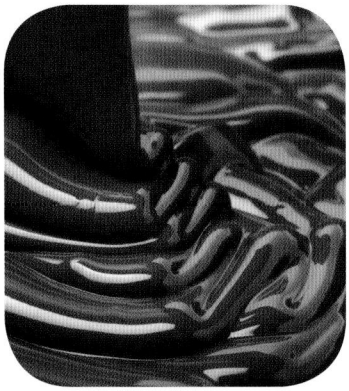

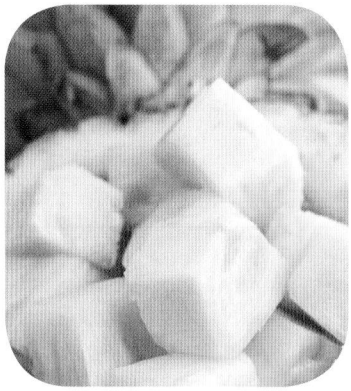

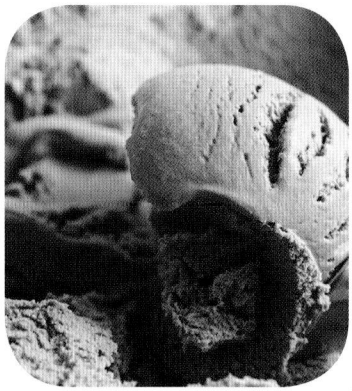

Candy

Gumdrops ❖ Butterscotch ❖ Lollipops ❖ Caramels ❖ Fudge ❖ Pastel Mint Patties ❖ Pralines ❖ Peanut Brittle ❖ Toffee Bars ❖ Rocky Road ❖ Peanut Butter Cups ❖ Marshmallows ❖ Candied Citrus Peels

Custards, Mousses and Puddings

Chocolate Pudding ❖ Panna Cotta ❖ Rice Pudding ❖ Bread and Butter Pudding ❖ Crème Brûlée ❖ Crème Caramel ❖ Chocolate Mousse ❖ Mango Mousse

Fruit Desserts

Brandied Peaches ❖ Dried Fruit Compote ❖ Wine Poached Pears with Strawberries ❖ Fruit Salad ❖ Chocolate-Dipped Strawberries

Ice Cream

French Vanilla Ice Cream ❖ Blueberry Ice Cream ❖ Peach Ice Cream ❖ Strawberry Ice Cream ❖ Honey Banana Ice Cream ❖ Coconut-Pineapple Ice Cream ❖ Rocky Road Ice Cream ❖ Rich Chocolate Ice Cream ❖ Chocolate Chocolate Chip Ice Cream ❖ Mint Chocolate Chip Ice Cream ❖ Peppermint Ice Cream ❖ Butter Pecan Ice Cream ❖ Ice Cream Cake

Frozen Yogurt

Lemon Frozen Yogurt ❖ Strawberry Frozen Yogurt ❖ Passion Fruit Frozen Yogurt

Ices, Granitas, Sherbets and Sorbets

Orange Ice ❖ Blood-Orange Champagne Granita ❖ Cappuccino Granita ❖ Kiwi Granita ❖ Peach Granita ❖ Lime Sherbet ❖ Strawberry Milk Sherbet ❖ Cassis Sorbet ❖ Citrus Sorbet ❖ Honeydew Sorbet ❖ Lemon Sorbet ❖ Raspberry Sorbet ❖ Strawberry Sorbet

Frozen Pops

Frozen Fruit Pops ❖ Fruity Frozen Yogurt Pops ❖ Chocolate Pops ❖ Strawberry Pops ❖ Tropical Pops ❖ Chocolate-Nut Frozen Bananas

Easy-to-Make Sweet Treats

Sometimes we all crave a little sweetness, so this chapter provides a collection of recipes for an array of sweet treats—candy, custards, fruity delights, irresistible ice creams, frozen yogurts and sorbets—that will more than satisfy that yearning.

What all these recipes have in common is that they are made with all-natural ingredients, with none of the fillers, stabilizers or artificial sweeteners that often give store-bought sweets that slightly artificial taste. Treats such as these are so astonishingly good when you make them yourself that you may never bother buying a package of candy or a supermarket sweet again. As an added bonus, treats you make at home won't cost nearly as much as store-bought alternatives.

Some people might be daunted by the idea of making their own candy, but our grandparents thought nothing of it, and it's really no more difficult than making cookies—sometimes even easier. And whether you're making marshmallows, lollipops or peanut brittle, they really do taste so much better than the wrapped products that now abound on supermarket shelves.

On the following pages you'll find hot and cold fruit desserts, along with custards and puddings. And when summer comes, you'll have a full assortment of ice creams, frozen yogurts, ices, granitas, sorbets and sherbets that you can try—topped perhaps with one of the dessert sauces from Chapter 1.

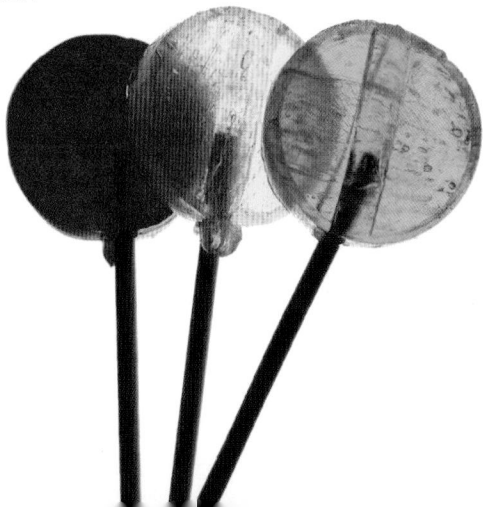

Candy

Gumdrops

3 envelopes (7 g each) powdered gelatin
1½ cups (330 g) sugar, plus extra, for coating
¼–½ teaspoon flavoring extract of your choice
2 food colorings of your choice

Makes about 1 lb (450 g)

These chewy goodies can be tailored to the occasion: For Christmas, use red and green food coloring and peppermint extract; for spring, try yellow and orange coloring and lemon or orange extract. Children will want to help make them.

1 Sprinkle the gelatin over ½ cup (125 ml) water and let stand for 5 minutes.
2 In a small saucepan, combine the sugar and ¾ cup (185 ml) water over medium heat. Bring the mixture to a boil, stirring constantly. Add the gelatin mixture, reduce the heat and simmer, stirring constantly, for 5 minutes. Remove from the heat and stir in the flavoring extract.
3 Divide the mixture between two small bowls. Add 2 to 4 drops of the desired color into each bowl and stir until the color is even.
4 Lightly grease two 8 x 4 x 2-inch loaf pans. Pour one colored gumdrop mixture into one loaf pan and the other mixture into the other pan. Chill until firm, about 3 hours.
5 Lightly coat a work surface with extra sugar and fill a small saucer with some more sugar. Cover a baking sheet with parchment paper. Using a sharp knife, loosen the edges of the gumdrop mixture from the side of the tins, then turn out onto the sugared surface. Cut each portion into ½-inch cubes, then roll each cube in the sugar in the saucer until completely coated.
6 Place the gumdrops on the baking sheet and leave at room temperature, uncovered, until they are dry on all sides, 3 to 4 hours; turn the gumdrops every hour to allow each side to dry. Cover with plastic wrap and store in the refrigerator.

Checking the candy thermometer

The one crucial item you need for making candy is a good-quality candy thermometer, which you should test before each use. To do this, in a saucepan bring some water to a boil and dip the thermometer in: It should read 212°F. Adjust your recipe temperature up or down based on your test.

Butterscotch

melted butter, for brushing
2½ cups (575 g) firmly packed light brown sugar
½ cup (110 g) light corn syrup or glucose syrup (optional)
¼ cup (90 g) honey
½ teaspoon salt
1 cup (250 g) butter, cut into cubes
½ teaspoon rum extract

Makes about 1½ pounds (650 g)

Butterscotch is very inexpensive to make. Rich and deliciously buttery, this recipe calls for a little rum extract to create its distinctive flavor.

1 Brush a 15 x 10 x 1-inch baking pan with the melted butter.
2 In a heavy saucepan, combine the sugar, syrup (if using) and ¾ cup (185 ml) water over medium heat. Cover and bring to a boil, without stirring. Remove the lid and continue to cook until a candy thermometer reads 270°F (soft-crack stage).
3 Add the honey, salt and butter cubes. Cook, stirring constantly, until the mixture reaches 300°F (hard-crack stage). Remove from the heat and stir in the rum extract.
4 Pour the butterscotch into the baking pan without scraping it; do not spread. Allow to cool until almost set, 1 to 2 minutes. Using a sharp knife, score the butterscotch into 1-inch squares and leave to cool completely.
5 Break the butterscotch squares along the scored lines. Store in an airtight container.

Lollipops

12 lollipop sticks
1 cup (220 g) sugar
2 tablespoons light corn syrup or glucose syrup
4–8 drops food coloring of your choice
2–3 drops flavoring oil of your choice

Makes 12 lollipops

Few goodies are as evocative of childhood as these brightly colored sweets on a stick. Flavoring oils can be purchased at health food stores—the flavor is more intense than flavor extracts, and as they are not alcohol-based, the flavor won't evaporate either.

1 Line a large baking sheet with foil. Arrange the lollipop sticks on the sheet, spacing them 4 inches apart.
2 In a heavy saucepan, combine the sugar, syrup and ½ cup (125 ml) water over medium heat. Cook, stirring, until the sugar has dissolved. Cover the saucepan, increase the heat to high and boil the mixture for 1 minute to wash down any sugar crystals. Remove the lid and boil the syrup until it registers 310°F on a candy thermometer. Immediately remove the saucepan from the heat and set it on a wire rack.
3 Let the syrup cool for 5 minutes, then add the food coloring and flavoring oil, stirring until the color is even.
4 Spoon the colored syrup over the top end of each lollipop stick, making a puddle about 2 to 3 inches in diameter. Leave the lollipops until they are completely cool and hardened. Wrap each lollipop in plastic wrap or cellophane and secure the wrapping.

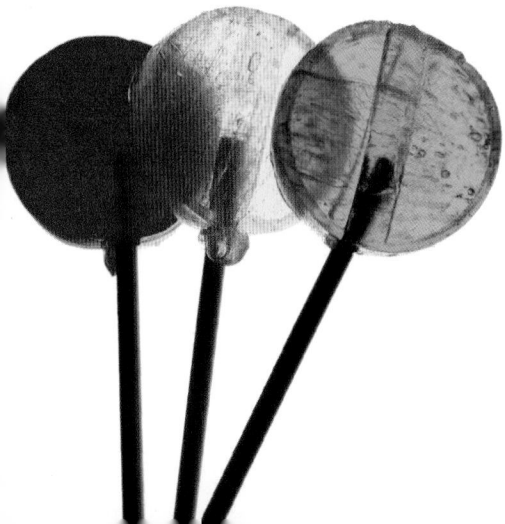

Caramels

melted butter, for brushing
1 cup (220 g) sugar
1 cup (220 g) dark corn syrup or glucose syrup (optional)
1 cup (250 g) butter
14 oz (400 ml) can sweetened condensed milk
1 teaspoon vanilla extract

Makes 64 pieces

Chewy, gooey and irresistible, homemade caramels make wonderful treats for Christmas stockings or as little gifts.

1 Line an 8-inch square baking pan with foil. Grease the foil with butter.
2 In a heavy saucepan, combine the sugar, syrup (if using) and butter over medium heat. Bring to a boil, stirring constantly, then reduce the heat slightly and boil slowly for 4 minutes without stirring.
3 Remove from the heat and stir in the condensed milk. Place back over medium-low heat and cook until a candy thermometer reads 238°F (soft-ball stage), stirring constantly. Remove from the heat and stir in the vanilla.
4 Pour the mixture into the baking pan and leave until cool. Remove from the pan and cut into 1-inch squares. Wrap each caramel individually in parchment paper, cellophane or plastic wrap, twisting the ends to seal.

Fudge

3⅓ cups (750 g) sugar
1 cup (185 g) firmly packed dark brown sugar
1 cup (250 g) butter
12 oz (400 ml) can evaporated milk
2 cups (350 g) semi-sweet chocolate chips
two 7 oz (200 g) milk chocolate bars, broken into pieces
⅓ cup (50 g) chopped semi-sweet cooking chocolate
1 teaspoon vanilla extract
2 cups (240 g) chopped pecans

Makes about 5½ lb (2 kg)

Not one but three kinds of chocolate make this a deep, rich, chocolatey dream of a fudge.

1 Grease a 15 x 10 x 1-inch baking pan.
2 In a large saucepan, combine the sugars, the butter and evaporated milk over medium heat. Cook, stirring, until the sugar has completely dissolved. Increase the heat to high and bring to a boil, then boil for 5 minutes, stirring constantly.
3 Remove from the heat. Add all the chocolate, place back over low heat and stir until melted. Fold in the vanilla and pecans until well blended.
4 Pour the mixture into the baking pan, spreading it evenly, then refrigerate until firm. Using a sharp knife, cut the cooled fudge into squares.

Pastel Mint Patties

3 tablespoons butter, softened
⅓ cup (75 g) light corn syrup or glucose syrup (optional)
½–1 teaspoon peppermint extract
4 cups (500 g) confectioners' sugar
2 food colorings of your choice
1 cup (220 g) sugar, approximately

Makes about 7½ dozen

Pretty confections perfect for a wedding or baby shower.

1. In a small bowl, combine the butter and syrup (if using). Add the peppermint extract and half the confectioners' sugar and beat until well blended. Add another 1 cup (125 g) confectioners' sugar and beat well.
2. Lightly coat a work surface with the remaining confectioners' sugar. Turn the mixture out onto the surface and knead until the confectioners' sugar is completely absorbed and the mixture is smooth.
3. Divide the mixture into three portions. Set aside one portion to remain white; tint the remaining portions by adding 1 to 2 drops of food coloring and kneading until each portion is the desired color.
4. Line a baking sheet with parchment paper. Place the sugar in a shallow bowl or saucer. Pinch off a walnut-sized piece of the peppermint mixture. Using your hands, roll it into a ball, then roll it in the sugar. Place on the baking sheet and flatten into a round, using a fork. Repeat with the remaining peppermint mixture. Leave to stand, uncovered, at room temperature for 1 day, then store in an airtight container.

Pralines

melted butter, for brushing
1 cup (220 g) sugar
1 cup (230 g) firmly packed brown sugar
1 cup (250 ml) milk
8 large Marshmallows (page 210)
2 cups (240 g) roughly chopped pecans
2 tablespoons butter
½ teaspoon vanilla extract
pinch of ground cinnamon

Makes about 2 dozen

For the best-tasting pralines, select the freshest and finest-quality pecans you can find. Homemade pralines are an easy, inexpensive treat to share with friends.

1. Lightly brush two baking sheets with melted butter.
2. In a heavy saucepan, combine the sugars, the milk and marshmallows over low heat. Cook, stirring constantly, until the marshmallows are completely melted. Increase the heat to medium and cook, stirring occasionally, until a candy thermometer reads 234°F to 240°F (soft-ball stage). Without stirring or scraping, pour the hot mixture into a second heavy saucepan. Add the pecans, butter, vanilla and cinnamon. Stir rapidly until the mixture is thickened and creamy, about 3 minutes.
3. Using a tablespoon, drop the mixture onto the baking sheets, placing the pralines about 1 inch apart. Flatten them slightly and leave until set. Store in an airtight container.

Peanut Brittle

2¾ cups (600 g) sugar
3 tablespoons unsalted butter
1½ cups (250 g) lightly salted peanuts

Makes about 45 pieces

Crunchy with peanuts, melt-in-your-mouth delicious, this is a classic candy that the whole family can help to make and package as gifts. It's not nearly as much fun to buy it.

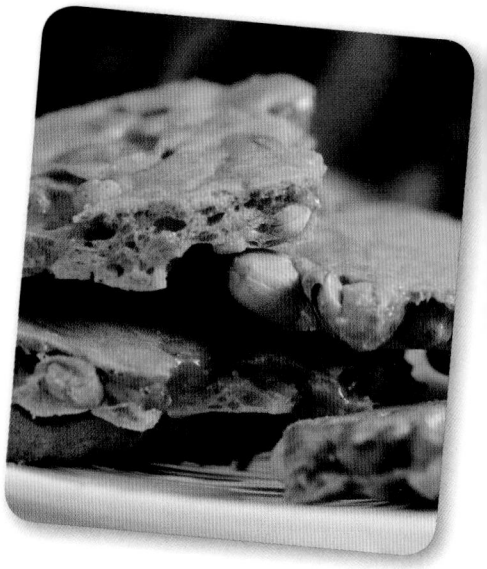

1 Grease a 9 x 13-inch baking pan and line with foil.
2 In a large, heavy saucepan, combine the sugar, butter and ⅔ cup (170 ml) water over medium heat. Mix with a wooden spoon, then simmer, stirring occasionally, until the mixture becomes a golden-brown syrup, about 25 minutes. Once the darkened mixture begins to bubble, remove the saucepan to a cool surface.
3 Add the peanuts to the syrup and stir until evenly distributed. Pour the mixture into the baking pan, spreading it evenly and ensuring that the peanuts are distributed equally.
4 Leave to cool and set completely, about 30 minutes.
5 Using a knife handle, break the peanut brittle into bite-sized pieces. Store in an airtight container in a cool, dry place for up to 1 month.

Toffee Bars

melted butter, for brushing
1¾ cups (435 g) butter, softened
2 cups (440 g) sugar
1 tablespoon light corn syrup or glucose syrup (optional)
1 cup (120 g) chopped pecans
¼ teaspoon salt
1 lb (450 g) milk chocolate

Makes about 2¼ lb (1 kg)

A crunchy confection that's sure to delight.

1 Brush a 15 x 10 x 1-inch baking pan with some melted butter.
2 In a heavy saucepan, melt the softened butter over medium heat. Add the sugar and syrup (if using) and stir until a candy thermometer reads 295°F (soft-crack stage). Remove from the heat, then stir in the pecans and salt.
3 Quickly pour the toffee mixture into the baking pan. Leave to stand for 5 minutes. Using a sharp knife, score the top of the toffee into bars, then leave at room temperature until cool. Break or cut the toffee into bars along the score lines.
4 Line one or two baking sheets with parchment paper. In a heavy saucepan over low heat, melt the milk chocolate, stirring often.
5 Dip each toffee bar into the chocolate until it is completely coated, then place on the baking sheets. Leave to stand at room temperature until the chocolate has set.

Rocky Road

14 oz (400 g) chocolate chips or chocolate block
2 cups (320 g) dry-roasted peanuts, or 9 oz (250 g) broken sweet cookies
9 oz (250 g) package of marshmallows, roughly chopped
3½ oz (100 g) package of glace cherries, chopped

Makes 40 squares

Chocolate and cherries and light-as-air marshmallows molten together appeal to the inner child in us all.

1 Grease a 9 x 13-inch baking sheet or sheet-cake pan and line it with parchment paper.
2 In the top of a double boiler, melt the chocolate over low heat, stirring occasionally until smooth. Transfer to a large bowl and stir in the remaining ingredients, combining well and breaking up any big bits of cookie, if using.
3 Pour into the baking sheet and chill until firm. Cut into squares and store in an airtight container.

Peanut Butter Cups

1 milk or dark chocolate candy bar (7 ounces/200g), broken into pieces
¼ cup (60 g) butter
1 tablespoon shortening
¼ cup (60 g) creamy Peanut Butter (page 33)

Makes 1 dozen cups

This is a tantalizing combination of chocolate and peanut butter.

1 Line the cups in a miniature muffin pan with paper or foil baking cups.
2 In a heavy saucepan over low heat or in a microwave-safe bowl following the manufacturer's directions, combine the chocolate, butter and shortening. Stir until the mixture is smooth.
3 In a second heavy saucepan over low heat or in a microwavesafe bowl following the manufacturer's directions, heat the peanut butter until it has melted.
4 Pour 1 tablespoon of the chocolate into each of the prepared cups. Drop 1 tablespoon of peanut butter onto the chocolate in each cup. Pour the remaining chocolate, divided equally, into the cups, covering the peanut butter.
5 Place the muffin pan in the refrigerator until the cups are set, about 30 minutes. Store in an airtight container in the refrigerator.

Marshmallows

¼ cup (30 g) confectioners' sugar
¼ cup (30 g) cornstarch
1½ tablespoons powdered gelatin
½ cup (110 g) sugar
⅔ cup (150 g) light corn syrup or glucose syrup (optional)

Makes about 36 marshmallows

An electric stand mixer makes these marshmallows quick and easy to whip up. They cost less than the commercial ones and children will love the process.

1 Line a 13 x 9 x 2-inch baking pan with parchment paper. In a small sieve, combine 1 tablespoon of the confectioners' sugar and 1 tablespoon of the cornstarch and sift the mixture over the baking pan.
2 Pour ⅓ cup (80 ml) water into a heatproof bowl. Sprinkle the gelatin over and let stand for 5 minutes.
3 Place the bowl in a large saucepan of simmering water and stir until the gelatin has dissolved. Add the sugar and stir until the sugar has dissolved. Remove the bowl from the water and add the syrup (if using). Using an electric mixer, beat until the mixture is creamy and thick, 10 to 15 minutes. Leave to cool.
4 Using a wet spatula, spread the mixture into the baking pan, smoothing the top. Leave to cool and set, about 20 minutes.
5 Carefully lift the marshmallow mixture onto a cutting board. Put another 1 tablespoon of the remaining confectioners' sugar and cornstarch in the sieve and lightly dust over the top. Using a sharp knife, cut the marshmallow into small squares.
6 Combine the remaining confectioners' sugar and cornstarch in a cup. Dip each marshmallow square into the mixture until completely coated. Store in an airtight container in a cool, dry place for 1 to 2 weeks.

If you run out of corn syrup

If a recipe calls for 1 cup (220 g) light corn syrup and you don't have any on hand, you can use glucose syrup. Alternatively, combine 1 cup (220 g) sugar and an additional ¼ cup (60 ml) of the liquid used in the recipe and stir until blended.

Candied Citrus Peels

3 firm ripe lemons or oranges
¼ cup (55 g) sugar

Makes about 1 cup

Dip these zesty citrus strips in chocolate for an easy confection, or use them as exquisite decorations on cakes, ice cream and other desserts.

1 Using a swivel-bladed vegetable peeler, remove the peel from the citrus fruit, avoiding the bitter white pith. Using a sharp knife, cut the peel into strips. For decorations, cut it into matchstick-thin strips; for dipping in chocolate, cut it into larger strips.
2 Put the citrus strips in a small saucepan and add enough cold water to cover. Bring to a boil over high heat, then immediately drain the strips and rinse under cold running water.
3 Return the strips to the saucepan. Add the sugar and ½ cup (125 ml) water. Over medium heat, cook the mixture until the liquid has evaporated and the strips are bright and shiny.
4 Spread a sheet of foil over a work surface. Transfer the candied peel to the foil to cool, keeping the strips separate. Refrigerate in an airtight container for up to 6 months.

Custards, Mousses and Puddings

Chocolate Pudding

¾ cup (165 g) sugar
1½ tablespoons cornstarch
pinch of salt
2 cups (500 ml) milk
⅓ cup (50 g) chopped semi-sweet chocolate
1 egg
2 tablespoons butter
1 teaspoon vanilla extract

Makes 4 to 6 servings

Like a grilled cheese sandwich, chocolate pudding is pure comfort food. You can make it from a package or take a few more minutes and make a much better one from scratch.

1 In a saucepan, combine the sugar, cornstarch and salt. Add the milk and stir until smooth. Add the chocolate and stir constantly over medium heat until the mixture boils and thickens. Reduce the heat and simmer, stirring constantly, for 2 minutes. Remove the saucepan from the heat.
2 Beat the egg in a bowl until foamy, using electric beaters. Gradually stir in about ½ cup (125 ml) of the hot milk mixture, then pour the egg mixture into the remaining hot milk mixture. Cook over low heat, stirring constantly, for 2 minutes longer.
3 Remove the saucepan from the heat and stir in the butter and vanilla. Immediately pour the pudding into a bowl or individual dessert dishes. Leave to cool to room temperature, then refrigerate.

Panna Cotta

2 cups (500 ml) milk
1 tablespoon powdered gelatin
⅓ cup (80 g) superfine sugar
3 oz (100 ml) whipping cream
1 strip orange zest
1 vanilla bean, split

RHUBARB AND STRAWBERRY COMPOTE
14 oz (400 g) rhubarb, trimmed and cut into 2 in (5 cm) lengths
juice of 1 orange
2 tablespoons superfine sugar
1 lb (450 g) ripe strawberries, hulled and sliced

Makes 4 servings

The traditional recipe for this "cooked cream," from the Piedmont region of Italy, is made with rich double cream. This lighter version, served with a pretty rhubarb and strawberry compote, is delightfully smooth and creamy yet much lower in fat. Prepare it the day before serving, if possible.

1 Pour 5 oz (150 ml) of the milk into a saucepan. Sprinkle the gelatin over and leave to stand for 5 minutes.
2 Stir in the sugar, then set the pan over low heat. Warm gently, without boiling, until the sugar and gelatin have completely dissolved, stirring frequently.
3 Remove the pan from the heat and add the remaining milk, the cream and orange zest. Scrape the seeds from the vanilla bean into the milk. Add the vanilla bean to the milk and leave to infuse for 10 minutes while preparing the compote.
4 In a saucepan, combine the rhubarb, orange juice and sugar. Bring just to a simmer, then cook gently until the rhubarb is tender but still holding its shape, 3 to 4 minutes. Spoon the rhubarb into a serving dish using a slotted spoon. Boil the juice remaining in the pan to reduce it slightly until syrupy. Pour the juice over the rhubarb and gently stir in the sliced strawberries. Leave to cool.
5 Strain the milk mixture through a fine sieve into a jug, then pour into four ⅔ cup (170 ml) molds, cups or ramekins. Allow to cool, then cover and chill for at least 3 hours, until set.
6 To serve, run the tip of a knife around the edge of each ramekin. Place an inverted serving plate over the top of each ramekin and turn them upside down, holding the two firmly together. Lift off the ramekin. Spoon some of the compote around the panna cotta and serve the remaining compote separately.

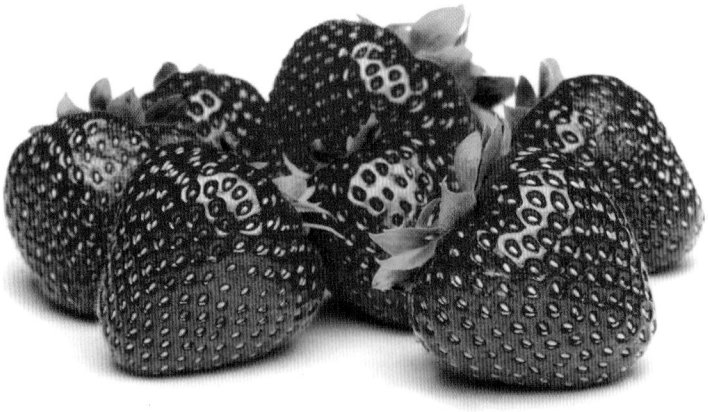

Rice Pudding

melted butter, for brushing
3½ cups (875 ml) milk
½ cup (100 g) long-grain white rice
⅓ cup (75 g) sugar
½ teaspoon salt (optional)
½ cup (60 g) raisins
1 teaspoon vanilla extract
ground cinnamon, for sprinkling (optional)

Makes about 6 servings

You can buy commercially made rice pudding, but it just isn't as beautifully textured and creamy as homemade. Rice pudding thickens on cooling, so if serving cold, stir in a little extra milk, or serve with summer berries.

1. Preheat the oven to 325°F. Brush a 6-cup (1.5 liter) baking dish with melted butter.
2. In a saucepan, combine the milk, rice, sugar and salt, if using. Bring to a boil over medium heat, stirring constantly. Pour into the baking dish, then cover and bake for 45 minutes, stirring every 15 minutes.
3. Stir in the raisins and the vanilla. Cover again and bake for 15 minutes longer. Remove from the oven and sprinkle with cinnamon, if desired. Serve warm or chilled.

Bread and Butter Pudding

2 cups (500 ml) milk
1¼ cups (310 ml) heavy cream
1 vanilla bean, split lengthwise
1 day-old light fruit loaf, cut into slices ½-inch (1 cm) thick
⅓ cup (90 g) unsalted butter, softened
⅓ cup (40 g) golden seedless raisins
6 egg yolks
½ cup (115 g) superfine sugar
1 tablespoon freshly grated nutmeg
⅓ cup (75 g) raw sugar or soft brown sugar

FOR THE SAUCE
1 cup (230 g) superfine sugar
6 egg yolks
1¼ cups (310 ml) dry cider

Makes 6 servings

The homely appeal of bread baked in custard is timeless. In this version, fruit loaf is used for extra flavor and a frothy cider sauce adds its own tang.

1. In a saucepan, gently heat the milk and cream with the vanilla bean until almost boiling. Remove from the heat, cover and leave to infuse for 30 minutes.
2. Meanwhile, spread each slice of bread liberally with butter and cut them in half diagonally. Overlap the slices attractively in a buttered, shallow, ovenproof dish, scattering raisins over the pieces as you go.
3. In a large bowl, whisk the egg yolks and superfine sugar until pale and creamy. Strain the infused milk and cream onto the egg mixture and whisk well. Pour evenly over the buttered fruit bread and leave to soak for 20 minutes.
4. Meanwhile, preheat the oven to 350°F. Sprinkle the nutmeg and raw sugar evenly over the pudding and set the dish in a roasting pan. Pour in enough boiling water to come halfway up the side of the baking dish. Bake until the custard is just set and the top is golden and crisp, about 45 minutes.
5. About 15 minutes before the pudding is due to come out of the oven, start making the sauce. Put the sugar and egg yolks in a heatproof bowl and place snugly over a pan of barely simmering water, making sure that the bottom of the bowl does not touch the water. Whisk until the mixture is pale and creamy and the sugar has dissolved. Still whisking, slowly pour in the cider and continue to whisk for 5 minutes, or until the mixture froths up to a creamy mousse. Whisk for another 5 to 10 minutes, or until the sauce is light and foamy.
6. Pour the sauce into a jug and serve with the hot pudding.

Crème Brûlée

3 cups (750 ml) milk
¾ cup (165 g) sugar
1 vanilla bean, split lengthwise
4 strips (each ½ x 3 inch/1 x 7.5 cm) orange zest
3 strips (each ½ x 2 inch/1 x 5 cm) lemon zest
3 strips (each ½ x 2 inch/1 x 5 cm) lime zest
¼ teaspoon salt
3 eggs, plus 3 egg yolks
¾ cup (165 g) firmly packed light or dark brown sugar

Makes 8 servings

Who can resist a smooth, rich and elegantly turned-out custard when it's hiding under a fine layer of brittle but gooey sweet caramel? You don't need to splash out on fancy restaurants to enjoy this creamy classic when it's simple enough to make at home.

1 Set eight ungreased ¾-cup (185 ml) ramekins on a folded dish towel in a large baking pan, spacing the ramekins well apart.
2 In a saucepan, combine the milk with ¼ cup (55 g) of the sugar, the vanilla bean, citrus zest strips and salt. Bring to a simmer over medium heat, then remove from the heat, cover and leave to infuse for 30 minutes.
3 Preheat the oven to 325°F. In a large bowl, whisk the eggs, egg yolks and remaining sugar until just blended. Set a large sieve over the bowl and pour the milk mixture through into the egg mixture. Whisk until the ingredients are blended.
4 Spoon the custard into the ramekins. Pour enough water into the baking pan to come halfway up the side of the ramekins. Bake, uncovered, until a knife inserted into the center of a custard comes out clean, about 45 minutes. Remove the ramekins from the baking pan to wire racks.
5 Preheat the broiler to high. Sprinkle 1½ teaspoons of the brown sugar over the top of each custard. Set the ramekins in the broiler 6 to 8 inches from the heat source and broil until the sugar melts, about 45 seconds.
6 Remove the ramekins to wire racks and allow to cool to room temperature. Serve at room temperature or slightly chilled, but do not refrigerate too long or the crust will begin to soften.

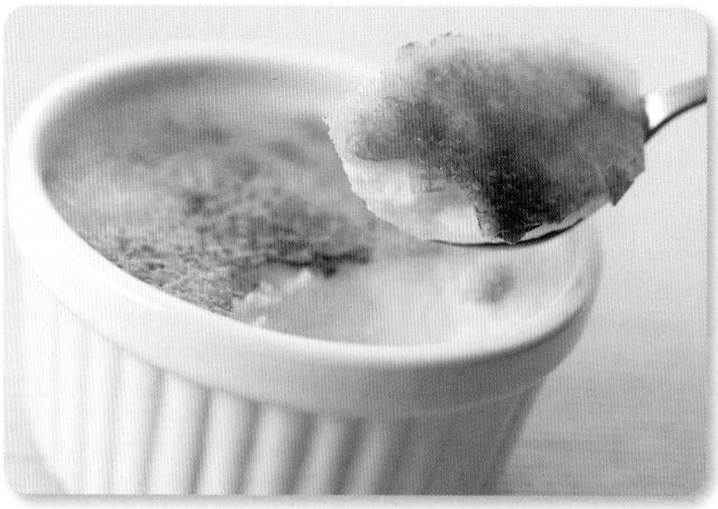

Crème Caramel

CARAMEL
½ cup (110 g) sugar
½ cup (125 ml) water

CUSTARD
3 cups (750 ml) milk
¾ cup (165 g) sugar
1 vanilla bean, split lengthwise
4 strips (each ½ x 3 inch/1 x 7.5 cm) orange zest
3 strips (each ½ x 2 inch/1 x 5 cm) lemon zest
3 strips (each ½ x 2 inch/1 x 5 cm) lime zest
¼ teaspoon salt
3 eggs, plus 3 egg yolks

Makes 8 servings

A close relative of the revered Crème Brûlée (opposite), the sauce of a crème caramel dribbles deliciously down the sides of the custard when the whole creation is inverted onto the plate. To make a lower-fat version, substitute 3 cups (750 ml) evaporated skim milk for the whole milk, 1½ cups (350 g) egg substitute (available from health food stores) for the whole eggs and yolks, and reduce the sugar in the custard to ⅔ cup (140 g).

1. To prepare the caramel, combine the sugar and water in a small saucepan over medium-high heat. Bring to a boil and continue to boil until the sugar turns amber in color, about 5 minutes.
2. Pour the caramel into eight ungreased ¾-cup (185 ml) ramekins. Tilt each ramekin so the caramel coats the bottom and about 1 inch of the sides. Place the ramekins on a folded dish towel in a baking pan that is large enough to hold them all without touching.
3. To make the custard, combine the milk in a saucepan with ¼ cup (55 g) of the sugar, the vanilla bean, citrus zest strips and salt. Bring to a simmer over medium heat, then remove from the heat, cover and leave to infuse for 30 minutes.
4. Preheat the oven to 325°F. In a large bowl, whisk the eggs, egg yolks and remaining sugar until just blended. Set a large sieve over the bowl and pour the milk mixture through into the egg mixture. Whisk until the ingredients are blended.
5. Spoon the custard into the caramel-coated ramekins. Pour enough water into the baking pan to come halfway up the side of the ramekins. Bake, uncovered, until a knife inserted into the center of a custard comes out clean, about 45 minutes.
6. Remove the ramekins to wire racks and allow the custards to cool to room temperature; refrigerate until ready to serve.
7. To serve, run a knife around the edge of the custards to loosen them, then invert the ramekins onto rimmed dessert plates or shallow dessert bowls. Allow the caramel to run down the custards and form a pool around them.

Tips for making custard

Although it is easy to make, custard requires a bit of cooking know-how. The main rule is don't overmix the eggs. More egg yolks make for a smoother texture, which in turn requires a slower cooking time; the container used for baking will determine the cooking time, so it's safest to stick to the one specified in the recipe. If you remember these simple principles you'll get great custard every time.

Chocolate Mousse

1½ cups (225 g) chopped semi-sweet chocolate
3 eggs, separated
¾ cup (185 ml) heavy cream
½ cup (110 g) sugar
1 teaspoon vanilla extract

Makes 8 servings

The ultimate mousse experience—and the finer the quality of chocolate you use, the more outstanding the final result. Expensive at a gourmet store or restaurant, chocolate mousse can be made at home for much less and tastes even better.

1 In the top of a double boiler, melt the chocolate over low heat, stirring occasionally until smooth.
2 Meanwhile, beat the egg yolks in a bowl until thick, using electric beaters. Pour a little of the melted chocolate into the egg yolks, whisking constantly, then whisk all the egg yolk mixture back into the double boiler.
3 Add ¼ cup (60 ml) of the cream and whisk until well blended. Cook, stirring constantly, until the mixture thickens and reaches 160°F on a candy thermometer, about 4 minutes. Remove the top of the double boiler and allow the mixture to cool to room temperature, whisking often.
4 In a small saucepan, combine the sugar and ¼ cup (60 ml) water. Bring to a boil over medium heat. Using a pastry brush dipped in water, brush down the sides of the saucepan, then cook the syrup without stirring until it reaches 238°F on a candy thermometer, about 5 minutes.
5 In a heatproof bowl, beat the egg whites until frothy, using electric beaters on medium speed. Place the bowl in a larger saucepan of boiling water (double-boiler style). With the beaters on low speed, gradually whisk the boiling sugar syrup into the egg whites until the meringue peaks stiffly and a candy thermometer inserted at the center reaches 160°F. Whisk a few tablespoons of the hot meringue into the chocolate mixture, then fold in the remaining meringue.
6 In a small bowl, beat the remaining cream until it forms soft peaks, using electric beaters on high speed. Beat in the vanilla. Fold the whipped cream into the chocolate mixture until no white streaks remain.
7 Spoon into individual serving dishes or glasses, then cover and refrigerate for at least 1 hour, or until serving.

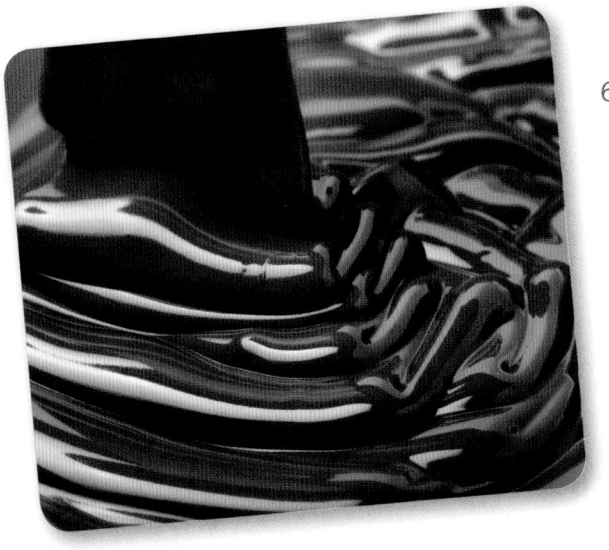

Mango Mousse

3 mangoes (about 2 lb/1 kg in total), peeled, pitted and sliced
¼ cup (60 ml) lime juice
½ teaspoon ground ginger
3 teaspoons powdered gelatin
2 tablespoons sugar
½ cup (125 g) light sour cream

Makes 6 servings

Nothing signals the arrival of summer more than the presence of juicy mangoes. Prepare this light mousse for friends and bask in the warmth of their admiration.

1. Reserve 12 small mango slices. In a food processor, puree the remaining mango with the lime juice and ginger. Leave in the food processor and set aside.
2. Sprinkle the gelatin over ½ cup (125 ml) water and let stand for 5 minutes.
3. In a small saucepan, combine the sugar and ½ cup (125 ml) water and bring to a boil. Add the gelatin mixture and stir until well dissolved.
4. Add the syrup mixture to the mango puree and process until well combined. Add the sour cream and process again briefly just to blend.
5. Spoon into dessert bowls or glasses and top with the reserved mango slices. Cover and refrigerate for 2 hours, or until the mousse has chilled and set.

Fruit Desserts

Brandied Peaches

2 cups (440 g) sugar
½ cup (125 ml) brandy
1 tablespoon whole cloves
2 cinnamon sticks
zest of 1 lemon, slivered
zest of 1 orange, slivered
4 peaches, peeled, pitted and halved

Makes 4 servings

You can buy brandied peaches in jars at gourmet stores, but you can just as easily—and much more cheaply—delight your loved ones by making your own.

1. Pour 3 cups (750 ml) water into a large, heavy saucepan. Add the sugar, brandy, cloves, cinnamon sticks and citrus zest and bring to a strong boil over high heat.
2. Reduce the heat to medium. Prick the peach halves several times with a fork and add them to the saucepan. Cover and reduce the heat to the lowest simmer. Gently poach until the peaches are just cooked but still firm, about 20 minutes.
3. Serve the brandied peaches hot, warm or chilled.

Dried Fruit Compote

1¼ cups (275 g) pitted prunes
⅔ cup (85 g) golden seedless raisins
½ cup (80 g) dried figs
½ cup (90 g) dried apricots
1½ cups (375 ml) orange juice
⅓ cup (80 ml) water
¼ cup (55 g) sugar
1 cinnamon stick, broken
¼ teaspoon ground ginger
pinch of ground cloves
pinch of freshly ground black pepper
¾ teaspoon vanilla extract (optional)

Makes 6 servings

For a fast and fantastic dessert, keep these dried fruits on hand in your pantry, then simply poach them as required. They're soft and enticingly spicy.

1 In a saucepan, combine all the ingredients except the vanilla. Bring to a boil over high heat, then reduce the heat to low. Cover and simmer until the fruit is tender, 25 to 30 minutes.
2 Remove the saucepan from the heat. Remove and discard the cinnamon sticks. Allow the mixture to cool to room temperature, then stir in the vanilla, if using.
3 Serve at room temperature or chilled. The compote can be refrigerated in an airtight container for up to 3 days.

Wine Poached Pears with Strawberries

4 cups (1 liter) red wine
1 cup (220 g) sugar
3 tablespoons thinly sliced fresh ginger
2 cinnamon sticks
zest of 1 lemon, slivered
zest of 1 orange, slivered
4 firm ripe pears, such as bosc or bartlett, peeled and cored with stems intact
2 cups (300 g) strawberries, hulled

Makes 4 servings

This is a restaurant dessert you can make at home for a modest sum and enjoy extravagantly. Serve them with a drizzle of homemade Custard (page 59).

1 In a large, heavy saucepan, combine the wine, sugar, ginger, cinnamon sticks and citrus zest slivers. Bring to a strong boil over high heat.
2 Reduce the heat to medium and add the pears. Cover and reduce the heat to the lowest simmer. Gently poach until the pears are just cooked but still firm, about 15 minutes.
3 Remove from the heat and allow to cool for 5 minutes, then stir in the strawberries. Using a slotted spoon, remove the pears and strawberries to a serving platter or individual bowls.
4 Return the saucepan to high heat and bring the poaching liquid to a boil; boil until the liquid is reduced to about 1½ cups (375 ml). Pour the hot poaching liquid over the pears and strawberries and serve.

Fruit Salad

1 large mango, peeled, pitted and sliced
9 oz (250 g) cherries, pitted
⅔ cup (120 g) seedless green grapes
9 oz (250 g) strawberries, hulled and cut in half
3 large apricots, halved, pitted and sliced
¾ cup (65 g) desiccated coconut
2 teaspoons superfine sugar
generous pinch of ground cayenne pepper
generous pinch of mustard powder
pinch of salt

Makes 6 servings

This recipe is easily adapted to showcase other summer fruits and berries. Mustard and cayenne pepper add a subtle spicy heat.

1 Place all the fruit in a large serving bowl.
2 Finely grind the desiccated coconut in a spice mill or using a pestle and mortar. Add the sugar, spices and salt and mix well.
3 Add the coconut mixture to the fruit and stir well to combine.
4 Cover and refrigerate for at least 2 hours, preferably overnight, to allow the flavors to blend and develop. Serve cold.

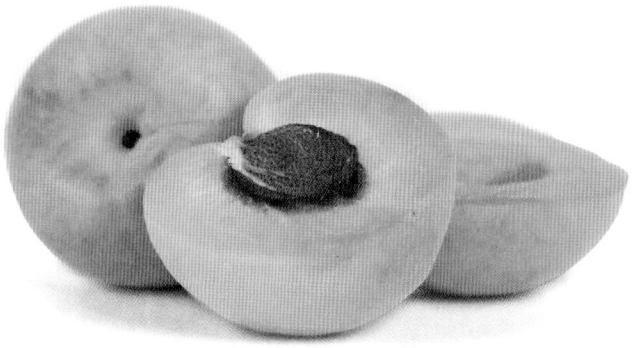

Chocolate-Dipped Strawberries

1 cup (150 g) chopped good-quality dark chocolate
12 large strawberries, hulls left on
finely chopped nuts or sprinkles (optional)

Makes 12

These are so simple to make and cost a mere fraction of the bought ones. You can substitute white chocolate if you prefer, or make a mixture of white and dark.

1 Line a baking sheet with parchment paper.
2 In the top of a double boiler, melt the chocolate over low heat, stirring occasionally until smooth.
3 Holding the strawberries by their leaves, dip them one at a time into the melted chocolate, allowing the excess chocolate to run back into the pan. Dip into some finely chopped nuts or sprinkles, if desired.
4 Place on the baking sheet and stand in a cool place until set.

Ice Cream

French Vanilla Ice Cream

1¾ cups (440 ml) milk
2½ cups (625 ml) heavy cream
1 cup (220 g) sugar
1 vanilla bean, split lengthwise
¼ teaspoon salt
6 egg yolks

Makes 1 quart (1 liter)

This is the real thing—rich, creamy and full of the strong, wonderful scent of vanilla.

1 In a large saucepan, combine the milk, cream, ½ cup (110 g) of the sugar, the vanilla bean and salt. Scald the mixture over medium heat just until small bubbles appear.
2 In a bowl, whisk the egg yolks and remaining sugar until well blended. Gradually whisk a little milk mixture into the egg mixture, then pour both mixtures into the saucepan. Cook over low heat, whisking constantly, until the custard coats the back of a spoon, about 15 minutes.
3 Remove from the heat and allow to cool to room temperature. Remove the vanilla bean and scrape the seeds into the custard; discard the pod. Cover the saucepan and refrigerate until the custard is cold, 1 to 2 hours.
4 Transfer the custard to an ice-cream maker and freeze according to the manufacturer's instructions.

Churn it yourself: ice-cream makers

Few pleasures in life compare with homemade ice cream—or frozen yogurt. But to make it, you need an ice-cream maker. As a general rule, homemade ice cream costs much less than commercial varieties. An ice-cream maker will pay for itself in no time. Keep an eye out at discount sales.

❖ **Hand crank churns** These old-fashioned machines use a combination of rock salt and ice packed around the churn to freeze the cream mixture. As the handle is cranked, the interior paddles stir the cream mixture while it is freezing. Naturally, the harder the ice cream gets, the harder it is to turn the handle, so you get a good workout before the delicious reward. This machine works well for family gatherings or parties, where people can trade off on the cranking but everyone enjoys the results.

❖ **Electric ice-cream makers** These handy machines are more costly up front but much easier on you, so you are likely to end up using them more frequently than a hand-churned model. Larger electric makers do both the freezing and the churning for you. A less costly version requires a freezer for the insert to be frozen ahead of time, but still does the arm-tiring churning for you.

Blueberry Ice Cream

2 cups (300 g) blueberries, washed and stemmed if necessary
1⅓ cups (300 g) sugar
4 strips (each ½ x 2 inch/1 x 5 cm) lemon zest
½ teaspoon ground white pepper
½ teaspoon ground ginger
1¾ cups (440 ml) milk
2½ cups (625 ml) heavy cream
1 vanilla bean, split lengthwise
¼ teaspoon salt
6 egg yolks

Makes 1 quart (1 liter)

When blueberries come into season, toward the end of summer, indulge in this glorious concoction served in glass bowls so everyone can admire the color as well as the taste.

1 In a saucepan, combine the blueberries, ⅓ cup (75 g) of the sugar and the lemon zest. Cook over medium heat, stirring very frequently, until the blueberries are very soft, 4 to 5 minutes.
2 Place a fine sieve over a bowl. Pour the blueberry mixture through the sieve, pressing with the back of a wooden spoon to extract all the juice; discard the solids. Stir in the pepper and ginger and set aside.
3 In a large saucepan over medium heat, combine the milk, cream, ½ cup (110 g) of the sugar, the vanilla bean and salt. Scald the mixture just until small bubbles appear.
4 In a bowl, whisk the egg yolks and remaining sugar until well blended. Gradually whisk a little milk mixture into the egg mixture, then pour both mixtures into the saucepan. Cook over low heat, whisking constantly, until the custard coats the back of a spoon, about 15 minutes.
5 Remove from the heat and allow to cool to room temperature. Remove the vanilla bean and scrape the seeds into the custard; discard the pod. Cover the saucepan and refrigerate until the custard is cold, 1 to 2 hours.
6 Pour the reserved blueberry mixture into the custard and stir until well blended. Transfer to an ice-cream maker and freeze according to the manufacturer's instructions.

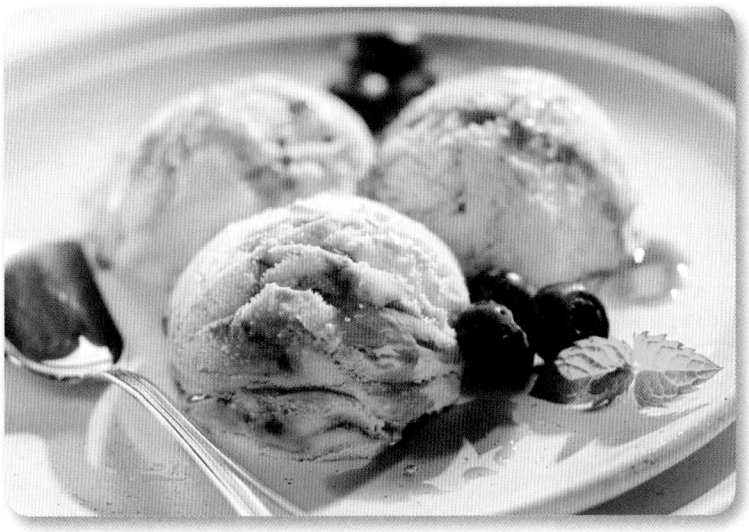

Peach Ice Cream

2 large, ripe peaches
⅓ cup (55 g) firmly packed light brown sugar
1 tablespoon lemon juice
¼ teaspoon ground ginger
1¾ cups (440 ml) milk
2½ cups (625 ml) heavy cream
1 cup (220 g) sugar
1 vanilla bean, split lengthwise
¼ teaspoon salt
6 egg yolks

Makes 1 quart (1 liter)

Ripe, juicy peaches are a true taste of summer, so how could they be any better? In a luscious ice cream that you've made yourself!

1. Blanch, peel and pit the peaches, then finely chop them. Place in a bowl with the brown sugar, lemon juice and ginger and toss until well blended. Set aside.
2. In a large saucepan, combine the milk, cream, ½ cup (110 g) of the sugar, the vanilla bean and salt. Scald the mixture over medium heat just until small bubbles appear.
3. In a bowl, whisk the egg yolks and remaining sugar until well blended. Gradually whisk a little milk mixture into the egg mixture, then pour both mixtures into the saucepan. Cook over low heat, whisking constantly, until the custard coats the back of a spoon, about 15 minutes.
4. Remove from the heat and allow to cool to room temperature. Remove the vanilla bean and scrape the seeds into the custard; discard the pod. Cover the saucepan and refrigerate until the custard is cold, 1 to 2 hours.
5. Pour the reserved peach mixture into the custard and stir until well blended. Transfer to an ice-cream maker and freeze according to the manufacturer's instructions.

Lowering the fat in homemade ice cream

We love the richness and texture of full-fat ice cream, but our bellies and thighs are not always so appreciative. Fortunately, it is not hard to lower the fat in homemade ice cream—and since it is home-churned as well, you should still have satisfyingly creamy results. The trick is to substitute an equal amount of evaporated skim milk for the whole milk and ¾ cup (180 g) egg substitute for the egg yolks when making a 1-quart (1 liter) batch.

Strawberry Ice Cream

1¾ cups (440 ml) milk
2½ cups (625 ml) heavy cream
1⅓ cups (300 g) sugar
1 vanilla bean, split lengthwise
¼ teaspoon salt
6 egg yolks
4 strips (each ½ x 3 inch/1 x 7.5 cm) orange zest
2 cups (300 g) strawberries

Makes 1 quart (1 liter)

Celebrate the start of summer with homemade ice cream studded with sweet fresh strawberries.

1 In a large saucepan, combine the milk, cream, ½ cup (110 g) of the sugar, the vanilla bean and salt. Scald the mixture over medium heat just until small bubbles appear.
2 In a bowl, whisk the egg yolks and another ½ cup (110 g) sugar until well blended. Gradually whisk a little milk mixture into the egg mixture, then pour both mixtures into the saucepan. Add the orange zest strips and cook over low heat, whisking constantly, until the custard coats the back of a spoon, about 15 minutes.
3 Remove from the heat and allow to cool to room temperature. Remove the vanilla bean and scrape the seeds into the custard; discard the pod. Remove and discard the orange zest strips. Cover the saucepan and refrigerate until the custard is cold, 1 to 2 hours.
4 Rinse and hull the strawberries. Place the strawberries in a food processor or blender with the remaining sugar and puree to the desired consistency.
5 Stir the strawberries into the custard and stir until well blended. Transfer to an ice-cream maker and freeze according to the manufacturer's instructions.

Honey Banana Ice Cream

6 egg yolks
2 cups (500 ml) milk
½ cup (175 g) honey
2 teaspoons vanilla extract
2 cups (500 ml) heavy cream
3 ripe bananas, mashed

Makes about 5 to 6 cups (1.25 liters)

Gingersnaps (page 130) make a perfect partner for this smooth number.

1 In the top of a double boiler set over simmering water, combine the egg yolks and milk. Whisk until well blended, then stir in the honey and vanilla. Cook over medium heat, whisking constantly, until the mixture coats the back of a spoon and registers 170°F on a candy thermometer.
2 Pour into a large bowl, then cover and refrigerate until the mixture is chilled, about 1 hour.
3 Add the cream and mashed bananas to the mixture and stir until well blended. Transfer to an ice-cream maker and freeze according to the manufacturer's instructions.

Coconut-Pineapple Ice Cream

1⅓ cups (330 ml) milk
3 eggs
1 cup (220 g) sugar
½ cup (30 g) flaked coconut
2 teaspoons vanilla extract
1 lb (450 g) can crushed pineapple, drained
1⅓ cups (330 ml) heavy cream

Makes about 1 quart (1 liter)

A taste of the tropics in every bite, this coconut-pineapple ice cream is rich and cooling—a piña colada in a bowl!

1 In a small, heavy saucepan, scald the milk over medium-high heat just until tiny bubbles appear.
2 In a heavy saucepan, combine the eggs and sugar over low heat. Pour the scalded milk into the egg mixture, whisking constantly. Cook, whisking constantly, until the mixture coats the back of a spoon and registers 170°F on a candy thermometer.
3 Set a fine sieve over a large bowl. Pour the custard through the sieve; discard the solids. Whisk in the coconut and vanilla until well blended, then stir in the pineapple and cream. Cover and refrigerate until the custard is cold, 1 to 2 hours.
4 Transfer the custard to an ice-cream maker and freeze according to the manufacturer's instructions.

Rocky Road Ice Cream

5⅔ cups (1.4 liters) milk
⅓ cup (90 g) butter, melted
9 oz (275 g) semi-sweet chocolate
2¾ cups (600 g) sugar
¾ teaspoon salt
6 cups (1.5 liters) heavy cream
3 cups (150 g) miniature marshmallows
2¼ cups (375 g) mini chocolate chips
1½ cups (180 g) chopped pecans
1½ tablespoons vanilla extract

Makes about 4½ quarts (4.5 liters)

Chocolate chips, marshmallows and pecans come together in this popular ice cream creation. Once you've made your own, you'll wonder how you could have spent so much money on commercially prepared ice cream.

1 In a large, heavy saucepan, combine the milk and butter over medium-high heat. Cook, stirring constantly, until the mixture registers 175°F on a candy thermometer. Add the chocolate, sugar and salt and stir until the chocolate has melted and the sugar has dissolved completely.
2 Remove the saucepan from the heat and place it in a large bowl of ice water to cool the mixture quickly; stir and chill for 2 minutes. Remove the saucepan and allow to cool completely.
3 Pour the mixture into a large bowl. Then add the cream, marshmallows, chocolate chips, pecans and vanilla and stir until well blended. Cover and refrigerate until the mixture is cold, 30 minutes.
4 Working in batches, transfer the mixture to an ice-cream maker and freeze according to the manufacturer's instructions. Keep the remaining mixture refrigerated until ready to freeze; stir well before adding to the ice-cream maker.
5 Leave in the ice-cream maker or place in the freezer to firm for 2 to 4 hours before serving.

Rich Chocolate Ice Cream

1¼ cups (310 ml) milk
3 eggs
¾ cup (165 g) sugar
⅓ cup (50 g) finely chopped unsweetened chocolate
2 teaspoons vanilla extract
¼ teaspoon salt
2 cups (500 ml) heavy cream

Makes about 1 quart (1 liter)

A rich, thick chocolate custard is the base for this decadent delight.

1 In a small, heavy saucepan, scald the milk over medium-high heat just until tiny bubbles appear.
2 In a heavy saucepan, combine the eggs and sugar over low heat. Whisking constantly, pour the scalded milk into the egg mixture. Cook, whisking constantly, until the mixture coats the back of a spoon and registers 170°F on a candy thermometer.
2 Set a fine sieve over a large bowl. Pour the custard through the sieve; discard the solids. Whisk in the chocolate, vanilla and salt until well blended. Stir in the cream. Cover and refrigerate until the custard is cold, 1 to 2 hours.
4 Transfer the custard to an ice-cream maker and freeze according to the manufacturer's instructions.

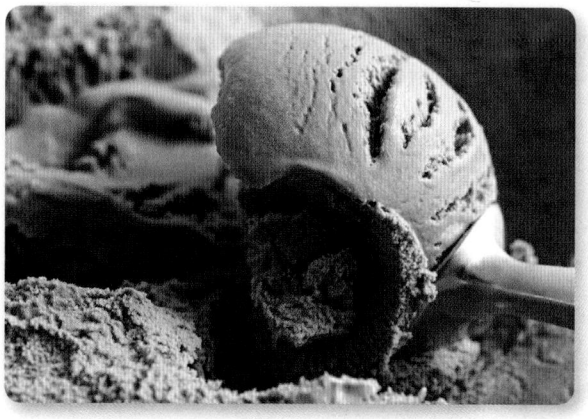

Chocolate Chocolate Chip Ice Cream

1¾ cups (440 ml) milk
2½ cups (625 ml) heavy cream
1 cup (230 g) firmly packed light brown sugar
¼ teaspoon salt
6 egg yolks
¼ cup (30 g) cocoa powder
1 teaspoon vanilla extract
½ cup (85 g) mini chocolate chips

Makes 1 quart (1 liter)

What could be better than chocolate? More chocolate! Remember, however, that just because homemade ice cream is cheaper, it doesn't have fewer calories!

1 In a large saucepan, combine the milk, cream, ½ cup (110 g) of the sugar and the salt. Scald the mixture over medium heat just until small bubbles appear.
2 In a bowl, whisk the egg yolks and remaining sugar until well blended. Whisk in the cocoa until well combined. Gradually whisk a little milk mixture into the egg mixture, then pour both into the saucepan. Cook over low heat, whisking constantly, until the custard coats the back of a spoon, about 15 minutes.
3 Remove from the heat and allow to cool to room temperature. Whisk in the vanilla. Cover the saucepan and refrigerate until the custard is cold, 1 to 2 hours.
4 Add the chocolate chips and stir until evenly distributed. Transfer the custard to an ice-cream maker and freeze according to the manufacturer's instructions.

Mint Chocolate Chip Ice Cream

1¾ cups (440 ml) milk
2½ cups (625 ml) heavy cream
1 cup (80 g/1 bunch) fresh mint, leaves rinsed, picked off and pureed
1 cup (220 g) sugar
¼ teaspoon salt
6 egg yolks
1 teaspoon vanilla extract
½ cup (85 g) mini chocolate chips

Makes 1 quart (1 liter)

Mint and chocolate are a natural combination and this is a popular flavor for ice cream, made using fresh mint. You won't find ice cream this lovely in a tub!

1. In a large saucepan, combine the milk, cream, mint, ½ cup (110 g) of the sugar and the salt. Scald the mixture over medium heat just until small bubbles appear.
2. In a bowl, whisk the egg yolks and remaining sugar until well blended. Gradually whisk a little milk mixture into the egg mixture, then pour both mixtures into the saucepan. Cook over low heat, whisking constantly, until the custard coats the back of a spoon, about 15 minutes.
3. Remove from the heat and allow to cool to room temperature. Whisk in the vanilla. Cover the saucepan and refrigerate until the custard is cold, 1 to 2 hours.
4. Add the mini chocolate chips and stir until evenly distributed. Transfer to an ice-cream maker and freeze according to the manufacturer's instructions.

Peppermint Ice Cream

4 egg yolks
1⅓ cups (330 ml) milk
1½ oz (45 g) butter, melted
¾ cup (165 g) sugar
¼ teaspoon salt
2 cups (500 ml) heavy cream
1–1½ tablespoons vanilla extract
1¼ cups (200 g) crushed peppermint candy

Makes 1 quart (1 liter)

Here's a cute concoction that you won't come across in stores every day!

1. In a large, heavy saucepan, combine the egg yolks, milk, melted butter, sugar and salt over low heat. Cook, stirring constantly, until the mixture coats the back of a spoon and registers 160°F on a candy thermometer.
2. Remove the saucepan from the heat and place it in a large bowl of ice water to cool the mixture quickly; stir and chill for 2 minutes. Stir in the cream and vanilla. Remove from the heat and let the mixture cool completely.
3. Cover the saucepan with plastic wrap and refrigerate for several hours or overnight, until the mixture is very cold.
4. Stir in the crushed peppermint candies until evenly distributed. Transfer to an ice-cream maker and freeze according to the manufacturer's instructions.
5. Leave in the ice-cream maker or place in the freezer to firm for 2 to 4 hours before serving.

Butter Pecan Ice Cream

¾ cup (90 g) chopped pecans
3 tablespoons butter, melted
pinch of salt
¼ cup (55 g) plus 1 tablespoon sugar
½ cup (115 g) firmly packed brown sugar
2 tablespoons cornstarch
2 eggs, beaten
⅓ cup (80 ml) maple syrup
2½ cups (625 ml) milk
1 cup (250 ml) heavy cream
2 teaspoons vanilla extract

Makes about 2 quarts (2 liters)

Toasting the pecans really brings out their flavor. Maple syrup adds extra goodness!

1 Preheat the oven to 350°F. Spread the pecans in a single layer in a baking pan. Drizzle with the melted butter, sprinkle with the salt and 1 tablespoon of the sugar and toss to coat. Toast in the oven for 15 minutes, then stir and toast for 15 minutes longer. Remove from the oven and allow to cool completely.
2 In the top of a double boiler set over simmering water, combine the remaining sugar, brown sugar, cornstarch, eggs and maple syrup. Stir until well blended, then gradually stir in the milk. Increase the heat to high and cook, stirring constantly, until the mixture thickens and coats the back of a spoon.
3 Remove from the heat and let the custard cool to room temperature. Cover the saucepan and refrigerate until the custard is cold, for several hours or overnight.
4 Add the toasted pecans, cream and vanilla and stir until evenly distributed. Transfer to an ice-cream maker and freeze according to the manufacturer's instructions.
5 Leave in the ice-cream maker or place in the freezer to firm for 2 to 4 hours before serving.

Ice Cream Cake

1½ cups (185 g) crumbled chocolate sandwich cookies or Oreo cookies
2 tablespoons butter, melted
3 cups (750 ml) ice cream flavor of your choice, softened
¾ cup (185 ml) Chocolate Sauce (page 60)
3 cups (750 ml) another ice cream flavor of your choice, softened
½ cup (60 g) grated chocolate or toasted slivered almonds

Makes 8 to 10 servings

This frozen cake is perfect for a summer birthday—or any time you need an easy but sensational dessert. Use whatever ice cream combination takes your fancy.

1 In a small bowl, combine the cookie crumbs and melted butter and toss until well blended. Press the mixture over the bottom and halfway up the side of an 8-inch springform pan. Place the pan in the freezer for 30 minutes.
2 Spoon your first ice cream variety into the springform pan, spreading it in an even layer over the crust. Freeze again until the ice cream is firm, about 30 minutes.
3 Pour the chocolate sauce into the pan, spreading it evenly over the ice cream layer. Freeze until firm, about 15 minutes.
4 Spoon the second ice cream variety into the pan, spreading it evenly over the hardened chocolate sauce. Using a knife or spatula dipped in hot water, smooth the top of the cake, then sprinkle with either the grated chocolate or almonds. Cover with plastic wrap and freeze for at least 1 hour.
5 To serve, wipe the bottom of the pan with a hot, damp cloth, then carefully release and remove the sides. Cut the cake using a sharp knife dipped in hot water.

Frozen Yogurt

Lemon Frozen Yogurt

4 cups (32 oz/1 kg) low-fat natural yogurt
1⅔ cups (360 g) sugar
⅓ cup (80 ml) lemon juice
1 tablespoon grated lemon zest
4 drops yellow food coloring (optional)

Makes 5 cups (1.25 liters)

Light and refreshing, the tang of lemon really comes through in this homemade frozen yogurt. Try a scoop with fresh berries.

1 In a bowl, combine the yogurt, sugar, lemon juice and lemon zest; stir until well blended. If a brighter yellow color is desired, stir in the food coloring.
2 Transfer the mixture to an ice-cream maker and freeze according to the manufacturer's instructions.
3 Leave in the ice-cream maker or place in the freezer to firm for 2 to 4 hours before serving.

Strawberry Frozen Yogurt

2 cups (16 oz/500 g) low-fat natural yogurt
2 cups (500 ml) pureed fresh strawberries
14 oz (400 ml) can sweetened condensed milk
1 cup (250 ml) milk
3 teaspoons vanilla extract

Makes 1.5 quarts (1.5 liters)

Fresh strawberries add just the right touch of sweetness to this simple, speedy frozen yogurt.

1 In a large bowl, combine all the ingredients and stir until well blended.
2 Working in batches if needed, pour the mixture into an ice-cream maker, filling it two-thirds full; store the remaining yogurt in the refrigerator until ready to freeze. Following the manufacturer's instructions, freeze the yogurt. Leave in the ice-cream maker or place in the freezer to firm for 2 to 4 hours before serving.
3 Remove from the freezer 30 to 45 minutes before serving to soften slightly.

Passion Fruit Frozen Yogurt

½ cup (125 ml) milk
1 teaspoon powdered gelatin
5 passion fruit
¾ cup (165 g) sugar
1 teaspoon lemon juice
1½ cups (375 g) Greek-style yogurt
1 egg white
⅓ cup (35 g) full-cream powdered milk

Makes about 1 quart (1 liter)

Fresh passion fruit adds a deliciously tangy note to frozen yogurt. Use full-cream milk and yogurt here for best results.

1 Pour the milk into a small saucepan and stir in the gelatin. Let stand for 1 minute, then stir over low heat until the gelatin has dissolved. Set aside.
2 Cut each passion fruit in half. Scoop the pulp and seeds into a bowl, discarding the shells. Stir in the sugar, lemon juice and dissolved gelatin until combined, then stir in the yogurt.
3 In another bowl, beat the egg white, powdered milk and ⅓ cup (80 ml) water until stiff but not dry, using electric beaters. Fold gently into the yogurt mixture and transfer to an ice-cream maker. Following the manufacturer's instructions, churn until frozen. Serve immediately or transfer to the freezer.

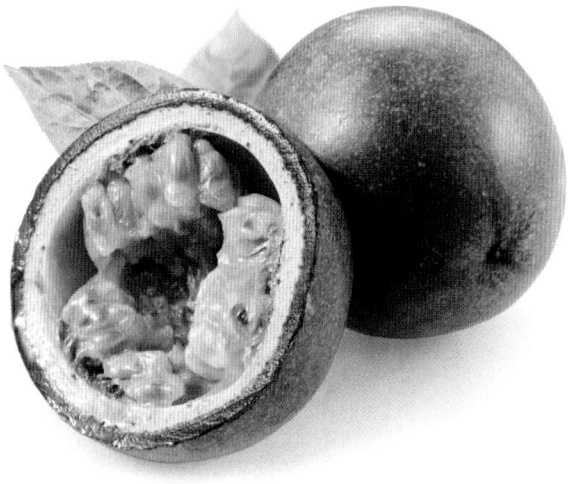

Frozen yogurt: an alternative to ice cream

Once only the province of health food aficionados, frozen yogurt has grown wildly in popularity. Generally lower in fat and calories (though not always) than ice cream, frozen yogurt combines the slight tanginess associated with yogurt with the cool creaminess of ice cream. For the most healthy results, use nonfat or reduced-fat yogurt when making it. You'll need an ice-cream maker to prepare it.

Ices, Granitas, Sherbets and Sorbets

Orange Ice

1 cup (220 g) sugar
12 oz (350 g) frozen orange juice concentrate, thawed
2 tablespoons lemon juice
4 oz (115 ml) milk
1 tablespoon melted butter

Makes 10 to 12 servings

This lovely treat requires only five ingredients and no ice-cream maker!

1 In a saucepan, combine the sugar and 1 cup (250 ml) water over high heat. Boil, stirring frequently, until the sugar has completely dissolved, about 1 minute.
2 Remove from the heat and stir in the orange juice concentrate, lemon juice and 2 cups (500 ml) water. Stir until well blended. Pour into a large bowl, cover and freeze until firm.
3 Remove the bowl from the freezer and beat the mixture until smooth, using electric beaters. Add the milk and melted butter and beat again until well blended. Cover and return to the freezer.
4 Leave to stand at room temperature for 20 minutes to soften before serving.

Blood-Orange Champagne Granita

1½ cups (330 g) sugar
2 cups (500 ml) blood-orange juice
2 cups (500 ml) Champagne or sparkling wine
pinch of salt

Makes 12 servings

If blood oranges are unavailable, substitute ruby red or pink grapefruit.

1 In a saucepan, combine the sugar and 1 cup (250 ml) water over medium heat, stirring constantly until the sugar has dissolved. Bring to a boil, reduce the heat and simmer for 3 minutes. Remove from the heat and leave until the syrup is cool, about 1 hour.
2 Pour the syrup into a large bowl. Stir in the orange juice, Champagne and salt until well blended.
3 Pour the mixture into a large, shallow pan. Cover with plastic wrap and place in the freezer. As the granita freezes, stir it with a fork every 45 minutes, two or three times, to break up the ice and create an icy, flaky texture. Cover with plastic wrap and freeze for 8 hours, or overnight.
4 When ready to serve, soften the granita in the refrigerator for 15 minutes. Then, using an ice-cream scoop or large spoon, scrape across the top to bring up the granita in thin shavings. Serve in chilled glasses or bowls.

Cappuccino Granita

1¼ cups (310 ml) brewed strong black coffee or espresso
¼ cup (55 g) sugar
5 tablespoons (100 ml) Kahlúa or other coffee-flavored liqueur
1 cup (250 ml) heavy cream
1 tablespoon confectioners' sugar
cocoa powder, for dusting

Makes 6 to 8 servings

An Italian specialty, this granita goes well with a few chocolate-covered coffee beans.

1. In a small bowl, combine the coffee, sugar and ¼ cup (60 ml) of the Kahlúa.
2. Pour the mixture into a large, shallow pan. Cover with plastic wrap and place in the freezer. As the granita freezes, stir it with a fork every 45 minutes, two or three times, to break up the ice and create an icy, flaky texture. Cover with plastic wrap and freeze for 8 hours, or overnight.
3. In a bowl, beat the cream, confectioners' sugar and remaining Kahlúa until soft peaks form, using electric beaters.
4. To serve, use an ice-cream scoop or large spoon to scrape across the top of the granita to bring up thin shavings. Place the granita in individual chilled serving bowls and top each with a dollop of the Kahlúa cream. Sprinkle with a dusting of cocoa powder and serve.

Kiwi Granita

2 cups (440 g) sugar
juice of 2 lemons
6 large, ripe kiwis, peeled and chopped

Makes about 4 cups (1 liter)

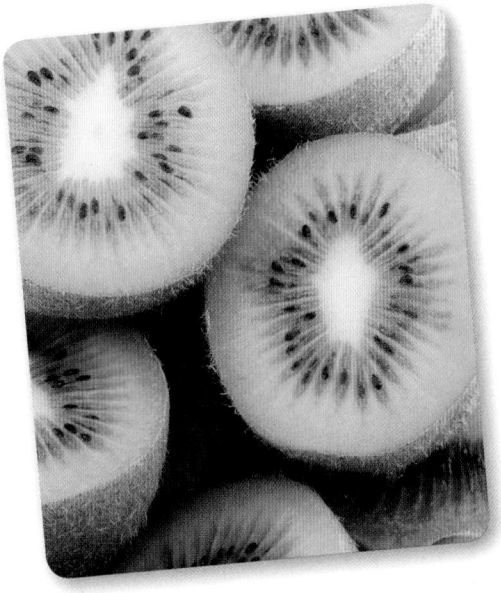

A lovely green with a lively, tart taste, this granita would be a fitting finale to a rich meal.

1. In a saucepan, combine the sugar, half the lemon juice and 1 cup (250 ml) water over medium heat, stirring constantly until the sugar has dissolved. Bring to a boil, reduce the heat and simmer for 3 minutes. Remove from the heat and leave until the syrup is just warm.
2. Puree the kiwis in a food processor or blender. Add the remaining lemon juice and blend. Pour the kiwi puree into the sugar syrup and mix well.
3. Pour the mixture into a large, shallow pan. Cover with plastic wrap and place in the freezer. As the granita freezes, stir it with a fork every 45 minutes, two or three times, to break up the ice and create an icy, flaky texture. Cover with plastic wrap and freeze 6 hours, or until solid.
4. When ready to serve, soften the granita in the refrigerator for 15 minutes. Then, using an ice-cream scoop or large spoon, scrape across the top to bring up the granita in thin shavings. Serve in chilled glasses or bowls.

Peach Granita

½ cup (110 g) sugar
4 ripe peaches, peeled, pitted and chopped
1 tablespoon peach schnapps or other fruit liqueur

Makes about 4 cups (1 liter)

An out-of-this-world cooler for a hot summer's day, this granita is an easy home project.

1. In a saucepan, combine the sugar and 1 cup (250 ml) water over medium heat, stirring constantly until the sugar has dissolved. Bring to a boil, reduce the heat and simmer for 3 minutes. Remove from the heat and leave until the syrup is cool, about 1 hour.
2. In a food processor or blender, puree the peach pieces. Add the syrup and schnapps and blend.
3. Pour the mixture into a large, shallow pan. Cover with plastic wrap and place in the freezer. As the granita freezes, stir it with a fork every 45 minutes, two or three times, to break up the ice and create an icy, flaky texture. Cover with plastic wrap and freeze for 6 hours, or until solid.
4. When ready to serve, soften the granita in the refrigerator for 15 minutes. Then, using an ice-cream scoop or large spoon, scrape across the top to bring up the granita in thin shavings. Serve in chilled glasses or bowls.

Lime Sherbet

4¼ cups (950 g) sugar
2 tablespoons grated lime zest
1½ cups (375 ml) lime juice
3 tablespoons lemon juice
7½ cups (1.9 liters) milk
½ cup (125 ml) buttermilk
1 drop green food coloring (optional)

Makes about 2½ quarts (2.5 liters)

Refreshingly tart, this homemade sherbet is better than any you can buy and costs much less.

1. In a large bowl, combine the sugar, lime zest, lime juice and lemon juice and stir until the sugar has dissolved. Gradually stir in the milk and buttermilk. If a brighter green color is desired, stir in the food coloring.
2. Working in batches if needed, pour the mixture into an ice-cream maker, filling it two-thirds full; store the remaining mixture in the refrigerator until ready to freeze. Following the manufacturer's instructions, freeze the sherbet. Leave in the ice-cream maker or place in the freezer to firm for 2 to 4 hours before serving.
3. Remove the sherbet from the freezer 10 minutes before serving to soften slightly.

Strawberry Milk Sherbet

1 pint (300 g) strawberries, rinsed and hulled
1 cup (250 ml) milk
1 cup (220 g) sugar

Makes about 2 cups

Smooth as ice cream but made with milk for a lighter treat, this sherbet is easy to make at home and an inexpensive treat whenever you want it.

1. In a food processor or blender, puree the strawberries until just smooth.
2. In a saucepan, combine the milk and sugar over high heat and bring to a boil. Remove from the heat and leave until the milk mixture is just warm.
3. Pour the milk mixture into a bowl. Add the strawberry puree and whisk until well blended.
4. Pour the mixture into an ice-cream maker and freeze according to the manufacturer's instructions.

Cassis Sorbet

½ cup (110 g) sugar
1 cup (250 ml) cassis (black-currant liqueur)

Makes about 2 cups

A black-currant liqueur, cassis has a smooth, strong flavor that makes this sorbet particularly delicious as a formal dinner dessert—one that makes both your guests and your hip pocket happy.

1. In a saucepan, combine the sugar and 1½ cups (375 ml) water over high heat. Bring to a boil, stirring constantly until the sugar has dissolved. Remove from the heat and leave until the syrup is just warm.
2. Pour the syrup into a bowl. Add the cassis and stir until the mixture is well blended.
3. Pour the mixture into an ice-cream maker and freeze according to the manufacturer's instructions.

Citrus Sorbet

½ cup (110 g) sugar
1¼ cups (310 ml) orange juice
¼ cup (60 ml) lemon juice
¼ cup (60 ml) lime juice

Makes about 2 cups

Oranges, lemons and limes all lend their distinctive notes to this refreshing sorbet. This is one you're not likely to find in a store!

1. In a saucepan, combine the sugar and 1 cup (250 ml) water over high heat. Bring to a boil, stirring constantly until the sugar has dissolved. Remove from the heat and leave until the syrup is just warm.
2. Pour the syrup into a bowl. Add all the citrus juice and stir until well blended.
3. Pour the mixture into an ice-cream maker and freeze according to the manufacturer's instructions.

Honeydew Sorbet

6 cups (1 kg) honeydew melon cubes
¾ cup (165 g) sugar
¼ cup (60 ml) Midori or other melon-flavored liqueur

Makes about 2 cups

Serve a scoop of this delicate sorbet in a wedge of fresh honeydew. Or try substituting your favorite melon in this recipe.

1 Place all the ingredients in a food processor or blender and puree until blended to a smooth consistency. Refrigerate until completely chilled.
2 Pour the mixture into an ice-cream maker and freeze according to the manufacturer's instructions.

Lemon Sorbet

1½ cups (330 g) sugar
1 tablespoon grated lemon zest
1½ cups (375 ml) lemon juice

Makes about 1 quart (1 liter)

Wonderfully tart, this classic sorbet works either as a dessert or as a palate cleanser between courses. As a variation, add ½ cup (10 g) fresh mint leaves to the syrup before it cools, then strain before freezing.

1 In a saucepan, combine the sugar and 3 cups (750 ml) water over high heat. Bring to a boil, stirring constantly until the sugar has dissolved. Remove from the heat and leave until the syrup is just warm.
2 Pour the syrup into a bowl. Add the lemon zest and lemon juice and stir until well blended.
3 Pour the mixture into an ice-cream maker and freeze according to the manufacturer's instructions. Leave the sorbet in the ice-cream maker or place in the freezer to firm for 2 to 4 hours before serving.
4 Remove the sorbet from the freezer 10 minutes before serving to soften slightly.

Raspberry Sorbet

10 oz (300 g) package frozen raspberries, thawed
1 cup (220 g) sugar
1 tablespoon lemon juice

Makes about 2 cups

Since it uses frozen raspberries, you can make this sorbet any time of the year. Try drizzling with a little Chocolate Sauce (page 60) before serving.

1 In a food processor or blender, puree the raspberries until smooth.
2 In a saucepan, combine the sugar and 1 cup (250 ml) water over high heat. Bring to a boil, stirring constantly until the sugar has dissolved. Remove from the heat and leave until the syrup is just warm.
3 Pour the syrup into a bowl. Add the raspberry puree and lemon juice and stir until well blended.
4 Pour the mixture into an ice-cream maker and freeze according to the manufacturer's instructions.

Strawberry Sorbet

6 cups (1 kg) strawberries, rinsed and hulled
1¾ cups (300 g) sugar
2 cups (500 ml) orange juice, strained
2 tablespoons Grand Marnier or other orange-flavored liqueur

Makes about 3 cups

Look for really ripe, firm red strawberries for their extraordinary flavor and ravishing color. This sorbet is another treat you can make much better and more frugally at home.

1. Cut the strawberries in half and place in a small bowl with the sugar and orange juice. Mix gently and leave to stand for 1 hour.
2. In a food processor or blender, puree the strawberry mixture until smooth. Add the liqueur and pulse until well blended.
3. Pour the mixture into a large, shallow pan and freeze until just firm but not hard, 1 to 2 hours.
4. Spoon the mixture back into the food processor and pulse until the mixture becomes slushy. Refreeze, then repeat. Return the mixture to the pan and freeze until solid.
5. Before serving, place the pan in the refrigerator and let the sorbet soften slightly for about 15 minutes.

Frozen Pops

Frozen Fruit Pops

3 oz (85 g) package fruit-flavored gelatin
10–12 plastic pop molds or 3 oz (100 ml) paper cups
10–12 frozen pop sticks or plastic spoons

Makes 10 to 12 pops

These treats are delicious on a hot summer's day.

1. In a bowl, combine the gelatin and 1 cup (250 ml) boiling water, stirring until completely dissolved. Stir in 7 oz (200 ml) cold water.
2. Pour the gelatin mixture into the molds or paper cups and freeze until the pops are almost firm, about 2 hours.
3. Insert a frozen pop stick or spoon into the center of each pop. Freeze until firm, 4 to 8 hours.
4. To serve, unmold or tear the paper cup from the pop.

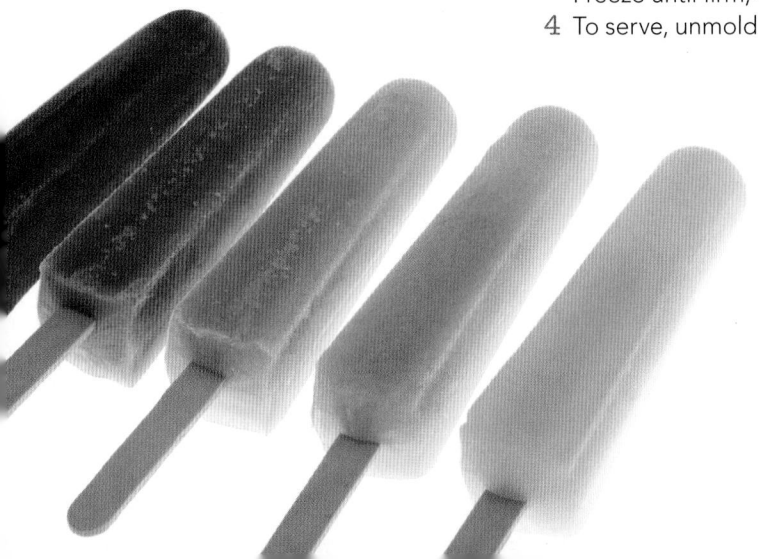

Fruity Frozen Yogurt Pops

3 oz (85 g) package fruit-flavored gelatin
1½ cups (375 g) vanilla or natural yogurt
10 oz (300 g) chopped fruit, such as mango, strawberries or raspberries
10–12 frozen pop molds or 3 oz (100 ml) paper cups
10–12 frozen pop sticks or plastic spoons

Makes 10 to 12 pops

Whip up these creamy, fruit-flavored frozen yogurts at home—they go down very nicely on a hot day.

1 In a bowl, combine the gelatin and 1 cup (250 ml) boiling water, stirring until completely dissolved. Stir in 7 oz (200 ml) cold water. Cool the mixture to room temperature.
2 Whisk in the yogurt, then stir in the fruit.
3 Spoon the mixture into the molds or paper cups and freeze until almost firm, about 2 hours.
4 Insert a frozen pop stick or spoon into the center of each yogurt. Freeze until the yogurts are firm, 2 to 4 hours.
5 To serve, unmold or tear away the paper cup from the pop.

Chocolate Pops

3.4 oz (100 g) package instant chocolate pudding mix
3 cups (750 ml) milk
¼ cup (55 g) sugar
½ cup (125 ml) whipping cream
12–13 frozen pop molds or 3 oz (100 ml) paper cups
12–13 frozen pop sticks or plastic spoons

Makes 12 to 13 pops

A great way to enjoy chocolate when the going gets hot!

1 In a saucepan, combine the pudding mix, milk and sugar over medium heat. Bring to a boil and cook, stirring constantly, for 2 minutes. Remove from the heat and leave to stand for 30 minutes, stirring several times, until the mixture is cool.
2 In a small bowl, whip the cream until soft peaks form, using electric beaters. Fold the whipped cream into the milk mixture until well blended and no streaks of white remain.
3 Pour the mixture into the molds or paper cups and freeze until almost firm, about 2 hours.
4 Insert a frozen pop stick or spoon into the center of each pop. Freeze until the pops are firm, 2 to 4 hours.
5 To serve, unmold or tear away the paper cup from the pop.

Strawberry Pops

2 pints (600 g) strawberries, rinsed and hulled
½ cup (125 ml) apple juice concentrate
8 frozen pop molds or 3 oz (100 ml) paper cups
8 frozen pop sticks or plastic spoons

Makes 8 pops

Fresh strawberries make these pops extra special—much lovelier than any sold in stores.

1 In a large bowl, mash the strawberries roughly, leaving some chunks of strawberry intact. Add the apple juice concentrate and stir until well blended.
2 Spoon or pour the mixture into the molds or paper cups and freeze until the pops are almost firm, about 2 hours.
3 Insert a frozen pop stick or spoon into the center of each pop. Freeze until the pops are firm, 4 to 8 hours.
4 To serve, unmold or tear away the paper cup from the pop.

Tropical Pops

6 cups (1 kg) chopped fresh tropical fruit, such as pineapples, papayas and/or mangoes, peeled and cored as needed, cut into bite-sized pieces, reserving any juices
24 small frozen pop molds, or ½ cup (125 ml) paper cups
3 cups (750 ml) mixed tropical fruit punch, or orange or pineapple juice
24 frozen pop sticks or plastic spoons

Makes 24 pops

If you can't be sipping tropical drinks, you can at least keep your cool with these inexpensive tropical ices. This recipe makes 24 little pops, but you could make them in larger molds or paper cups.

1 In a large bowl, combine the fresh fruit with any juices collected during their preparation. Stir well to distribute the fruits equally.
2 Spoon the fruit mixture into the molds or paper cups, filling them three-quarters full.
3 Pour some of the fruit punch or juice into each mold or cup, leaving room at the top for the liquid to expand. Freeze until the pops are almost firm, about 2 hours.
4 Insert a frozen pop stick or spoon into the center of each pop. Freeze until the pops are firm, 4 to 8 hours.
5 To serve, unmold or tear away the paper cup from the pop.

Chocolate-Nut Frozen Bananas

8 wooden skewers, with the sharp ends cut off
8 small bananas, peeled
8 oz (225 g) dark chocolate
3 tablespoons margarine
1 cup (125 g) chopped walnuts, toasted
1 cup (125 g) chopped macadamia nuts, toasted

Makes 8 servings

Bananas are one of those versatile fruits that can be frozen and eaten out of hand. But for a special treat, try dipping them in chocolate and nuts!

1 Line a baking sheet with plastic wrap.
2 Insert one skewer into each banana, about halfway down the length of the fruit. Place the bananas on the baking sheet, cover with plastic wrap and freeze until frozen solid, about 8 hours.
3 Place a small heatproof bowl over a saucepan of simmering water, ensuring the base of the bowl does not touch the water. Add the chocolate and margarine and melt, stirring occasionally. Remove the bowl from the heat.
4 On a shallow plate, combine the walnuts and macadamia nuts and toss to mix well.
5 Remove the bananas from the freezer. Holding one banana by the skewer over the bowl of chocolate, spoon the chocolate over the banana, coating it completely. Then hold the banana over the nuts and sprinkle them over the banana to coat the chocolate. Return the banana to the baking sheet. Repeat to coat all the bananas.
6 Return the baking sheet to the freezer until the chocolate hardens. Wrap each banana separately in plastic wrap, then place in a large, self-sealing freezer-safe plastic bag and store in the freezer.

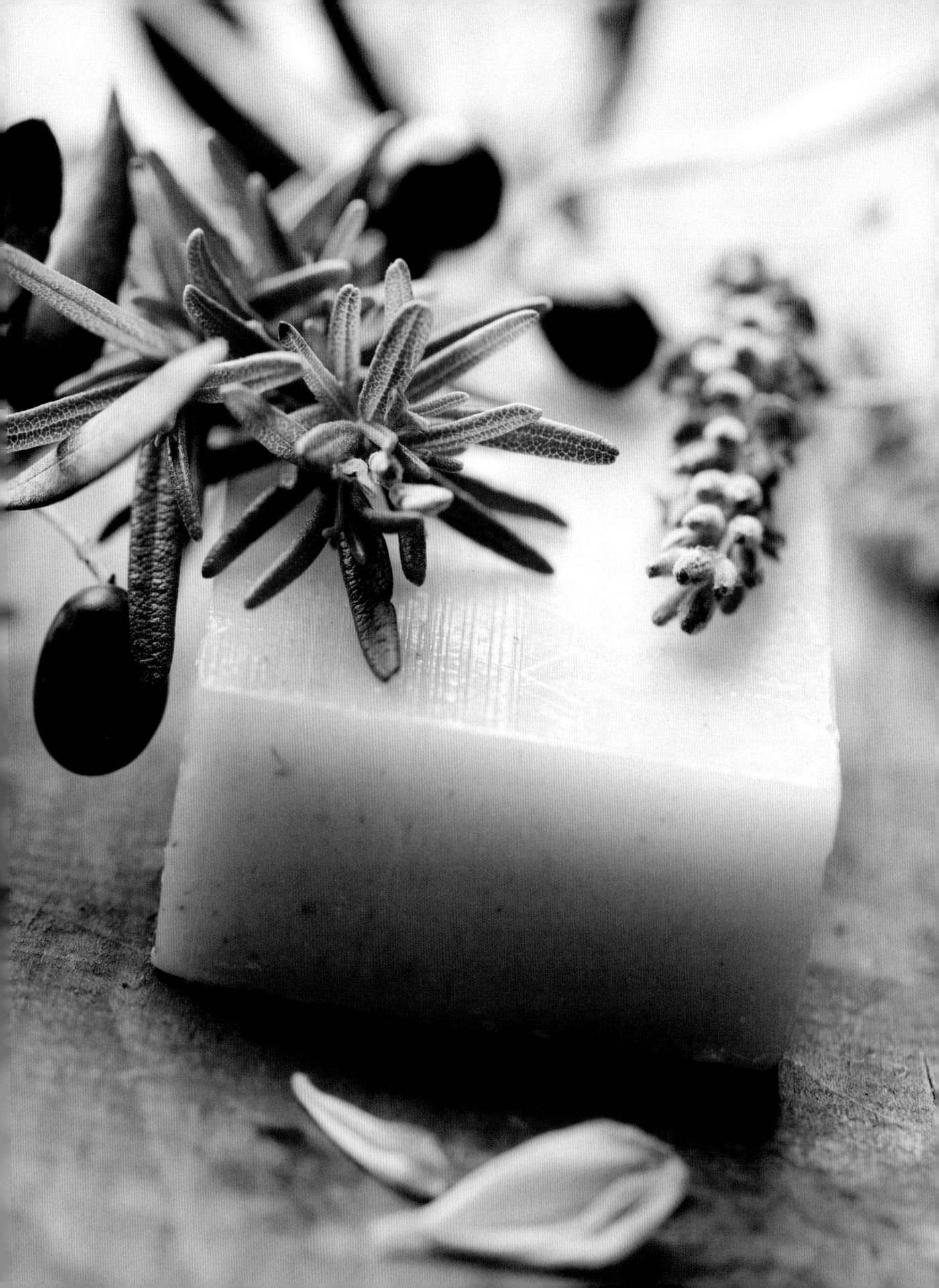

Part 2

Health and Beauty Care

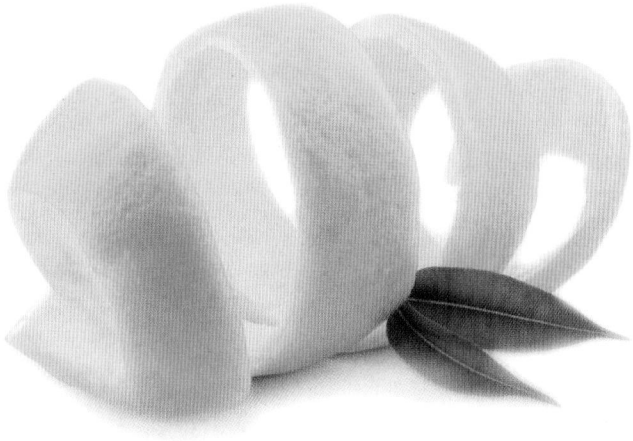

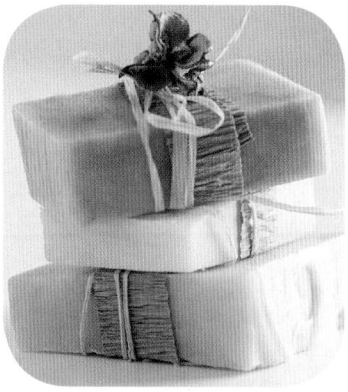

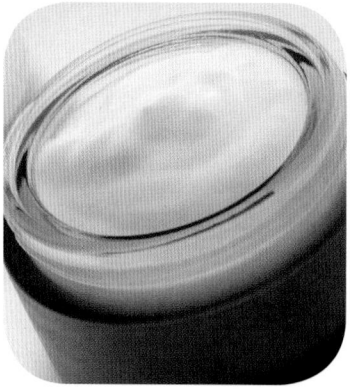

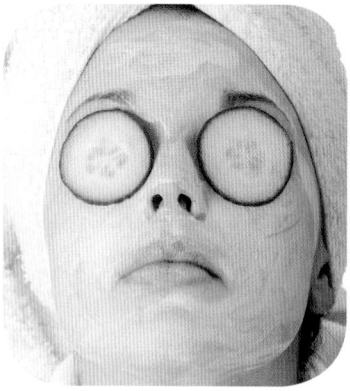

Face Care

Anti-Wrinkle Eye Cream ❖ Tired Eye Remedy ❖ Simple Eye Makeup Remover ❖ Rich Neck Moisturizer ❖ Artichoke Facial ❖ Basic Skin Toner ❖ Peachy Complexion Cream ❖ Cucumber Astringent ❖ Egg-White Toner ❖ Lemon Skin Toner ❖ Facial Cleansing Mask ❖ Green Clay Purifying Face Mask ❖ Deep-Cleansing Facial ❖ Almond Mayonnaise Scrub ❖ Honey Mask ❖ Banana, Sour Cream and Honey Face Mask ❖ Youthful Skin Face Mask ❖ Oatmeal Exfoliant ❖ Mask for Oily Skin ❖ Galen's Cold Cream ❖ Strawberry Yogurt Mask

Care for Lips and Mouth

Honey Lip Balm ❖ Cocoa Lip Balm ❖ Chocolate Chip Lip Balm ❖ Refreshing Mouthwash ❖ Spicy, Minty Mouthwash ❖ Bacteria-Fighting Citrus Mouthwash ❖ Toothpaste

Shampoos, Conditioners and Rinses

Beer Shampoo ❖ Dandruff Treatment ❖ Highlighting Rinse ❖ Chamomile Shampoo ❖ Instant Dry Shampoo ❖ Thick Hair Conditioner for Everyone ❖ Nourishing Conditioner ❖ Natural Head Lice Treatment

Body Care Treatments

Warm Herbal Body Treatment ❖ Citrus Moisturizing Treatment ❖ Green Aloe Moisturizing Lotion ❖ Shaving Gel for Women ❖ Summer Body Splash ❖ Simple Fragrant Body Splash ❖ Citrus Cologne Splash ❖ Cellulite Massage Oil ❖ Almond Exfoliating Body Scrub ❖ Simple Sugar Scrub for Dry Skin ❖ Cranberry Sugar Scrub ❖ Body Powder ❖ Body Spray ❖ Deodorant

Bath Products

Bubble Bath for Kids ❖ Conditioning Bubble Bath ❖ Bath Gel ❖ Liquid or Gel Soap ❖ Almond Rose Soap ❖ Cinnamon Soap ❖ Strawberries and Cream Bath Bags ❖ Herbal Bath Bag ❖ Cinnamon Oatmeal Milk Bath ❖ Gentle Milk Bath ❖ Zingy Citrus Bath Salts ❖ Bath Cookies ❖ Basic Bath Powder ❖ Easy Bath Powder ❖ Delicately Scented Bath Powder

Nail, Hand and Foot Care

Gardener's Hand Cream ❖ Cuticle Cream ❖ Warm Oil Hand Treatment ❖ Cornmeal Hand Scrub ❖ Love Your Feet Cream ❖ Soothing Footbath ❖ Eucalyptus Foot Lotion ❖ Strawberry Foot Scrub ❖ Refreshing Foot Spray ❖ Leg Massage Cream

Just for Men

Rosemary Shaving Soap ❖ Lightly Scented Aftershave ❖ Shaving-Cut Lotion ❖ Aloe Aftershave Gel ❖ Muscle Rub

Your Own Beauty Products

Some of the most seductive ads on television and in magazines are for beauty products—scents and skin care products in beautiful packages.

They are all very intriguing and inviting until you read the small print and realize that you don't know what all those ingredients are or what they are designed to do. And, although you may feel that the price doesn't matter, you just might want to know what is going onto your skin.

Making your own beauty products is neither difficult nor mystifying. With just a little time and effort, you can even give yourself spa treatments that will benefit your spirits as well as your skin—with face masks, exfoliants and wrinkle fighters. Your wallet will be spared. You might even want to involve friends in the making and using of these recipes for special spa treatment sessions.

For everyday use, you can make cleansers, moisturizers and toners; toothpaste and gargles; shampoos and hair rinses; shaving gels and refreshing splashes—with or without scent. For your bath, you can prepare lovely bath gels from soap slivers; almond, rose or cinnamon soap; and several bath scrubs and milk baths. For hands and feet, there are special creams and soaks. There is also a selection of recipes for homemade men's toiletries: shaving soap, aftershaves, a shaving cut lotion and a muscle rub.

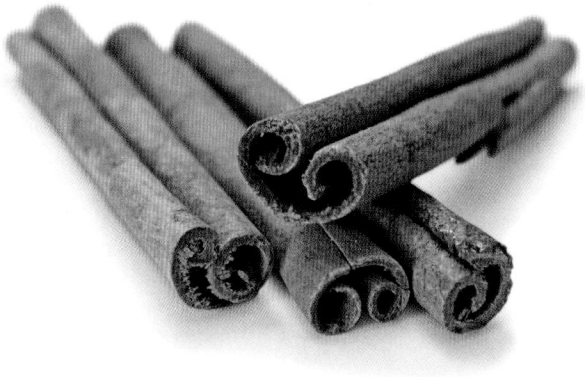

Face Care

Anti-Wrinkle Eye Cream

2 tablespoons (30 ml) elder flower water
¼ cup (60 ml) avocado oil
2 tablespoons (30 ml) almond oil
4 teaspoons (20 ml) wheat germ oil
2 tablespoons (30 ml) lanolin
2 tablespoons (30 ml) glycerine
2 drops geranium essential oil
1 vitamin E capsule, 500 IU

Apply this cream with a gentle touch around the eye, using light, circular strokes. It is especially geared for the soft tissue under and around the eyes.

1 Warm the elder flower water in a nonreactive saucepan over low heat.
2 In the top of a double boiler set over simmering water, warm the avocado, almond and wheat germ oils. Stir in the lanolin until melted. Remove from heat.
3 Gradually beat in the warmed elder flower water. Stir in the glycerine and geranium essential oil. Pierce the vitamin E capsule with a needle, squeeze out the contents, and stir in.
4 Pour the mixture into a clean widemouthed 6 oz glass jar with a tight-fitting lid. Store in a cool, dark place.

Tired Eye Remedy

1 cup (250 ml) boiling water
2–3 rose petals

Here's a simple soak you can apply to soothe irritated or inflamed eyes. The price is just a few rose petals from your garden.

1 Pour the boiling water over the rose petals into a bowl. Steep for about 10 minutes. Cool and strain out the petals.
2 Soak two large cotton balls in the rose tea and apply over closed eyelids. Rest and relax.

Simple Eye Makeup Remover

1 teaspoon glycerine
3 teaspoons distilled water
4 teaspoons (20 ml) olive, jojoba or baby oil

Why should you spend good money on eye makeup remover when you can make a pure and gentle but very effective solution in your own kitchen?

1 Shake all the ingredients in a small glass bottle.
2 Apply a little solution to makeup remover pads or a cotton wool ball, press against the eyelid for a minute to loosen makeup, then gently wipe the makeup away.

Fast relief with witch hazel eye compresses

We give our eyes a constant workout while reading, watching TV and staring at the computer screen. Here's a basic eye care remedy that costs very little and provides a very valuable service. Just keep a small jar of witch hazel in the refrigerator. Soak two cotton pads in the chilled liquid, lie down, cover both eyelids, and relax for 5 minutes.

Rich Neck Moisturizer

1 teaspoon dried chamomile
1¼ cups (310 ml) boiling water
3 tablespoons (45 ml) avocado oil
3 tablespoons (45 ml) almond oil
2 teaspoons jojoba oil
1 oz (30 g) shaved or grated cosmetic-grade beeswax
2 teaspoons glycerine
20 drops lemon essential oil

In your beauty regimen, don't forget the neck, which can show the first signs of aging. Products like this often sell at beauty counters for a considerable amount of money, but you can make it quite inexpensively with natural ingredients. This recipe uses oils to keep the skin supple. Use a small amount and massage from the neckline all the way to the chin.

1. Place the chamomile in a large cup and add the boiling water. Cover and allow to steep for 15 minutes. Strain the liquid into another cup.
2. In the top of a double boiler set over simmering water, warm the avocado, almond and jojoba oils. Add the beeswax. Stir until melted. Remove from heat and beat in 1 ounce (2 tablespoons) of the warmed chamomile infusion, drop by drop until the mixture thickens and cools. Thoroughly mix in the glycerine and lemon essential oil.
3. Spoon into a sterilized, widemouthed, 6-ounce glass or ceramic jar with a tight-fitting lid. Store in a cool, dark place.

Know your skin type

To pick the best products for your skin, you need to know your skin type. Most people have a combination of skin types—particularly on the face—where oily areas around the chin, nose and forehead are different from the normal or dry skin around the eyes and on the cheeks. There are four basic skin types:

❖ **Normal skin** is clear, supple and soft. It is neither too dry nor too oily, and it is not overly sensitive to sun, humidity or the environment.
❖ **Dry skin** looks dull, feels tight after washing and needs sun protection and frequent moisturizing to prevent flaking.
❖ **Oily skin** feels soft and supple, but it looks shiny and needs cleaning several times a day. Oily skin tends to support large pores and is more prone to pimples and blackheads than dry or normal skin.
❖ **Sensitive skin** is easily burned by the sun and irritated by chemicals found in many commercial skin products that may cause rashes or blotching.

Artichoke Facial

1 fresh artichoke heart, well cooked, or canned hearts in water, not oil
2 teaspoons light oil (avocado, olive or canola)
1 teaspoon vinegar or fresh lemon juice

Artichoke conditions dry or damaged skin. It reduces flaking and restores suppleness. Enjoy making this recipe in your kitchen laboratory.

1. Mash the artichoke heart in a ceramic bowl. Mix in the oil and vinegar or lemon juice. Stir well until a smooth paste is formed.
2. Massage on your face and neck. Let sit for 10 to 15 minutes. Rinse off with warm water and pat dry.

Basic Skin Toner

1 teaspoon dried chamomile
⅓ cup (80 ml) boiling water
2 drops essential oil

A gentle cleanser or first step in your daily ritual. You can custom-design this basic skin toner to suit your skin type. See the box on page 259 to choose the essential oils that are right for you.

1. Place the chamomile and boiling water in a cup. Cover and allow to steep for 15 minutes. Strain the liquid through a fine sieve into a sterile ½ cup (125 ml) glass bottle that has a tight-fitting lid. When cool, add the essential oil and shake well to mix. Allow to stand for 48 hours, shaking periodically.
2. Pour the liquid through a paper coffee filter into a sterile glass bottle. Cap the bottle and store in a cool, dark place.
3. Apply daily with a cotton ball.

Peachy Complexion Cream

1 ripe peach
heavy cream

This wonderful rich combination is easily made. You'll find it helps give your complexion that fabled glow. And you can't find anything like it in stores.

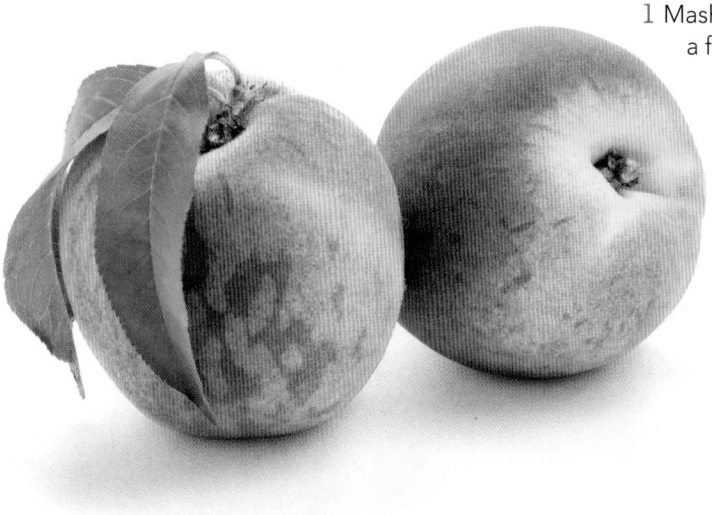

1. Mash the peach by hand or puree it in a food processor.
2. Add enough cream to the pulp to give you a soft, creamy mixture. Spoon into a clean glass jar with a tight-fitting lid and store in the refrigerator.
3. Once a day, apply the mixture to your face and massage in.

Fixed oil vs. essential oil

Olive oil, almond oil and vegetable oils are all derived primarily from seeds. They are "fixed oils" that are nonvolatile. Essential oils, distilled from leaves or flowers, are volatile and flammable. They evaporate even at low temperatures, and they are potentially toxic if they are inhaled or used incorrectly.

Most essential oils must be diluted in a fixed, or "carrier," oil before they are applied to the skin. The exceptions are lavender and tea tree essential oils, but even they should be used sparingly.

Cucumber Astringent

1 cucumber

Straight from your garden or the grocer's counter, you can make this skin bracer in a jiffy. In summer, this is a refreshing and light treat for your skin. But any time of year, a simple cucumber astringent will perk you up.

1. Peel the cucumber and puree it in a food processor. Apply the puree to your skin using a cotton pad, gently swathing your face. Rinse off with cool water.
2. Refrigerate any leftovers in a clean, covered container. The mixture should keep for 1 to 2 days.

Egg-White Toner

1 egg white

For the price of an egg, you can make this one-ingredient toner that leaves your skin feeling tight and silky smooth.

1. Clean your face thoroughly using any natural cleanser.
2. Whisk the egg white just before applying it to your face. Leave it on for about 15 minutes.
3. Wash off with tepid water and pat skin dry.

Lemon Skin Toner

¼ cup (60 ml) lemon juice
½ cup (125 ml) distilled water
⅓ cup (80 ml) witch hazel

You can toss this toner together in just a few seconds from items you have in your pantry. Total cost to you: small change.

1. Combine all the ingredients. Pour into a clean bottle or decorative cosmetics container. Shake well before using. Apply with a clean cotton ball.
2. Keep in the refrigerator indefinitely.

Facial Cleansing Mask

1 package (7 g) dry yeast
3 drops lemon juice
2 teaspoons water

This simple recipe is aimed at deep cleansing and is especially suited for young faces and the treatment of oily skin.

1. In a small bowl, mix the yeast, lemon juice and water vigorously until a thick paste forms. If necessary, add more water to achieve the correct consistency for applying to the face.
2. Pat the mixture on the face, avoiding the eyes. Allow to sit for 10 to 15 minutes. Rinse off with warm water. Pat skin dry.

Green Clay Purifying Face Mask

1 teaspoon apricot kernel oil
2 drops palmarosa
3 teaspoons bentonite or green clay powder
warm water

Green clay—also known as bentonite—is the most commonly used clay in face masks. It can absorb large quantities of water. In this mask, it is used to draw out excess sebum and dirt from deep down, making the mask suited to oily complexions. Green clay powder can be purchased online or in health food stores and is a much cheaper option than commercially prepared masks. Palmarosa is an essential oil available at health food or "new age" stores.

1. Clean your face thoroughly using any natural cleanser. In a small dish, mix the apricot oil and the palmarosa together. Put the green clay in a small bowl and stir in the apricot oil mixture. Add just enough warm water to make a spreadable paste. With your fingers, work the mixture thoroughly to incorporate all the ingredients.
2. Apply the mask immediately, avoiding the eyes. Let it sit for 10 to 15 minutes. As the moisture evaporates, you will feel the mask tighten.
3. Rinse the mask off with warm water, pat skin dry and follow with an application of toner and then moisturizer.

Instant grape cleanser for your face

Here's a sweet way to clean and refresh your skin. Split 3 or 4 large green or red grapes, remove any seeds, and rub the fleshy interior on your face and neck. The grapes condition your skin and reduce dryness, restoring suppleness. Rinse with cool water and gently pat skin dry.

Deep-Cleansing Facial

3 teaspoons yogurt (any kind)
3 teaspoons finely ground oatmeal
½ teaspoon honey

Imagine! You can mix up this deep-cleansing face mask for less than the cost of a morning newspaper.

1. Before starting, clean your face thoroughly with any natural cleanser so that you can immediately apply the deep-cleansing facial mixture when it has been stirred together.
2. In a clean bowl, combine the yogurt and oatmeal and mix to a spreadable consistency. In a small glass bowl sitting in a larger bowl of hot water, warm the honey and pour it into the yogurt and oatmeal mixture. Using a spoon, blend.
3. Immediately apply the mask to your face, avoiding the eyes, and let it stay on for 10 to 15 minutes. Wash it off with warm water. Pat skin dry and apply a toner and moisturizer.

Almond Mayonnaise Scrub

¼ cup (40 g) whole, natural almonds
⅛ teaspoon mayonnaise
1 teaspoon red wine or cider vinegar
½ cup (125 ml) water

Don't be afraid of this one, but keep in mind that it is for very dry skin. Mayonnaise will nourish the face. Almonds will provide a mild exfoliation.

1. Clean your face thoroughly with any natural cleanser. Grind the almonds in a blender or food processor until they form a meal. Whirl in the mayonnaise. Set aside.
2. In a small bowl, combine the vinegar and water. Rinse your face with this mixture.
3. Now gently and thoroughly massage your face with the almond-mayonnaise scrub. Leave it on your skin for 10 minutes. Rinse off with warm water and pat skin dry.

Honey Mask

⅔ cup (85 g) instant oats
½ cup (125 ml) hot water
½ apple, cored but with peel on
2 heaping tablespoons (40 g) plain yogurt
2 tablespoons (30 ml) honey
1 egg white

The mask's ingredients would make up a solid breakfast, but they're nourishing for your skin, too. For the cost of a bowl of cereal, it's a good deal for a meal or a mask.

1. Clean your face thoroughly with any natural cleanser. In a small bowl, stir the oats into the hot water until you have a smooth mixture. Let stand for about 5 minutes or until the mixture thickens to a paste.
2. Put the apple, yogurt, honey, and egg white in a blender or food processor and pulse for 45 seconds just to mix. Now add the oat mixture and pulse for 20 seconds more.
3. Apply this mask evenly to the face, avoiding the eyes, and let sit for 15 minutes or until skin feels tight. Rinse thoroughly with warm water and pat skin dry.

Banana, Sour Cream and Honey Face Mask

½ banana
3 teaspoons honey
2 tablespoons (30 ml) sour cream

Although this recipe sounds somewhat like dessert, it's actually an enriching mask for your face. The banana is an astringent, the honey conditions and the sour cream binds them together in a mask. You could travel to a fancy spa for a treatment like this, but making it at home will cost you next to nothing. Enjoy!

1 Clean your face thoroughly with any natural cleanser. In a small bowl, mash the half-banana. Stir in the honey and sour cream.
2 Apply to your face, avoiding the eyes, and let set for 10 minutes. Gently wipe off with a damp washcloth. Rinse clean with warm water. Pat your skin dry.

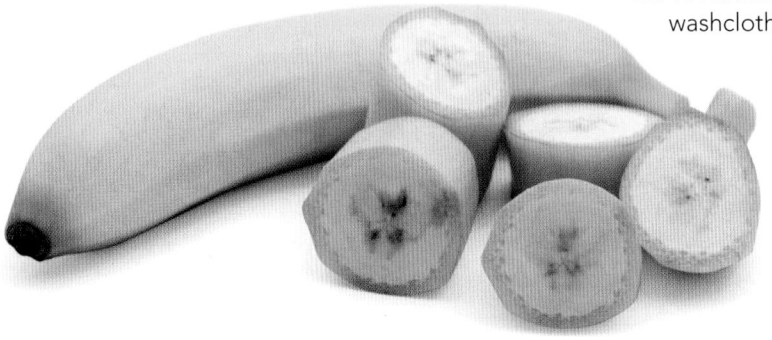

Youthful Skin Face Mask

¼ cup (60 ml) heavy whipping cream
1 medium banana
1 vitamin E capsule, 500 IU

In this variation of the banana facial mask, banana is again the astringent. It induces a tightening or tingling sensation and thereby gives the effect of decreasing the appearance of wrinkles.

1 Clean your face thoroughly with any natural cleanser. In a small bowl, mash together the cream and banana. Pierce the vitamin E capsule with a needle, squeeze out the contents, and stir in.
2 Smooth onto your face and neck. Leave on for 10 to 15 minutes. Remove with damp cloth. Rinse clean with warm water. Pat your skin dry.

When vitamin E is called for

Several of the recipes in this part of the book call for using vitamin E. You can buy vitamin E oil as a liquid at most pharmacies, but when you only need a small amount, it's sometimes more practical to use a 500 IU vitamin E capsule. Just pierce the capsule with a needle and squeeze out the contents.

A quick banana wrinkle fighter

Peel away the years with this easy facial treatment. Banana is an astringent that induces a tightening or tingling sensation on the skin, which helps decrease the appearance of wrinkles. When bananas are at their best and cheapest, this is a very reasonable facial treatment. Clean your face thoroughly with any natural cleanser. Mash one-quarter of a ripe banana until very creamy and spread it all over your face, avoiding the eyes. Leave on for 15 to 20 minutes. Rinse with warm water and then splash cold water on your face. Gently pat your skin dry.

Oatmeal Exfoliant

2 heaped teaspoons fine oatmeal
1 teaspoon baking soda
lukewarm water

Here's a treat for your face that might be part of a spa regimen. You can mix this up in a jiffy to use as a cleanser anytime you're in the mood. Cost to you: almost negligible.

1. Clean your face thoroughly with any natural cleanser.
2. In a small bowl, stir together the oatmeal and baking soda. (The oatmeal needs to be fine; if necessary, first pulse it in a food processor or blender.) Add enough lukewarm water to make a paste. Apply to face and rub gently. Rinse and gently pat the skin dry.

Mask for Oily Skin

1 teaspoon brewer's yeast
⅓ cup (90 g) yogurt, or as needed

The combination of brewer's yeast and yogurt deep-cleanses oily skin without overdrying. This inexpensive homemade mask leaves skin feeling fresh and revitalized.

1. Clean your face thoroughly with any natural cleanser. In a small bowl, mix the brewer's yeast with the yogurt to make a thin paste. Pat this mixture onto the oily areas of your face. Allow the mask to dry for 15 to 20 minutes.
2. Rinse with warm water. Splash with cool water. Gently pat dry.

Galen's Cold Cream

1 oz (30 g) cosmetic-grade beeswax, grated or shaved
⅓ cup (80 ml) light olive oil
2 tablespoons (30 ml) distilled water or rose water
3 drops geranium essential oil

This recipe for cold cream is believed to have been devised by the Greek philosopher and doctor Galen in the 2nd century AD. It is still every bit as effective today and will cost you very little compared to the name brands at cosmetics counters.

1 In the top of a double boiler over simmering water, melt the beeswax gently.
2 In a small saucepan over low heat, heat the oil slightly and then pour it into the melted wax. Using a fork, beat this mixture until combined.
3 Now heat the water or rose water in the saucepan and then stir it into the oil and wax mixture, one drop at a time. Remove from heat and stir until the mixture is cooled and thick. Stir in the essential oil.
4 Using a wooden spoon, put the mixture into a clean 5-ounce widemouthed jar with a tight-fitting lid. Store in a cool, dark place for several months.

How to apply a face mask

Women have used face masks for centuries to clean and tone the skin and give it a glowing vitality. Face masks give their best results if used regularly—once a week is not too often.

1 To make the process easier, sit or stand before a mirror. Cover your shoulders with a clean towel and have a damp washcloth or hand towel ready for wiping up any drips.
2 Apply the mask with a clean cotton ball or with your fingers. The mask should cover your face from the hairline to the chin, missing only the area around the eyes.
3 Leave the mask on for 15 minutes the first few times you use it. Later, if your skin is not irritated and you like the mask's effects, you can slowly increase the time to 30 minutes. To best enjoy the facial mask, lie down, shut your eyes, and relax while the mask is working.
4 When the time is up, remove the mask with your fingers over a basin. If the mask has dried, splash warm water on your face and try again to remove the mask with your fingers. Then use a wet washcloth to remove the last residue of the mask. Finally, splash your face with cool water, pat the skin dry, and apply a toner and moisturizer.

Strawberry Yogurt Mask

1 handful ripe strawberries
3 teaspoons ground almonds
2 tablespoons (30 g) yogurt

If you grow strawberries in your garden, pluck a few to use in this treatment. Your face will thank you for this gentle, delicious treat that leaves the skin smooth and refreshed.

1. Clean your face thoroughly with any natural cleanser. In a small bowl, mash the strawberries and almonds until completely blended together. Stir in the yogurt to make a spreadable paste.
2. Apply immediately or refrigerate and use within 1 day on a clean face.

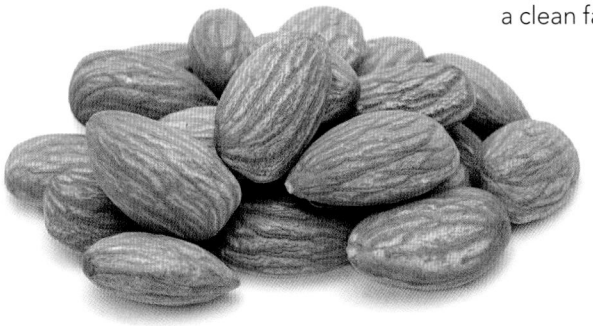

Care for Lips and Mouth

Honey Lip Balm

3 oz (90 g) cosmetic-grade beeswax, grated or shaved
½ cup (125 ml) extra virgin olive oil
1 oz (30 g) honey
½ capsule vitamin E, 500 IU

You'll get a kick out of making lip balm at home. You'll feel a little bit like a mad scientist and a little bit like a truly creative cook. The following three formulations are inexpensive to make and provide a lot of lip gloss or balm for the buck. Consider dividing the lip balm mixture into several small containers so that you can carry some with you.

1. In a microwave or the top of a double boiler, melt the beeswax and oil together. Do not boil. If the mixture starts to boil, remove from heat and allow it to cool. Once the beeswax and oil are blended, stir in the honey. Then pierce the vitamin E capsule with a needle, squeeze out half the contents, and stir in. Pour the resulting mixture into clean containers with tops.
2. Let the lip balm sit at room temperature for 48 hours until it arrives at the proper consistency for spreading. You can carry a small container of lip balm around with you during the day, but you may find it keeps better in the refrigerator overnight.

Cocoa Lip Balm

3 oz (90 g) cosmetic-grade beeswax, grated or shaved
½ cup (125 ml) extra virgin olive oil
½ teaspoon cocoa powder
½ capsule vitamin E, 500 IU

Remember, although this concoction smells sweet, it is not a food product. If you plan to give the balm to a child, label it accordingly and explain how to use it.

1. In a microwave or the top of a double boiler, melt the beeswax and oil together. Do not boil. If the mixture starts to boil, remove from the heat and allow it to cool. Once the beeswax and oil are blended, stir in the cocoa powder. Pierce the vitamin E capsule with a needle, squeeze out half the contents, and stir it in. Pour the resulting mixture into clean containers with tops.
2. Let the lip balm sit for 48 hours at room temperature until it arrives at the proper consistency for spreading. You can carry a small container of lip balm around with you during the day, but you may find it keeps better in the refrigerator overnight.

Chocolate Chip Lip Balm

3 oz (90 g) cosmetic-grade beeswax, grated or shaved
½ cup (125 ml) extra virgin olive oil
½ capsule vitamin E, 500 IU
3–6 chocolate chips

When you cook up this little treat in your kitchen, you may be tempted to eat it, but this yummy-smelling lip balm is not a food. Be sure to label it as lip balm and to supervise its use on children.

1. In a microwave or the top of a double boiler, melt the beeswax and oil together. Do not boil. If the mixture starts to boil, remove from the heat and allow it to cool. Once the beeswax and oil are blended, pierce the vitamin E capsule with a needle, squeeze out half the contents, and stir in. Stir in the chocolate chips and pour the resulting mixture into clean containers with tops.
2. Let the lip balm sit for 48 hours at room temperature until it arrives at the proper consistency for spreading. You can carry a small container of lip balm around with you during the day, but you may find it keeps better in the refrigerator overnight.

A fast, hard-working mouthwash

For fighting bacteria and removing food particles caught in your teeth, this inexpensive recipe is about as effective a mouthwash as you can get. It uses the standard 3 percent hydrogen peroxide sold in pharmacies. Hydrogen peroxide, however, may irritate sensitive teeth or delicate tissue in the mouth, so this rinse should not be used any more than three times a week. In a cup, mix 2 tablespoons (30 ml) hydrogen peroxide solution with 2 tablespoons (30 ml) water. Swish the mixture in your mouth for 30 seconds, then spit it out—don't swallow it.

Refreshing Mouthwash

1 cup (250 ml) water
2 tablespoons (15 g) angelica seeds
dash of peppermint oil or lemon verbena

For just a few cents or pence, you can cook up a potful of this rinse that tastes good and can be safely used as often as you like. Unlike more expensive commercial mouthwashes, it has no alcohol.

1. In a small saucepan over medium heat, bring the water to a boil. Remove from the heat. Stir in the angelica seeds and peppermint oil or lemon verbena. Let the mixture sit for 10 minutes. Strain off and discard the solids.
2. Store the liquid in a clean, covered container in the refrigerator and use every day. It should keep indefinitely.

Spicy, Minty Mouthwash

1 cup (250 ml) water
1 teaspoon whole cloves
1 teaspoon ground cinnamon
1 teaspoon peppermint extract
2 teaspoons finely chopped fresh parsley

This simple recipe offers a kick that will make your mouth feel wonderful for hours. Use it as often as you like—it's inexpensive and doesn't burn like some commercial mouthwashes with alcohol in them.

1. In a small saucepan, bring the water to a boil over medium heat. Remove the pan from the stove and stir in the cloves, cinnamon, peppermint extract and parsley. Let the mixture sit for 10 minutes. Strain off the solids.
2. Pour the liquid into a clean, tightly covered container and store in the refrigerator, where it will keep indefinitely. Use as a gargle and mouthwash.

Bacteria-Fighting Citrus Mouthwash

¾ cup (185 ml) vodka
30 drops lemon essential oil
25 drops bergamot essential oil
1¼ cups (310 ml) distilled water

Fight the damaging bacteria that dwell in your mouth with this lemon-tasting mouthwash with an alcohol base that acts as a disinfectant. Rinse and swish or gargle, but don't swallow the liquid.

1. Place the vodka and the lemon and bergamot essential oils in a sterilized 16-ounce glass bottle with a tight-fitting lid. Shake the mixture vigorously to combine.
2. Add the distilled water and shake until well blended. Leave in the refrigerator for 1 week to mature, shaking the bottle from time to time.
3. To use, shake the bottle and mix 1 part of the mixture with 3 parts lukewarm distilled water in a small drinking glass. Rinse, but do not swallow the mouthwash.

Toothpaste

½ cup (140 g) baking soda
2 teaspoons salt
3 teaspoons glycerine
10 or more drops peppermint or wintergreen flavoring
1 drop green or blue food coloring (optional)
warm water

Once you perfect your own homemade toothpaste recipe by adjusting the ingredients to your liking, you should be able to keep a family of four in toothpaste for a whole year for less than the cost of one commercial tube!

1. In a small bowl, mix the baking soda and salt. Add the glycerine, flavoring and, if desired, 1 drop food coloring. Add warm water, a drop at a time, until the texture and consistency seem right. Spoon the mixture into a clean squeeze bottle or any convenient, clean container with a tight lid.
2. You may have to adjust the amount of glycerine to arrive at a consistency that suits you. This toothpaste will keep indefinitely in a covered container.

Shampoos, Conditioners and Rinses

Beer Shampoo

¾ cup (185 ml) beer
1 cup (250 ml) shampoo (any kind)

This concoction will leave your hair with wonderful body. The proteins from the malt and hops in the beer coat the hair and build it up, helping to repair damage.

1. In a nonreactive pan, boil the beer until it reduces to ¼ cup (60 ml). Cool the beer and add it to the 1 cup of shampoo in a clean bottle with a tight cap.
2. Wash your hair as usual. Rinse thoroughly.

Dandruff Treatment

2 teaspoons dried rosemary
2 teaspoons dried thyme
⅔ cup (170 ml) boiling water
⅔ cup (170 ml) cider vinegar

Over-the-counter dandruff treatments can be costly. You can create this herbal remedy for considerably less than you'll pay for a commercial treatment.

1. Place the herbs in a heatproof ceramic bowl. Pour in the boiling water. Cover and allow to steep for 15 to 20 minutes.
2. Strain the liquid into a clean, 10-ounce bottle with a tight-fitting lid. Add the vinegar and shake. Store in a cool, dark place.
3. After shampooing, rinse hair thoroughly and then massage a small amount of the herbal treatment into the scalp. Between shampoos, massage a small amount into the scalp before going to bed.

A quick, sweet-smelling vinegar hair rinse

Pick up a bottle of raspberry or plum vinegar next time you go shopping. It's inexpensive in the supermarket and can do double duty in the kitchen. Use a few spoonfuls for this recipe and the rest for salad dressings.

Rather than prepare this rinse ahead of time, simply bring a clean 1- or 2- cup (250 or 500 ml) measuring cup containing 2 to 3 tablespoons (30–45 ml) scented vinegar into the shower. After shampooing, add water and rinse your hair with the solution. You can use this every time you shampoo, if you like.

Vinegar restores the proper acidic pH balance to hair. This rinse will remove remnants of shampoo and give your hair more shine.

Highlighting Rinse

juice of 1 lemon
2 teaspoons chamomile tea

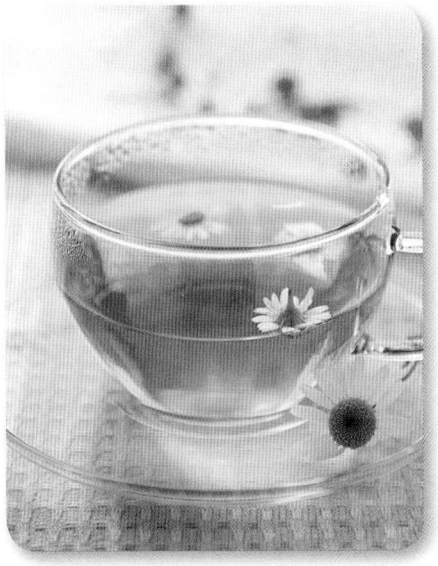

This is a rich hair dressing that provides sheen and elegance to tired hair. People with light-colored hair will find that it helps them get clean, honest-looking highlights. It can also be used as a pressing solution for hair straightening.

1. In a small bowl, mix the lemon juice and tea. To achieve blonde highlights, use an inexpensive straw hat with lots of holes in it. Pull strands of hair you would like to lighten through the holes with a crochet hook or pencil.
2. Douse the strands with the rinse. Sit in the sun for 1½ hours, protecting your body from the sun's rays, of course.

What herbs in hair rinses do

- **Chamomile** Keeps scalp and hair follicles healthy
- **Comfrey** Soothes scalp irritations
- **Elderberries** Traditionally used to add color to gray hair
- **Lemongrass** Tones scalp
- **Nettle** An astringent that helps relieve skin irritations and itching
- **Parsley** Helps to relieve skin irritations
- **Rosemary** Believed to enhance color of dark hair and help control dandruff
- **Sage** An astringent for oily hair and a benefit for damaged or fragile hair
- **Thyme** Has antiseptic, tonic and astringent properties
- **Yarrow** Acts as a tonic for the hair

Chamomile Shampoo

1 handful fresh or dried chamomile flowers
1¼ cups (310 ml) boiling water
3 tablespoons (15 g) pure soap flakes or leftover slivers of soap
3 teaspoons glycerine
5 drops yellow food coloring

This mild shampoo leaves your hair clean and healthy. The recipe gives you a chance to use those leftover slivers of soap that you wonder why you save. Forget those well-advertised, costly shampoos—you need only 3 teaspoons of this inexpensive shampoo per washing.

1 Place the flowers in a heatproof bowl and add the boiling water. Let stand for 15 minutes, then strain into another heatproof bowl.
2 Clean out the first bowl. Combine the soap flakes and the chamomile mixture and let them stand until the soap softens—a few minutes. Beat in the glycerine and food coloring until well blended.
3 Pour the mixture into a clean 14-ounce bottle with a tight-fitting lid. Keep in a cool, dark place.

Instant Dry Shampoo

3 teaspoons cornstarch or finely ground oatmeal

This home-style, penny-pinching recipe is tailor-made for that moment when you need a quick pick-me-up or you haven't got time to wash your hair.

1 Sprinkle small amounts of cornstarch or oatmeal onto the hair, lifting it up in sections to let the powder get to the scalp. Rub the dry shampoo through the hair to absorb excess oil.
2 Comb the hair to remove tangles, then spend 5 to 10 minutes brushing (depending on the length and thickness of the hair) to remove all traces of the powder and prevent the suggestion of dandruff. Shake and blow on your hairbrush to clean it while you brush your hair.

Thick Hair Conditioner for Everyone

½ ripe avocado
¼ cup (60 ml) coconut milk, or as needed

This two-ingredient conditioner offers a protein boost for your hair that in turn will make it feel thicker and more luxuriant. You don't need to go to an expensive hair salon to revitalize your hair.

1 In a small bowl, mash the avocado with a spoon. Mix in the coconut milk to form a thick gel-like substance.
2 Apply entire recipe to clean hair and comb through. Leave the conditioner on the hair for 10 to 15 minutes. Rinse thoroughly.

Nourishing Conditioner

2 tablespoons (30 ml) olive oil
3 teaspoons lemon juice
½ teaspoon apple cider vinegar
1 egg

Use this to leave your hair feeling cleansed and enriched at a fraction of the cost of salon treatments.

1. In a blender, combine the ingredients and whirl until blended. Alternatively, whisk vigorously until combined.
2. Use entire recipe to condition hair after a regular shampoo. Leave on the hair for 10 to 15 minutes. Rinse clean.

Natural Head Lice Treatment

¼ cup (60 ml) olive oil
20 drops tea tree oil
15 drops rosemary essential oil
15 drops lemon essential oil
15 drops thyme essential oil
small amount of regular shampoo (any kind)

Try this herbal remedy for an effective, gentler alternative to those harsh commercial treatments.

1. Combine the olive oil and essential oils in a small bowl, add a small amount of shampoo and mix well.
2. Massage into dry hair, making sure it is thoroughly covered.
3. Cover the hair with a towel, plastic wrap or a shower cap and leave for 1 hour.
4. Shampoo the mixture out of the hair, then comb the hair carefully with a nit comb to remove any dead lice and nits.

Body Care Treatments

Warm Herbal Body Treatment

8 cups (2 liters) water
4 chamomile tea bags or other gentle herbal tea
3 peppermint tea bags
sprigs of fresh rosemary or sage (optional)

This warm, scented spa-style treatment will relax and rejuvenate you—for the cost of a few tea bags!

1. In a large saucepan, bring the water to a boil. Remove from heat and add the tea bags and herbs. Cover pan and steep for 10 to 15 minutes. Once the tea has cooled to a comfortably warm temperature, remove the tea bags and herbs.
2. Drop several clean but dispensable hand towels into the tea until saturated, then wring them out. Wrap your upper arms and legs with the tea-soaked towels. You may also place a soaked towel on your torso, but don't put one on your face.
3. Lie down on a protected bed, couch or pad and rest for 10 to 15 minutes. Remove the towels and relax while cooling off for another 10 to 15 minutes. Shower off the residue.

Caution: Heat treatments such as this are not recommended for people with high blood pressure or heart problems.

Citrus Moisturizing Treatment

1 egg yolk
2 tablespoons (30 ml) lemon juice
1 cup (250 ml) olive oil

This creamy moisturizer will leave your skin soft and silky, while barely leaving a mark on your grocery bill.

1. In a medium bowl, whisk the egg yolk, lemon juice and olive oil together until the mixture reaches a creamy consistency. Thin with more lemon juice as desired.
2. Massage into your skin as an intense moisturizing treatment before a shower or bath. Apply a light coating on your hands, arms, legs and face. Gently massage into nails and cuticles. Apply about 1 tablespoon to each foot. Gently massage your toes, one by one, and then the arch of your foot, moving to the heel. Relax and allow the moisturizer to soak in for 10 to 15 minutes. Wipe away the excess and then step into the shower or tub to complete the treatment.
3. Store any leftovers in the refrigerator for a day or two.

Green Aloe Moisturizing Lotion

1 cup (250 ml) aloe vera gel
1 teaspoon vitamin E oil (if necessary, break several 500 IU capsules)
5–10 drops essential oil of your choosing
¾ oz (25 g) cosmetic-grade beeswax, grated or shaved
½ cup (125 ml) vegetable oil

It takes no time and very little money to cook up this delightful body lotion that has aloe vera, an antioxidant, as its primary ingredient. You scoop the gel out of aloe vera leaves or you can buy it at a health food store.

1. In a medium bowl, stir together the aloe vera gel, vitamin E and essential oil. Set aside.
2. In the top of a double boiler over simmering water, melt together the beeswax and vegetable oil. Stir until smooth and well blended. Remove from heat.
3. Slowly and continuously pour the melted mixture into the bowl with the aloe vera mixture, using a handheld electric mixer at slow speed to combine. Run a clean rubber spatula around the rim of the bowl to incorporate all the ingredients. Continue mixing until all the ingredients are blended.
4. Pour the final mixture into one sterilized 13-ounce jar or two sterilized 6-ounce jars with tight-fitting lids. You can use sterilized jam jars, if you have them. Keep the lotion in the refrigerator for up to 6 weeks.

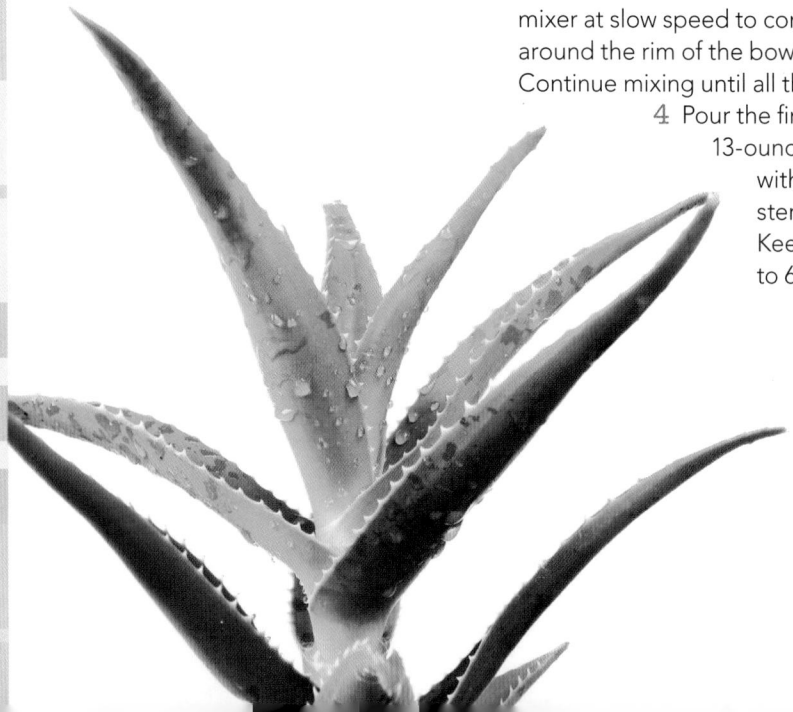

The best body oil for your skin type

To make body oil, put 4 teaspoons almond oil in a small sterile glass jar with a tight-fitting lid. Add the appropriate drops of essential oils listed below for your skin type, shake and pour a little into your palm so that you can apply it to the rest of your body. Each blend will give you four body rubs.

Normal skin	Dry skin	Oily skin	Sensitive skin
8 drops lavender	8 drops patchouli	10 drops lemon	3 drops geranium
6 drops geranium	4 drops geranium	6 drops geranium	2 drops patchouli
2 drops chamomile	2 drops carrot	4 drops sandalwood	

Shaving Gel for Women

- 2 tablespoons (30 ml) conditioner
- 2 tablespoons (30 ml) shampoo (preferably the same brand as the conditioner used)
- ½–1 teaspoon baby oil
- 1 teaspoon hand cream

Using just four ingredients you probably already have at home, you can make your very own gel for shaving legs and underarms. It's a good recipe to make in a pinch, but it will also help you cut one more expense from your weekly shopping bill.

1. Start with a clean bottle with a secure cap. Pour the conditioner into the bottle, then add the shampoo. Mix together. Add the baby oil and then the hand cream. Secure the top and shake until all the ingredients are well blended. Let mixture sit for about 1 hour before using.
2. Lather legs or underarms with the gel, shave and rinse skin thoroughly. The shaving gel should keep for about 1 month in the bathroom. If the mixture separates, just shake it up before you use it.

Summer Body Splash

- ⅓ cup (80 ml) vodka
- 10 drops lavender essential oil
- 5 drops lime essential oil
- 5 drops lemon essential oil
- 5 drops lemongrass essential oil
- 2 cups (500 ml) distilled or boiled water

Refresh yourself with a splash of this delicate mixture of fruit and flower scents just perfect for hot summer days and nights.

1. Pour the vodka and essential oils into a sterilized 20-ounce bottle with a tight-fitting stopper. Stopper the bottle and shake for several minutes. Add the distilled or boiled water and shake for several minutes more. Set aside for at least 48 hours or up to 3 weeks.
2. Place a paper coffee filter in a sieve and drip the liquid through the filter into a ceramic or glass bowl. Pour the liquid back into the large bottle or into a few smaller sterilized bottles. Keep one bottle in the refrigerator and store the others in a cool, dark place until needed.

What is a cool, dark place?

When you make home remedies and beauty products, you are usually told to store them in a cool, dark, dry place. Where is that?

If you seal things in amber or opaque containers, that takes care of dark (most homemade preparations are weakened by exposure to sunlight). A cool, dry place could be the linen cupboard or a shelf in a closet that is not near any hot pipes, or a garage cupboard if the garage is dry. A safe last resort is the refrigerator.

Simple Fragrant Body Splash

1 cup (250 ml) water
5–7 drops perfume oil

If you have a favorite perfume oil that you'd like to wear in a lighter concentration, you'll love this easy recipe. Keep this spritzer in your purse for a pick-me-up on a warm day.

1. Have on hand a clean 8-ounce spray bottle. Pour the water into the bottle and drip the perfume oil drops into the water. Cover the top with your thumb and shake well.
2. Screw the top on and your body splash is ready.

Citrus Cologne Splash

1 lime
½ cup (125 ml) rubbing alcohol
3 teaspoons lemon extract or orange extract

Make this cooling scent at home for spare change.

1. Juice the lime and strain out the pulp. Combine the rubbing alcohol, lime juice and lemon or orange extract in a clean bottle with a tight-fitting lid. Shake well.
2. Dab on pulse points. You may also transfer the splash to a spray bottle. Store the splash in the refrigerator.

Cellulite Massage Oil

2 tablespoons (30 ml) almond oil
½ teaspoon jojoba oil
½ teaspoon carrot oil
14 drops geranium essential oil
6 drops lemongrass essential oil
4 drops cypress essential oil

Include this massage oil—along with regular exercise and a healthy diet—in your tool kit to help lessen cellulite. A regular massage with this oil may help increase circulation and break down fatty deposits.

1. Combine all the ingredients in a 1½- to 2-ounce sterilized glass jar with a tight-fitting lid. Shake vigorously.
2. After a bath or shower, pat your skin dry and massage a small amount of the oil on cellulite-affected areas, using circular movements. Use ¼ to ½ teaspoon, depending on the size of the area you are treating. Apply only once a day.

Almond Exfoliating Body Scrub

¼ cup (60 g) coarse sea salt
¼ cup (60 ml) baby oil
½ teaspoon almond extract, vanilla extract, or lightly scented perfume oil

Scented, gritty body scrubs are all the rage. Here's a recipe you can make at home for next to nothing.

1 In a small bowl, stir the salt and baby oil together until the oil is thoroughly incorporated into the salt. Add the extract and stir until it, too, is incorporated.
2 Use in the shower, after you are thoroughly wet. Apply with your hands, a washcloth or a body puff scrubber. Massage in and rinse off.

Simple Sugar Scrub for Dry Skin

1 cup (220 g) sugar
½ cup (125 ml) olive, grapeseed or other oil
2 drops vanilla or almond extract (optional)

Here's another yummy body scrub that costs less than a cup of coffee for three or four uses.

1 In a medium bowl, combine the sugar and oil. Mix with a wooden spoon until you achieve a pastelike blend. Add extract if desired and stir until incorporated.
2 Transfer to a clean, airtight glass container to slow breakdown of the oil.
3 In the shower, massage this mixture gently over damp skin. It will exfoliate and moisturize at the same time. Do not use on broken, irritated or scarred skin. Avoid the eyes. This is an especially oily mixture, so it is really best for dry skin.
4 Store the mixture in the refrigerator for 6 months to 1 year.

Cranberry Sugar Scrub

½ cup (80 g) frozen cranberries
1 teaspoon glycerine
¼ cup (60 ml) sweet almond oil
¼ cup (55 g) sugar
2 drops orange essential oil
2 tablespoons (15 g) oat powder (grind oatmeal in blender if needed)

The beauty of sugar scrub recipes is the way they offer up scent while managing to exfoliate, nourish and polish the skin. Here is another spa-quality product you can make in your own kitchen.

1 In the container of a food processor, combine cranberries, glycerine and almond oil and process for 30 seconds—just enough to blend the ingredients without turning the berries to pulp. You want to keep the mixture thick.
2 Transfer the mixture to a bowl and stir in the sugar. Stir in the essential oil. Add just enough of the oat powder to create a cohesive mixture that you can apply to your skin.
3 In the shower, rub the mixture on your skin. Massage in and remove with warm water.

Body Powder

½ cup (75 g) arrowroot
2 tablespoons (20 g) white cosmetic clay powder
7 drops lavender essential oil
5 drops clary sage essential oil
2 drops patchouli essential oil

This fresh-smelling and silky after-shower powder can be used every day. For a more feminine product, use just lavender and rose essential oils.

1 In a medium bowl, mix the arrowroot with the white cosmetic clay. Add the essential oils and mix well with your fingers.
2 Store in a tightly covered container for a couple of days to allow the powder to absorb the oils, then use all over your body as desired.

Body Spray

3 teaspoons finely chopped orange peel
3 teaspoons finely chopped lemon peel
3 tablespoons (45 ml) vodka
3 teaspoons witch hazel
1 cup (250 ml) water
5 drops lemon verbena essential oil
10 drops bergamot essential oil
10 drops orange essential oil

This citrusy mixture smells good, tones the skin, and feels delightfully cool.

1 In a small jar with a tight top, add orange and lemon peels to the vodka. Cover and leave for 1 week in a cool, dark place.
2 Strain the liquid into a clean spray bottle. Add the witch hazel, water and the essential oils. Shake well and use as needed. Store in the refrigerator for up to 2 weeks.

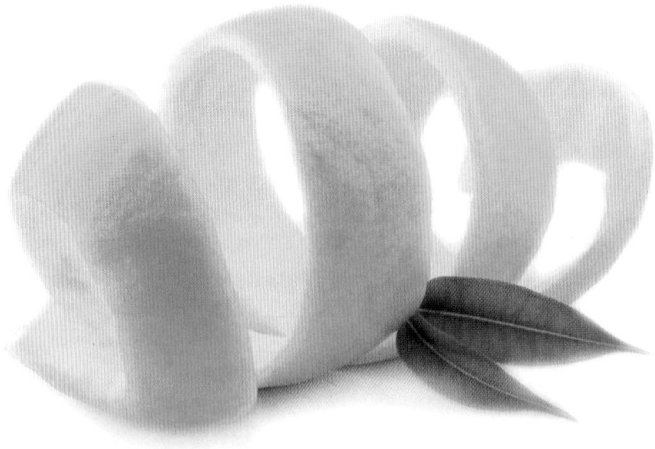

Deodorant

¼ cup (60 ml) distilled witch hazel
1 oz (30 ml) sage alcohol-based herbal extract
10 drops grapefruit-seed extract
10 drops clary sage essential oil
5 drops patchouli essential oil

Here's a serious homemade underarm deodorant that won't stain your clothes or strain your wallet.

1 In a small spray bottle, combine all the ingredients.
2 Shake well and spray under arms as needed.

Bath Products

Bubble Bath for Kids

½ cup (125 ml) shampoo
¾ cup (185 ml) water
¼ teaspoon table salt

This simple recipe provides a scented, bubbly bathful of suds that you know are safe for your child and, as a bonus, helps you recycle extra shampoo. As always, parents should supervise children's use of such products. Beware of slippery tubs. Bubble baths are fun, but children shouldn't use them daily. Too much of a good thing could irritate sensitive skin.

1 In a medium bowl, mix the shampoo and water. Gently stir until blended. Add the salt. Stir until the mixture thickens.
2 Pour through a funnel into a clean bottle with a tight cap. This bubble bath will keep safely for months in the bathroom.

Conditioning Bubble Bath

¼ cup (60 ml) gentle dishwashing liquid
5–6 cups (1.25–1.5 liters) water
1 oz (30 ml) glycerine

For an inexpensive, fun and squeaky-clean bubble bath, this recipe gives you lots of bubbles and cleans up the tub as well. To be extra safe, test the solution on your child's inner arm to make sure he or she is not allergic to the solution. As always, parents should handle bubble bath products. Keep out of children's reach.

1 In a small bucket, swish all the ingredients together, altering the balance as you see fit. Pour into a bathtub of warm water for long-lasting bubbles. You may want to bring a bubble wand to the tub.
2 Keep an eye on children in the tub, which may be extra slippery with the bubble bath. Infants and very young children should not take bubble baths.

Bath Gel

½ cup (125 ml) distilled or bottled water (not tap water)
one package (10 g) unflavored gelatin
½ cup (125 ml) baby shampoo

This recipe is especially suited for children or adults with sensitive skin. It's easy to make and costs very little for an 8-ounce jar. Wrap a grosgrain ribbon around the jar and you've got a delightful homemade gift.

1. In a small saucepan, bring the water to a boil. Add the gelatin and stir until it is dissolved. Remove the mixture from heat. Slowly stir in the baby shampoo. Let this mixture cool until it's tepid enough to put in a clean, decorative widemouthed jar with a tight-fitting lid.
2. Place the jar in the refrigerator to set the gel.
3. Use a few teaspoons of gel per bath. Bath gel should keep for up to 1 month in the refrigerator.

Liquid or Gel Soap

2 cups (200 g) pure soap flakes or grated bar soap
8 cups (2 liters) water
2 tablespoons (30 ml) glycerine

This bath or hand soap is easy to cook up and is a good way to use up old slivers of bar soap. Transfer the liquid soap to an empty pump container and you can supply your bathroom for just a portion of the price you'd pay at the store.

1. In a large pot or Dutch oven, combine all the ingredients. Cook over low heat, stirring occasionally, until the soap flakes have dissolved.
2. Transfer the mixture to a clean ½-gallon container and cover tightly. For a thinner gel soap, increase the water to 1 gallon.

Almond Rose Soap

2 tablespoons (5 g) dried red rose petals
2½ cups (250 g) pure soap flakes
⅔ cup (170 ml) boiling water
½ cup (125 ml) rose water
2 tablespoons (20 g) ground almonds
9 drops geranium essential oil

Here's a simple method of soap-making that uses just a few basic tools. You'll create a fragrant soap that gently cleans and exfoliates.

1. Pound the rose petals with a mortar and pestle. In a large bowl, combine the ground petals, soap and water and stir until smooth. If the soap starts to solidify, place the bowl over near-boiling water.
2. Stir in the rose water and ground almonds. Allow to cool. Stir in the essential oil.
3. Shape the mixture into 6 balls and flatten them slightly. Allow the soap to harden between sheets of parchment paper. Keep any unused soap in a cool, dark place until needed.

Cinnamon Soap

2 lb (1 kg) leftover soap (or buy bulk bars)
3 teaspoons spring water
1 teaspoon glycerine
½ teaspoon cinnamon essential oil
3 teaspoons sweet orange essential oil
10 drops clove bud essential oil (optional)

You'll enjoy making this rich, spicy soap, which gives you another opportunity to use up leftover soap scraps.

1. Coarsely grate the scraps of soap into a large mixing bowl. Add the spring water, glycerine and essential oils. Mix well.
2. Cover the bowl with a clean cloth and allow it to stand for about 15 minutes, until the soap is slightly soft and pliable. (If your soap scraps are fairly new, they may be soft and not need much softening time.)
3. Scoop the mixture up by the handful and press or roll it into small balls. Compress it tightly. Place on parchment paper. Allow the soap balls to dry and harden for 1 to 2 days.

Strawberries and Cream Bath Bags

½ cup (60 g) oats (regular or quick)
½ cup (50 g) powdered milk
4 tablespoons (40 g) almond meal (if necessary, grind almonds in blender, coffee grinder or food processor)
16 drops strawberry essential oil

Here's a charming idea you can make that provides a relaxing and soothing bath. The oatmeal mixture may help relieve dry or itching skin. For extra-sensitive skin, reduce or eliminate the essential oil. Dress up this bath product by scooping it into attractive cloth bags bought at a crafts store to create your own inexpensive version of exclusive bath goodies.

1. In a small bowl, combine the oatmeal, powdered milk and almond meal, stirring to mix well. Stir in the essential oil until blended. Divide the mixture among three pretty cloth bags, and tie them at the top. Tie a generous loop of string or ribbon to the top of each bag.
2. When ready to use, hang the bag from the tub faucet by its loop. When you fill the bath, the water will run over the mixture inside the bag, dispersing it into the bath.
3. Keep the bath bags in a cool, dark place until ready to use.

Herbal Bath Bag

1 large handful mixed herbs (rosemary, lovage, lavender, lemongrass, sage, parsley or peppermint)
cheesecloth

This is a simple luxury for your bath. It makes you smell good afterward, but it is also delightful while you soak.

1. Place herbs of your choice in a doubled square of cheesecloth. Gather up the corners and tie securely.
2. Toss the herb bag into a hot bath to soften and scent the water. Once you're in the bath, rub it all over your skin, paying particular attention to areas where odor is a problem.

Cinnamon Oatmeal Milk Bath

1 cup (100 g) powdered milk
½ cup (140 g) baking soda
½ cup (60 g) finely ground oatmeal
2 teaspoons cornstarch
1 teaspoon cream of tartar
1 teaspoon cinnamon

Mixing up this pleasantly scented bath will give you a double benefit. You'll gain as much pleasure making the concoction as you will from soaking in it. The combination of powdered milk, oatmeal and cornstarch will leave you feeling silky and soft. The cinnamon will gently warm you and offer up a soothing aroma.

1. Place all the ingredients in a food processor and whirl to combine. Transfer into a clean, tightly covered, moisture-proof container, where it will keep indefinitely.
2. Add about ½ cup (75 g) of the milk bath to a full tub of warm water and enjoy the soak.

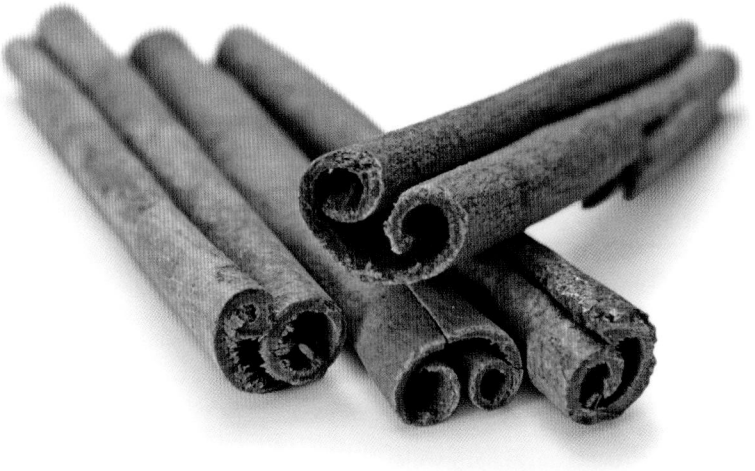

Gentle Milk Bath

⅓ cup (35 g) powdered milk
¼ cup (30 g) cornstarch
drops essential oil of your choice

You can shake up a soothing milk bath anytime you want to escape into a warm tub. Milk will leave your skin smooth and silky.

1. Pour the powdered milk and cornstarch into a clean jar with a tight top. Shake well. Add the essential oil and shake to incorporate thoroughly. If the mixture starts to clump, use your fingers to dissolve the lumps.
2. For a bath, put the mixture under the running water. Splash around with your hand to disperse it in the tub.

Note: You may double or triple this recipe and store it indefinitely by omitting the oil. Store the combined powdered milk and cornstarch in an airtight container; use ½ cup (50 g) for each bath. Add the essential oil to the tub separately after swishing in the combined powders.

Zingy Citrus Bath Salts

2 cups (500 g) Epsom salts
½ cup (160 g) sea salt
1 teaspoon glycerine
12 drops mandarin orange essential oil (or more if you like a stronger fragrance)
12 or more drops orange food color

Mix up a large batch of colorful, soothing bath salts. They're every bit as good as any you'd find in boutiques or on pharmacy shelves, selling for a whole lot more than you'll pay here.

1. Gently stir all the ingredients in a large bowl until they are well combined and the color is evenly distributed. You might want to add more color for a stronger shade, but do it 1 drop at a time.
2. Transfer the salts to a pretty tight-lidded jar and label.
3. Use up to ½ cup (160 g) of bath salts per bath, adding it while the water runs.

Bath Cookies

2 cups (500 g) fine sea salt
½ cup (60 g) cornstarch, plus more for rolling dough
½ cup (140 g) baking soda
3 teaspoons dried, chopped lavender or sage (optional)
2 eggs
2 tablespoons (30 ml) vegetable oil
1 teaspoon vitamin E oil (if necessary, break open several 500 IU capsules)
8 drops essential oil or perfume oil of your choosing

If you like experimenting with recipes in the kitchen, you'll get a real kick out of making these "cookies" for the tub. Bakers will recognize the steps in dough-making, rolling and baking, but there's a twist! Make one batch for yourself and another for friends.

1. Preheat the oven to 350°F. In a large bowl, combine the salt, cornstarch and baking soda. Stir in the chopped herbs, if using. Stir in the eggs, vegetable oil, vitamin E oil and essential oil and keep stirring until you form a dough.
2. Rub cornstarch on a rolling pin and spread some on a work surface. Roll the dough out to about ¾ inch. Cut into shapes with cookie cutters or a biscuit cutter. Place your "cookies" on an ungreased cookie sheet about 1 inch apart. Bake for 10 to 12 minutes. Cool and store in a tight-topped cookie tin in a cool, dry place.
3. When ready to use, place one or two of your bath cookies into the tub as the water runs.

Basic Bath Powder

½ cup (140 g) baking soda
½ cup (60 g) cornstarch

For an after-bath or after-shower touch, this fragrance-free homemade powder is so natural, it's a safe bet that your great-grandmother used it. Keep a container of this mixture in your bathroom. Apply with a powder puff or sprinkle it on from a shaker-top jar.

In a small bowl, stir the ingredients to combine. Store the bath powder in a widemouthed glass jar or plastic container or keep in a shaker-top jar. The powder should keep indefinitely.

Easy Bath Powder

1 cup (150 g) powdered arrowroot
1 cup (125 g) cornstarch
¼ cup (70 g) baking soda

This simple combination creates a refreshing finish to the shower or bath and costs very little to make.

In a medium bowl, stir together all the ingredients. Store in an airtight container. The powder should keep indefinitely.

Delicately Scented Bath Powder

2 tablespoons (30 g) crumbled dried chamomile flowers
¼ cup (30 g) cornstarch
3 teaspoons ground orris root
½ teaspoon alum

This variation provides a lightly scented powder suitable for adults. While alum is used as an antiperspirant and deodorant for adults, it is best to use a simple sprinkle of cornstarch on children or babies.

1. Combine all the ingredients in a bowl and mix well. Let stand for a few days.
2. Sift mixture through a flour sifter. Pour into a powder shaker or other container. The powder should keep indefinitely.

Nail, Hand and Foot Care

Gardener's Hand Cream

3 tablespoons (30 g) cosmetic-grade beeswax, grated or shaved
½ cup (125 ml) sesame oil
3 teaspoons coconut oil
1 teaspoon honey
2 tablespoons (30 ml) calendula tea
3 drops lavender essential oil
½ teaspoon baking soda

This hand cream is especially good for hard-working hands. It costs very little to make the entire recipe, but because you are using unpreserved vegetable oils, if you don't have a cool, dark place to store the hand cream or a friend to share with, consider halving the recipe. To make calendula tea, pour a cup of boiling water over half a teaspoon of dried calendula flower petals and let it steep until cool.

1. In a small microwave-safe bowl, mix all the ingredients. Set the microwave to a medium heat and cook for 30 seconds or until the beeswax is melted. Remove from the oven with a pot holder and allow to cool.
2. Pour the mixture into a widemouthed, sterilized jar with a tight top. Store in cool, dark place until ready to use.

Cuticle Cream

3 tablespoons (30 g) paraffin wax
½ cup (125 ml) mineral oil (or baby oil)
3 teaspoons coconut oil
3 teaspoons glycerine

Here's a spa treatment that you can make in the comfort of your own kitchen.

1. In the top of a double boiler over simmering water, combine the paraffin with the oils. Stir until the paraffin is melted and the mixture is blended. Stir in the glycerine and remove the pan from the heat. Let the mixture cool.
2. Apply the cooled cream to the cuticle area. Rub in and allow to rest for 10 minutes or so.
3. Trim cuticles with a cuticle tool. Massage away the cream by applying a gentle body or hand lotion and rubbing lightly, then rinsing with warm water.

Warm Oil Hand Treatment

3 teaspoons olive or other cooking oil
1 teaspoon almond extract or 1 drop lavender essential oil (optional)
2 small plastic bags that will fit over your hands

Manicurists can charge a great deal for hot oil hand treatments. Here is a delightfully simple and effective recipe you can create from ingredients in the pantry.

1. Place the oil in a microwave-safe dish and heat it on medium-high for a few seconds until it is warmed, but not hot. Add the almond extract or lavender oil, if desired. Stir.
2. Rub the oil on your hands, massaging your fingers and palms. Cover your hands with the plastic bags and wrap a clean hand towel over the bags. Sit comfortably for about 5 minutes.
3. Remove the bags and rinse your hands with warm water, massaging away the oil. Gently pat dry with the towel and apply a light hand lotion.

Cornmeal Hand Scrub

¼ cup (35 g) cornmeal
3 tablespoons (45 ml) milk
1 drop almond oil (or almond extract)

This gentle massage scrub costs small change to make and leaves your hands smooth and soft.

1. In a small saucepan, mix the cornmeal with the milk. Heat the mixture over a low heat until it forms a paste. Remove from heat and stir in the almond oil. Allow to cool.
2. Spread the mixture on your hands and allow to sit for 10 minutes. Gently scrub your hands with the mixture and then rinse off with warm water.

Love Your Feet Cream

1 oz (30 g) cosmetic-grade beeswax, grated or shaved
¾ cup (185 ml) almond oil

Our feet take a lot of abuse. Here's a special treatment to apply to dry, cracked feet that will leave them soft and pretty and costs much less than a visit to the salon for a pedicure.

1. Place the beeswax and almond oil in the top of a double boiler over simmering water. Stir together until they are blended and the wax has melted. Remove from heat and pour into two 4-ounce sterilized containers with tight tops.
2. Allow mixture to cool before applying to feet. Spread on feet at night before bedtime. Wear a pair of clean cotton socks over the cream. In the morning, your feet will be much softer.

Soothing Footbath

3 teaspoons sea salt
2 drops lavender essential oil
1 drop rosemary essential oil
1 drop bay essential oil
1 drop geranium essential oil
rose petals (optional)

Gently soothe tired, sore feet by soaking them in this deliciously scented footbath. Relax in the knowledge you'll be saving a pretty penny by making it yourself. Use a large plastic bowl or baby bath if you don't have a special foot tub.

1. Fill a soaking pan or small tub with enough warm water to cover the feet.
2. Stir in the sea salt until it dissolves. Use your toes to stir, if you wish. Add the essential oils, mixing them well. Float the rose petals on the surface, if desired.
3. Soak your feet in the tub for 10 minutes, or until the water has cooled off. Pat your feet dry with a towel.

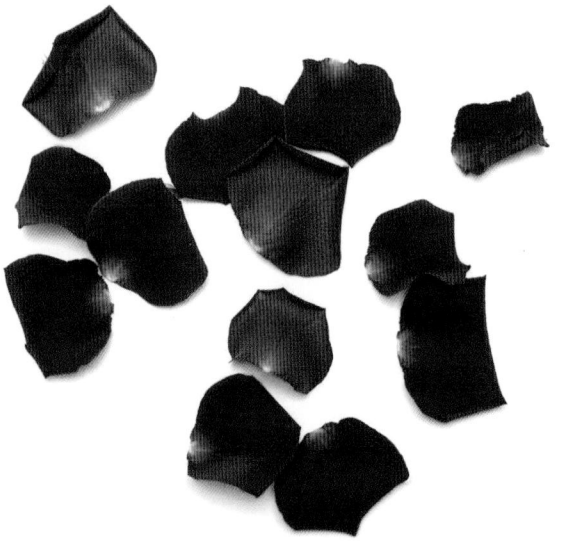

Eucalyptus Foot Lotion

3 teaspoons almond oil
1 teaspoon avocado oil
1 teaspoon wheat germ oil
10 drops eucalyptus essential oil

Use this rich and refreshing foot lotion to follow the Soothing Footbath (opposite) or simply to salve sore feet.

1. Put all the ingredients in a small, sterilized glass bottle with a tight-fitting stopper. Shake the liquid vigorously until it is completely combined.
2. Store the bottle in a cool, dark place. Shake well before using.

Strawberry Foot Scrub

2 teaspoons coarse salt
2 tablespoons (30 ml) olive oil
8 fresh strawberries

Can't get to the spa for a luxury treatment for those tired feet? Work this simple and sweetly scented natural scrub into your feet and feel like a queen.

1. Pour salt into a mixing bowl. Add the oil and stir to combine. Hull the strawberries and slice or chop them. Add strawberries to the salt and oil mixture and mash with a potato masher or fork. The resulting mixture should be chunky but well blended.
2. Rub this mixture onto your feet, massaging the balls of the feet and the heels. If desired, use a body puff or foot brush. Rinse off and coat feet with a gentle lotion.

Refreshing Foot Spray

3 tablespoons (45 ml) witch hazel
3 teaspoons rose water, orange blossom water or distilled water
⅛ teaspoon glycerine
10–15 drops essential oil of your choice

This clean, fresh blend is great for hot summer days. Carry a little spray bottle of it with you and spritz it on tired feet.

Pour all the ingredients into a clean spray bottle and shake. The spray will keep for 2 months in a plastic container.

Leg Massage Cream

3 tablespoons (45 ml) anhydrous (water-free) lanolin
3 tablespoons (45 ml) olive oil
2 tablespoons (30 ml) apricot oil

Treat yourself to a massage from your knees to your toes with this easy-to-make cream designed especially for the legs.

1. Put all the ingredients together in the nonreactive top of a double boiler over simmering water. Heat and stir with a wooden spoon until the lanolin has liquefied.
2. Pour the mixture into a sterilized 4-ounce jar with a tight-fitting lid and allow to cool. Keep in a cool, dark place.

Just for Men

Rosemary Shaving Soap

⅔ cup (170 ml) rose water
1¼ cups (125 g) pure soap flakes
4 drops rosemary essential oil
3 drops lemon essential oil
2 drops bay essential oil
1 drop sage essential oil

Rinse your face with fresh water, then lather up your beard with this fragrant soap before shaving. Be sure to rinse off the lather thoroughly.

1 Warm the rose water in a nonreactive saucepan over low heat. Place the soap flakes in the top of a double boiler over simmering water. Stir the warmed rose water into the flakes to moisten. Keep stirring the mixture until the soap has melted to a smooth gel (if necessary, use a potato masher to dissolve the soap). Remove from the heat and cool to lukewarm.
2 Stir in the essential oils and spoon the soap into a sterilized shallow 7-ounce glass jar with a tight-fitting lid. Set aside to harden for 3 to 5 days. Keep handy in a cool, dark place.

Lightly Scented Aftershave

½ cup (125 ml) witch hazel
½ cup (125 ml) rose water

Aftershave splashes serve two purposes: to soothe the just-shaved beard area and to offer a pleasant scent. Instead of purchasing costly scented aftershaves, make this at home for a fraction of the price.

Combine the witch hazel and rose water in a sterilized jar. Splash on the face directly after shaving. Keep tightly covered. The aftershave should keep indefinitely on the bathroom shelf.

Shaving-Cut Lotion

4 teaspoons (20 ml) witch hazel lotion
13 drops lavender essential oil
7 drops geranium essential oil

Apply a drop of this simple, inexpensive and effective lotion to stop bleeding and help prevent infection in the event of a razor nick.

Put all the ingredients in a sterilized 1-ounce glass bottle with a tight-fitting lid. Shake well to combine. Keep in a cool, dark place. Shake before using.

Aloe Aftershave Gel

½ cup (125 ml) aloe vera gel
1½ tablespoons (25 ml) distilled water
3 teaspoons witch hazel
10 drops essential or fragrance oils of your choice

This alcohol-free gel is suitable for men or women because it refreshes and is safe for sensitive skin. See if you don't love it as much as anything you can buy. Aloe vera gel is available in health food stores—or you can scoop it out of the leaves of a plant.

1 Combine all the ingredients in the container you're going to store the gel in. Stir until well mixed. Cover the container with a tight-fitting lid.
2 Keep in a cool, dark place. The gel should keep indefinitely.

Muscle Rub

1 teaspoon lanolin
1½ oz (45 ml) extra virgin olive oil
¼ oz (7 g) cosmetic-grade beeswax, shaved or grated
2–3 drops arnica essential oil
6 drops ginger essential oil
3–4 drops lemon essential oil

This salve really does wonders for hard-working muscles. Massage into stressed, stiff and aching shoulders, neck, back or feet. (While suitable for both men and women, this is not recommended for pregnant women.)

1 In a heatproof glass measuring cup with a pour spout, combine the lanolin, olive oil and beeswax. Place the cup in a hot-water bath until the wax is nearly melted. At this point, remove the cup from the water bath and stir the mixture with a clean utensil to evenly mix the ingredients.
2 Allow the mixture to cool. When the mixture begins to harden around the edges of the cup, add the essential oils and stir to incorporate them.
3 Pour into a sterile widemouthed jar and allow to cool before capping. Store in a cool, dark place for several months.

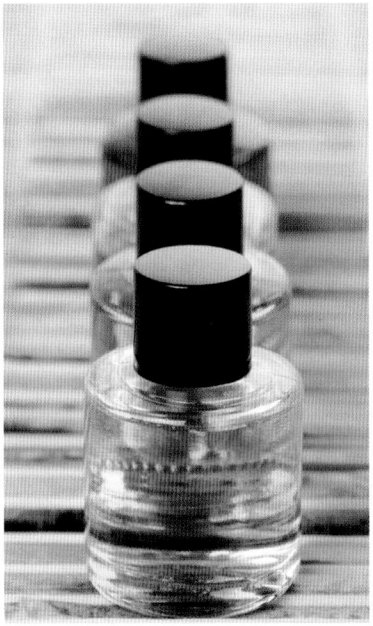

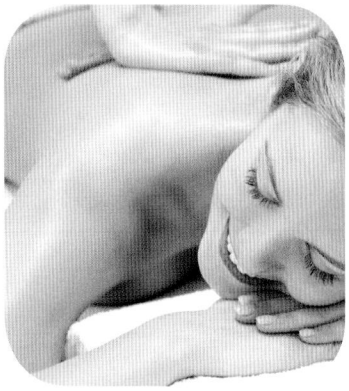

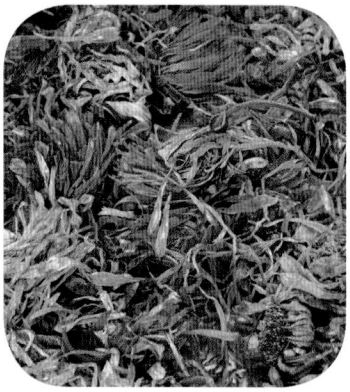

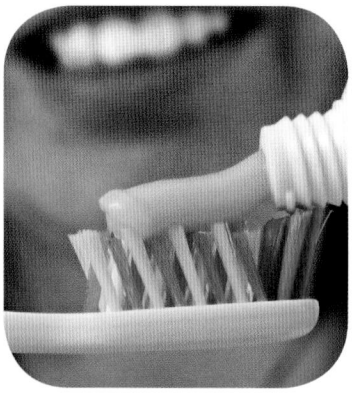

Digestive Distress

Soothing Tea for Heartburn ❖ Stomach-Calming Tea ❖ Settler for Motion Sickness ❖ Hiccup Reliever ❖ Anti-Diarrhea Tea ❖ Electrolyte Drink ❖ Laxative ❖ Herbal Tea for Flatulence ❖ Hemorrhoid Pads

Colds, Congestion and Fever

Chest Rub ❖ Chest Compress ❖ Mustard Seed Plaster ❖ Mustard Powder Plaster ❖ Cough Suppressant Tea ❖ Cough Suppressant ❖ Steam Cough Relief ❖ Cough Drops ❖ Gargle Solution ❖ Slippery Elm Tea ❖ Steam Treatment ❖ Sore-Throat Lozenges ❖ Decongestant Salve ❖ Herbal Inhalant ❖ Humidifier Booster ❖ Saline Spray for Sinuses ❖ Drops for Earache ❖ Fever Tea ❖ Spray for Fever

Bug Bites, Hives and Itching

Insect Repellent ❖ Soothing Gel for Insect Bites ❖ Essential Oil Itch Soother ❖ Poison Ivy Lotion ❖ Skin Rash Drying Paste ❖ Healing Oil Bath ❖ Healing Calendula Lotion ❖ Salve for Eczema or Dermatitis ❖ Honey Ointment ❖ Anti-Itching Solution for Hives ❖ Oatmeal Bath for Hives ❖ Anti-itch Wrap

Skin Outbreaks

Acne Facial Scrub ❖ Cleansing Liquid for Acne ❖ Acne Cleansing Pads ❖ Overnight Acne Cream ❖ Hot Compress for Boils ❖ Antibacterial Drawing Paste ❖ Antibacterial Oil ❖ Ringworm Paste ❖ Dandelion Wart Treatment ❖ Herbal Wart Treatment

Cuts, Bruises and Burns

First-Aid Antiseptic ❖ Calendula Ointment ❖ Healing Ointment ❖ Cleansing Soap ❖ Compress for Bruises ❖ Anti-Bruising Oil ❖ Oil Rub for Burned Skin ❖ Soothing Oil for Mild Burns ❖ Burn Spray ❖ Antiseptic Lotion for Burns ❖ Sunburn Cooler

Foot Care Products

Athlete's Foot Powder ❖ Antifungal Foot Ointment ❖ Antifungal Solution ❖ Corn Plaster ❖ Salicylic Acid Corn Remover

Lips and Mouth

Balm for Chapped Lips ❖ Cold Sore Ointment ❖ Mouthwash for Cold Sores ❖ Cold Sore Paste

Dental Care

Mouthwash ❖ Mints ❖ Toothpaste ❖ Gum Tonic ❖ Antibacterial Mouthwash ❖ Super Dental Floss ❖ Toothache-Relieving Rinse ❖ Toothache-Relieving Dental Paste

Joints and Muscles

Hot Pepper Rub ❖ Massage Cream ❖ Quick-and-Dirty Muscle Rub ❖ Muscle Soak ❖ Liniment ❖ Cold Pack for Strains and Sprains ❖ Castor Oil Rub for Back Pain

Women's Problems

Muscle Relaxant for Cramps ❖ Hot Compress for Cramps ❖ Anti-Cramp Tea ❖ Ginger Tea for Morning Sickness ❖ PMS Tea ❖ Yeast Infection Cream

Headaches

Headache Compresses ❖ Chamomile Tea ❖ Lemon Balm Tea ❖ Migraine Tea ❖ Headache Massage Oil ❖ Headache Oil with Vitamin E

Anxiety and Fatigue

Catnip Anti-Anxiety Tea ❖ Hops Anti-Anxiety Tea ❖ Calming Tea for Insomnia ❖ Sleep Pillow ❖ Herbal Milk Bath for Sleeplessness ❖ Relaxing Aromatic Bath ❖ Invigorating Oil for Fatigue ❖ Energy Tea for Fatigue

Healthy Home Remedies

In a time of increasing health care costs, it is comforting to know that you can often successfully treat many everyday health problems with homemade remedies.

As you use the recipes on the following pages, you will be happy to discover that they can make a real difference to how you or a family member feels and to when you start to improve without spending a small fortune at the drugstore.

From heartburn and motion sickness to constipation, colds and sore throats to sprains and muscle aches, and many more conditions, there are effective home remedies in this chapter that you can make and apply yourself.

Many of these homemade recipes use herbs and other natural ingredients that were known to our ancestors and have an honorable place in the history of healing. In many cases, modern medicines were discovered when scientists took plants that were recognized by herbalists as having special healing properties to the lab. The healing ingredients were then extracted and tested and later manufactured. So with many of these recipes, you are simply going back to the original natural source. However, if any symptoms persist, you should always seek medical treatment.

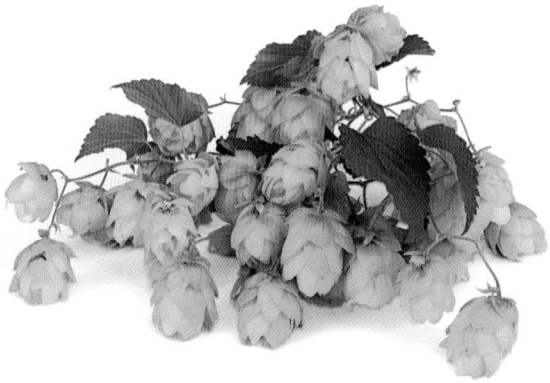

Digestive Distress

Soothing Tea for Heartburn

1 cup (250 ml) water
1 teaspoon grated licorice root
1 teaspoon chopped fresh ginger
1 teaspoon dried chamomile flowers

Licorice, ginger and chamomile are traditional, easy-to-make and inexpensive digestive tract soothers that still work wonders for occasional flare-ups of heartburn.

1. In a small pan, bring the water to a boil. Add the licorice and ginger. Simmer for 15 minutes. Remove from heat and add the chamomile. Cover and steep for 10 minutes.
2. Strain into a teacup and drink.

Stomach-Calming Tea

1 cup (250 ml) boiling water
1 teaspoon dried peppermint
1 teaspoon dried chamomile

If you have indigestion, this therapeutic infusion will help to tame your outraged stomach.

1. In a small pot, pour the boiling water over the dried peppermint and chamomile. Cover and steep for 10 minutes, then strain into a teacup.
2. Drink up to 3 cups a day to help ease intestinal cramps.

Quick antacid from your spice shelf

Some common kitchen spice seeds contain oils that soothe spasms in your stomach and relieve nausea—without costing too pretty a penny. Just chew 1 teaspoon of aniseed, dill or caraway seeds for 1 minute, then spit them out without swallowing any of them. Repeat three times a day.

Settler for Motion Sickness

juice of 1 lemon
1 cup (250 ml) boiling water
1 teaspoon honey
1 crushed sprig spearmint or peppermint

While over-the-counter motion-sickness remedies can make you sleepy, ours just helps to take away the sick feeling. This is a tummy-soothing drink.

1. In a large cup, combine the lemon juice, boiling water and honey. Stir to mix and add the spearmint or peppermint.
2. Sip as needed. Keep warm in a thermos when travelling.

Chew ginger to settle your stomach

Ginger is a traditional stomach settler for motion sickness, and crystallized ginger may save you a trip to the drugstore. Just chew on a lump of crystallized ginger as needed. Keep a package in the car or your purse so you always have it handy.

Hiccup Reliever

2–3 teaspoons sugar or dry drink mix (cocoa or Ovaltine)

You can't even find a remedy for hiccups in the drugstore, but you can make one yourself.

Swallow the dry sugar or drink mix, which isn't easy. Trying to get it down may short-circuit the hiccups.

Anti-Diarrhea Tea

2 teaspoons dried raspberry and/or blackberry leaves
boiling water

This tea settles the digestive system. If your diarrhea persists for more than 24 hours, however, see a doctor.

1. In a teacup, steep the berry leaves in freshly boiled water for at least 10 minutes. Strain.
2. Drink a small cup three times a day along with other fluids to prevent dehydration.

Electrolyte Drink

1 cup (250 ml) apple juice
2 cups (500 ml) water
½–1 teaspoon salt
juice from 1 lemon or 1 lime

Diarrhea can drain your body of fluid and electrolytes quickly and quite dangerously. This juice drink helps maintain your body's equilibrium. If your diarrhea persists for more than 24 hours, however, see a doctor.

1. In a jug, combine the apple juice, water, salt and the lemon or lime juice. Store in the refrigerator.
2. Drink throughout the day to maintain hydration and proper balance of electrolytes.

Making an infusion

Making an herbal infusion is similar to making a cup of tea. Place 3 rounded teaspoons (15 g) fresh herb leaves or 1 rounded teaspoon dried herb leaves in a teacup. Pour ½ cup (125 ml) boiling water over the leaves, cover with a saucer and let steep for 5 or 10 minutes. Strain the drink while still hot—or let it cool if you're going to use it as part of a lotion or gargle with it. Infusions may be stored in the refrigerator for up to 24 hours.

Laxative

1–3 teaspoons psyllium husks
1 cup (250 ml) warm water

You don't have to buy expensive psyllium husk fiber supplements to treat temporary constipation.

1. Stir the psyllium husks into the warm water and drink once a day. Follow with a glass of plain water.
2. Drink 6 to 8 additional glasses of water throughout the day.

Grandma's always-ready laxative

Here is an old-fashioned penny-pincher's remedy for constipation—it sounds simple because it is. Just take 1 to 2 teaspoons castor oil on an empty stomach. It should get things moving within 8 to 10 hours.

Herbal Tea for Flatulence

1 teaspoon dried chamomile
½ teaspoon dried peppermint
1 teaspoon dried catnip
1 teaspoon dried basil
2 crushed fennel seeds
½ teaspoon dried marjoram

It's embarrassing to have flatulence and embarrassing to have to buy something to treat it. Instead, make the following tea in the privacy of your home.

1. In a large cup, mix the herbs. Pour in ¾ to 1 cup (180 to 250 ml) boiling water and steep, covered, for 10 minutes. Strain and drink tea.
2. Drink 3 or more cups a day.

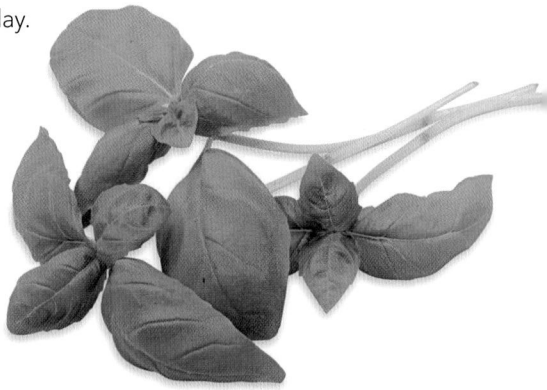

Hemorrhoid Pads

1 oz (30 ml) witch hazel
5 drops cypress essential oil
3 drops geranium essential oil
5 drops lavender essential oil
2 tablespoons aloe vera gel
cotton cosmetic pads

These pads are cool and soothing.

1. In an open-mouthed jar with a tight-fitting lid, combine the witch hazel, essential oils and aloe vera gel. Saturate several cotton cosmetic pads with the liquid and refrigerate for at least 1 hour.
2. Use a pad on the affected area when it burns and after each bowel movement. Store in the refrigerator for several days.

Colds, Congestion and Fever

Chest Rub

30 drops massage or carrier oil such as almond, jojoba or avocado oil
5–10 drops eucalyptus or wintergreen essential oil

The essential oils in this rub are therapeutic. Cover them with flannel and a hot pad to warm your chest and help you absorb the essential oil.

1 In a small bowl, mix the carrier oil with the essential oil. Rub the mixture onto your chest.
2 Cover your chest with a cotton towel or piece of flannel, then put a heating pad or hot-water bottle on top of the flannel and snuggle under the blankets.

Chest Compress

a handful of dried, chopped mullein or dried, chopped lobelia
1–2 cups (250–500 ml) boiling water

This warm, soothing compress will make you relax while it helps you breathe.

1 In a bowl, steep the mullein or lobelia in boiling water for 10 minutes.
2 Saturate a hand towel in the warm liquid, wring it out, and place it on your chest. Cover with a warm towel and place a heating pad on top of that.

Mustard Seed Plaster

2 or more tablespoons (30–45 ml) olive oil
⅓ cup (70 g) mustard seed
2 tablespoons (20 g) grated beeswax
cloth to cover chest

It's old-fashioned, but sometimes it's these kinds of remedies that are the best. And you are not risking the family fortune to try it.

1 Blend 2 tablespoons olive oil and the mustard seed in a blender. Continue adding olive oil until you have a nice, thick liquid.
2 Pour the mixture into the top of a double boiler over low heat; add the beeswax and heat, stirring, until the wax melts. Spread the cloth on a flat surface. Once the mustard-wax mixture is warm and can be spread, apply it to the cloth and let it cool to room temperature.
3 Place the cloth, salve-side-down, on your chest and cover with a T-shirt or old flannel, then apply external heat on top with a heating pad or hot-water bottle. You should start to feel warmth seeping into your chest in about 10 to 15 minutes. Leave on for another 15 minutes. You can store the plaster in the fridge for several days; when needed, remove and let warm to room temperature before using.

Mustard Powder Plaster

3 teaspoons mustard powder
2 tablespoons (20 g) flour

You can make an inexpensive, effective mustard plaster using a strong mustard powder.

1. In a small bowl, mix the mustard powder with the flour. Add enough water to make a paste.
2. Spread the paste over half of a dish towel. Then fold the towel in half, covering the paste, and apply to chest. Don't apply the mustard paste directly onto the skin. Check chest skin often and remove the mustard plaster if there are signs of irritation.

Cough Suppressant Tea

4 fresh sage leaves or
1 teaspoon dried
boiling water

Here's a nicer, cheaper alternative to commercial cough syrups, which may help you cope with a nagging cough.

In a standard teacup, steep the sage leaves in freshly boiled water for at least 20 minutes. Strain and drink hot or cold.

Cough Suppressant

1 large onion, finely diced
2 garlic cloves, finely diced
2 tablespoons (50 g) finely diced fresh ginger
honey

Gain a new appreciation of onions, garlic, ginger and honey after they conspire to stop your coughing.

1. In a small saucepan, combine the onion, garlic and ginger. Add honey to cover and cook over very low heat for 30 minutes. Then mash together and let cool. Strain and store in a clean jar with a tight-fitting lid in the refrigerator.
2. Take 1 teaspoon every 15 to 30 minutes.

Steam Cough Relief

4 cups (1 liter) water
2 drops thyme essential oil
4 drops eucalyptus essential oil
2 drops hyssop essential oil

Make your own herbal steam treatment to help relieve the symptoms of a persistent cough.

1. In a saucepan over medium heat, heat the water until nearly boiling (but don't boil). Pour into a heat-safe bowl and add the essential oils.
2. Hold your head about 8 inches above the water, drape a towel over your head and the bowl to make a tent, and breathe in deeply until the water cools. Make sure that you keep your eyes closed throughout.

Cough Drops

2 oz (60 g) dried or 6 oz (170 g) fresh horehound leaves
3½ cups (800 g) firmly packed dark brown sugar
20 drops eucalyptus essential oil
20 drops tea tree essential oil

Do a little steeping and straining, boiling and stirring, rolling and cooling. Voilà! Your very own cough drops at a fraction of the price of commercial ones. You need a candy thermometer to make these.

1. In a saucepan, pour 3 cups (750 ml) boiling water over the horehound leaves and steep for 30 minutes over low heat. Strain into another saucepan and add the brown sugar; stir until the sugar dissolves.
2. Bring the mixture to a boil and boil until it reaches 295°F on a candy thermometer. Stir in the eucalyptus and tea tree oils. Let cool slightly, then, using buttered hands, roll into small balls and let the balls harden on parchment paper. Wrap them individually in plastic wrap and use as needed.

Pepper spray for a raw throat

This quick and easy spray is an antiseptic and a painkiller that costs almost nothing to make. In a clean 8-ounce spray bottle, combine 3 teaspoons of ground cayenne pepper with just enough water to almost fill the bottle. Shake well and use as a spray to numb the back of your throat. You can also use it for gargling. Use the spray sparingly and don't get it near your eyes. Keep out of reach of children.

Gargle Solution

2 heaping tablespoons (40 g) brown sugar
½ teaspoon salt
¼ teaspoon baking soda
4 cups (1 liter) warm water

This old-fashioned gargle will make your throat feel much better, and it costs very little.

1. In a jar with a tight-fitting lid, combine all the ingredients. Shake well before using.
2. Gargle with up to ½ cup (125 ml) of this solution as often as needed.

Slippery Elm Tea

2 teaspoons powdered slippery elm bark
2 teaspoons powdered marshmallow root
⅔ cup (170 ml) boiling water

The combination of slippery elm and marshmallow root is soothing for a sore throat.

In a cup, place the slippery elm and marshmallow root. Pour in the boiling water and steep until cool. Strain into a teacup and drink. Store in the refrigerator and gently reheat as needed.

Steam Treatment

3 tablespoons (15 g) finely chopped fresh thyme, sage, peppermint, eucalyptus or pine needles
boiling water

Aromatic herbs and humidity can do wonders for a stuffed-up head—the results can be priceless!

1 Put the herbs in a medium bowl and add boiling water.
2 Drape a towel over your head and the bowl, lean over and inhale for 10 minutes. Repeat two or three times a day as needed.

Sore-Throat Lozenges

¼ cup (about 5 g) dried violet petals
¼ cup (about 5 g) dried rose petals
honey or maple syrup
1 teaspoon powdered marshmallow root
confectioners' sugar (optional)

These lozenges are made with dried plant ingredients. They are cheap, easy to make and very effective.

1 With a mortar and pestle, crush the violet and rose petals until you get a fine powder. Mix with just enough honey or maple syrup to form a ball and add marshmallow root. Add more herbs or confectioners' sugar until the mixture can hold its shape.
2 Form into pea-sized balls and place on a greased cookie sheet. Leave for 24 to 48 hours or until they harden, then wrap each individually in plastic wrap and store in a cool, dry place.

Decongestant Salve

½ cup (125 ml) olive oil
½ oz (15 ml) peppermint oil
½ oz (15 ml) eucalyptus oil
½ oz (15 ml) wintergreen oil
½ oz (15 g) grated beeswax
4 drops tincture of benzoin

This decongestant rub can be rubbed on the chest or under the nose for warm relief.

1 In the top of a double boiler over low heat, heat the oils. Add the beeswax and tincture of benzoin and stir until the beeswax is melted and the oils are well mixed.
2 Pour into a clean, widemouthed jar with a tight top and allow to cool. Put under your nose or rub on your chest. Keep this mixture in a cool, dark place for up to 2 weeks.

A quick decongestant to carry with you

The good news about this decongestant is that it doesn't come with a list of warnings! Just put 1 drop of tea tree, peppermint or rosemary essential oil on a clean handkerchief and carry the handkerchief with you. Inhale as needed.

Herbal Inhalant

¼–½ teaspoon rock salt
2–4 drops peppermint essential oil
2–4 drops each eucalyptus and wintergreen essential oils

Make your own quick inhalant for a blocked nose.

1 Put the rock salt in the bottom of a small glass bottle or jar with a tight-fitting lid. Add the oils.
2 Carry with you and sniff as needed.

Humidifier Booster

2–4 drops peppermint essential oil
2–4 drops eucalyptus essential oil
2–4 drops wintergreen essential oil
cotton ball

Getting a good night's sleep is probably the best thing you can do for a cold. This recipe will help you to breathe and sleep through the night.

1 In a small bowl, mix the oils. Dip a cotton ball into the mixture and put it near the vent of a steam humidifier.
2 Place the humidifier and the cotton ball near your bed when you have a cold.

Saline Spray for Sinuses

¼ teaspoon table salt
1 cup (250 ml) distilled water, warmed to a comfortable temperature

Why pay good money for something that is essentially salt and water? Make your own saline spray.

1 Add the salt to the distilled water and stir until it dissolves.
2 To get the solution into your nose, use an ear bulb syringe (available from pharmacies). Flush your nasal passages two to three times a day.

Drops for Earache

1 garlic clove, crushed
2 tablespoons (5 g) fresh or dried mullein flower
½ cup (125 ml) olive or almond oil

In winter weather, when earaches are more prevalent, keep these bargain ear drops close at hand in the refrigerator for emergencies. Always consult a doctor if earache persists.

1 In a clean jar with a tight-fitting lid, combine the garlic and mullein flower. Cover with the oil, seal the top and shake to blend. Store in a cool, dark place and shake daily.
2 Make sure the herbs remain under the oil for 2 weeks, then strain and store the oil in a clean jar with a tight-fitting lid in the refrigerator.
3 To treat an earache, let the oil come to room temperature or run it under warm water. Dispense 2 or 3 drops at a time with a sterile eye dropper. Gently massage the ear to help the oil make its way through the ear canal.

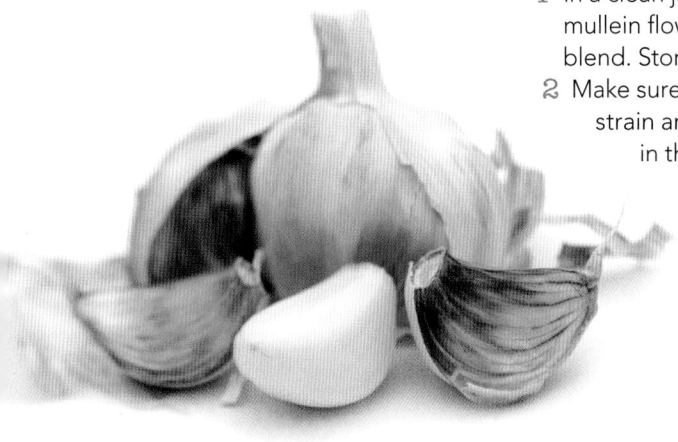

Fever Tea

yarrow
linden flowers
chamomile
spearmint
elder flowers
1 cup (250 ml) boiling water

Sip this tea to help reduce the symptoms of mild fever.

1. In a small bowl, mix equal amounts of dried, crushed yarrow, linden flowers, chamomile, spearmint and elder flowers.
2. Combine 3 teaspoons of this mix in a large cup and add boiling water.
3. Cover and steep for 10 to 15 minutes. Strain and drink hot. After drinking, get under the covers to induce sweating.

Spray for Fever

¼ cup (60 ml) rubbing alcohol
¼ cup (60 ml) witch hazel
3 drops peppermint essential oil
2 drops lavender essential oil

Spraying pulse points with a cool, soothing solution is said by many to help bring down a fever. It certainly feels great when you are hot and feverish. Pulse points are the places on the body where you can feel your heart rate when you touch them with your fingers—typically inside your wrists, just under each side of the jaw and the back of the knees.

1. In a clean spray bottle, combine the rubbing alcohol, witch hazel and essential oils. Shake the bottle to mix and then chill in the refrigerator.
2. Spray onto pulse points to reduce fever, taking care to avoid eyes and mouth.

Bug Bites, Hives and Itching

Insect Repellent

15–20 drops eucalyptus essential oil
15–20 drops lemon essential oil
15–20 drops lemongrass essential oil
15–20 drops citronella essential oil
1 oz (30 ml) carrier oil (olive oil or any massage oil)

The best way to treat bites is to avoid getting bitten in the first place. But forget spraying poisons on yourself. The essential ingredients of this insect repellent have been shown in studies to keep away stinging insects—notably, mosquitoes. Keep in mind, however, that if you live in an area with a high rate of mosquito-transmitted diseases, you may need stronger protection.

1. In a small jug, mix the essential oils with the carrier oil.
2. Put into a spray bottle and use as needed. Do not use on small children or infants.

Soothing Gel for Insect Bites

10–20 drops of a combination of lavender, tea tree, chamomile, cedarwood and/or eucalyptus essential oils
1 oz (30 ml) aloe vera gel or chamomile or calendula cream

Once you've been bitten, you need something to soothe the itch. This easy, inexpensive mixture will help.

1. In a small bowl, mix the essential oils into the gel or cream.
2. Smooth over the itchy/painful area. If you make more than you need, you can store the mixture in a clean jar in a cool, dark place for 1 week.

Essential Oil Itch Soother

1 drop lavender, rose, chamomile or tea tree essential oil
cold water

Instead of messy, expensive anti-itch salves, try this homemade soother, which can be made cheaply.

1. Fill a bowl with enough cold water to moisten a small washcloth or cotton pad. Swirl the essential oil through the water, then soak the cloth or pad.
2. Squeeze gently to remove any excess water and apply the cloth to the skin. Hold in place with your hand for as long as possible, or cover with plastic wrap and leave in place for about 1 hour.

Poison Ivy Lotion

½ teaspoon salt
½ cup (125 ml) water
bentonite or green clay powder
12 drops lavender essential oil
12 drops peppermint essential oil

The key to healing poison ivy is to dry it up. To make the process less annoying, a coating of a heavy lotion keeps them from itching. This may be just as messy as calamine lotion, but it is a lot cheaper.

1. In a small bowl, dissolve the salt in the water and add enough bentonite clay to make a creamy mixture. Stir in the lavender and peppermint essential oils.
2. Spread over the affected area.

Baking soda paste for itches

Here is an incredibly easy itch reliever that costs almost nothing. In a small bowl, mix ¼ teaspoon baking soda with a little iced water to make a paste. Then spread the paste over the bite area. Repeat as necessary.

Skin Rash Drying Paste

bentonite or green clay powder or finely ground oatmeal
10 drops of lavender, chamomile, cypress and/or geranium essential oils
water

This easily made, inexpensive paste will coat and stick to the skin, soothing skin rashes caused by exposure to stinging and itching plants, such as nettles.

1. In a small bowl, put enough bentonite clay or finely ground oatmeal to cover the affected area. For every 3 teaspoons of powder, stir in 10 drops of one or more of the essential oils. Moisten the mixture with water to allow for easy application and spread over the affected area.
2. Cover loosely and allow to dry. Then rinse off and reapply as needed.

Healing Oil Bath

6–8 drops pine, geranium or lavender essential oils

Dry, irritated skin is the greatest culprit with either eczema or dermatitis. Try a fragrant herb oil bath for simple relief.

1. Add essential oil to a hot bath. Swirl to disperse the oil, then get in and soak for about 10 minutes.
2. Carefully get out of the bath (it will be slippery) and massage in any oil still left on the skin. Don't take this bath more than once every 24 hours.

Healing Calendula Lotion

calendula flower petals

Be sure you have *Calendula officinalis* flowers from your garden or a health food store when making this lotion for treating eczema or dermatitis; they are the ones with the therapeutic effect.

1. Crush several calendula flower petals between your fingers (or with a mortar and pestle) until the petals are juicy.
2. Rub both petals and juice onto the skin.

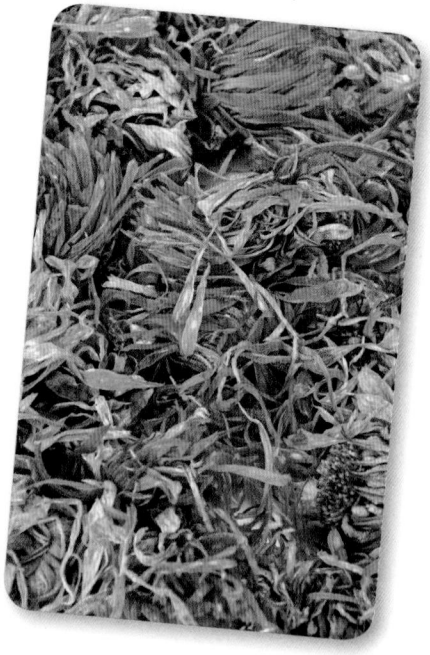

Salve for Eczema or Dermatitis

1 oz (30 g) grated beeswax
1 cup (250 ml) untoasted sesame oil
½ teaspoon tincture of goldenseal
½ teaspoon tincture of barberry root
8 drops tea tree essential oil
8 drops chamomile essential oil

Here is another gentle and natural treatment for rough, dry, irritated skin.

1. In the top of a double boiler over low heat, melt the beeswax, stirring occasionally. Stir in the sesame oil.
2. In a small dish, mix tincture of goldenseal and barberry root. Add the tea tree and chamomile essential oils.
3. Stir this mixture into the beeswax-oil mixture. Apply as needed.

Honey Ointment

1 oz (30 g) grated beeswax
1 cup (250 ml) untoasted sesame oil
⅓ cup (115 g) honey
1 capsule vitamin E, 500 IU
60 drops rose, geranium, chamomile, lavender or bergamot essential oils in any combination

The honey in this ointment serves as a humectant to draw in moisture, which helps to ease the skin irritation produced by eczema and dermatitis.

1. In the top of a double boiler over low heat, melt the beeswax, stirring occasionally. Stir in the sesame oil. Remove from heat and let cool slightly, then add honey. Pierce the vitamin E capsule and squeeze in contents. Add up to 60 drops of essential oils.
2. Pour the mixture into a clean jar or jars with tight-fitting lids and use as needed to keep skin smooth and hydrated.

Anti-Itching Solution for Hives

20–30 drops lavender essential oil
bowl of cold water

You can buy pricey salves at the drugstore to tame the itching of hives, but this easy solution is also effective.

1. Stir the lavender essential oil into the bowl of cold water.
2. Dip a cloth into the liquid and apply directly to the hives to reduce inflammation.

Oatmeal Bath for Hives

1 handful rolled oats
½ handful dry powdered milk
½ handful chamomile
¼ handful calendula and/or lavender
double-layer square of cheesecloth

Oatmeal bath products are famously good for soothing the skin. Now you can make your own.

1. Place the oats, milk, chamomile and calendula or lavender on the cheesecloth square. Tie the ends together to make a bag.
2. Run a warm (not hot) bath. Put the bag under the spout while the water is running. Leave it in the bath and allow the water to cool. (If the water is too hot, it will make the hives worse.)
3. Get into the tub and soak, squeezing the bag over your skin to reduce itching.

Using essential oil to soothe rashes

Lavender and tea tree essential oils have soothing properties that can alleviate as well as heal some rashes. Try this simple solution before buying expensive ointments. Put 1 drop of lavender or tea tree essential oil directly on the rash, gently smoothing it over the surface. To treat a large area, apply a blend made by mixing 3 drops of either essential oil in 2 teaspoons light olive oil.

Anti-Itch Wrap

¼ cup (60 ml) apple cider vinegar
¼ cup (60 ml) witch hazel
2 cups (500 ml) cold water
4 drops lavender essential oil
2 drops chamomile essential oil
2 drops bergamot essential oil
2 teaspoons baking soda
clean cloths

This herbal wrap solution will soothe irritating rashes. It will also help to relieve the itching associated with chicken pox.

1. In a large bowl, mix the vinegar, witch hazel and cold water. In a separate small bowl, mix the essential oils with the baking soda. Stir the baking soda mixture into the water mixture.
2. Soak a cloth in the cool solution and wrap it over the itchy area for 20 minutes at a time or until the cloth begins to dry. Keep the solution chilled in the refrigerator for up to 2 weeks.
3. May be repeated three times a day.

Skin Outbreaks

Acne Facial Scrub

2 cups (200 g) rolled oats
½ cup (80 g) almonds
2 tablespoons (5 g) dried lavender
3 teaspoons dried peppermint
3 teaspoons calendula leaf
½ cup (75 g) bentonite or green clay powder

For a homemade version of an acne-relieving exfoliant that won't break the bank, try this. For more information on green clay powder, see Green Clay Purifying Face Mask, page 246.

1. In a coffee grinder or blender, grind the oats, almonds, lavender, peppermint and calendula leaf.
2. Add the clay and mix thoroughly, then put in a clean covered container and keep in a cool place. You can keep this scrub for up to 3 months.
3. To use the scrub, in a small open dish, make a paste by mixing 1 teaspoon of the mixture with water. Massage the paste onto your skin. Let dry, then rinse well.

Cleansing Liquid for Acne

1 cup (250 ml) distilled water
1 teaspoon dried thyme
1 teaspoon dried calendula flowers
1 teaspoon dried lavender
1 teaspoon dried yarrow
¼ cup (60 ml) witch hazel
5–10 drops tea tree essential oil

Toners are primarily just water with a few other ingredients, yet they can cost far more than they should. Instead, make your own (see Making an Infusion, page 277). Dab an affected area three times a day, or use over your whole face after washing.

1. In a small pan, bring the distilled water to a boil. Add the thyme, calendula, lavender and yarrow. Remove from heat and steep, covered, until cool.
2. Strain and then mix the strained liquid with the witch hazel. Add the tea tree essential oil, shake and apply to affected areas with a cotton pad.
3. Store the leftover liquid in the refrigerator and use within 2 weeks.

Acne Cleansing Pads

2 cups (500 ml) distilled water
3 teaspoons dried yarrow
3 teaspoons dried chamomile
15 drops tincture of benzoin
6 drops peppermint or wintergreen essential oil
cosmetic pads

Forget those high-priced acne pads that come impregnated with the medicine. Just make your own!

1. In a small pan, bring the distilled water to a boil. Then add the yarrow and chamomile. Remove from heat after 2 to 3 minutes and steep, covered, for half an hour. Strain and add tincture of benzoin and peppermint or wintergreen essential oil. Mix well and pour into a sterilized jar with a tight-fitting lid.
2. Put several cosmetic pads in with the liquid. Refrigerate and use as needed.

Overnight Acne Cream

4 drops tea tree essential oil
1 teaspoon cosmetic clay

Antibacterial tea tree oil is the active ingredient in this easy homemade paste.

1. In a small dish, mix the tea tree oil and the cosmetic clay. Add just enough water to make a thick paste.
2. Dab onto blemishes and leave on overnight.

Hot Compress for Boils

4 teaspoons (20 ml) hot water
2 drops lavender, lemon, tea tree, sage or clove essential oil
1 cotton ball or gauze pad

This gentle treatment will help relieve the boil in a lovely, aromatic way.

1. In a bowl, pour the hot water. Swirl your chosen essential oil through the water, then soak the cotton ball or gauze pad in the solution.
2. Gently squeeze out excess liquid and apply the cotton ball or pad directly to the area of the boil. Cover with plastic wrap and secure with a bandage or tape. Leave in place for at least 1 hour. Repeat twice a day.

Antibacterial Drawing Paste

5 drops (in total) tea tree, lavender and/or spikenard essential oils
slippery elm powder or bentonite or green clay powder

This therapeutic paste works best if it is applied after putting a hot compress (above) on the boil for 15 minutes.

1. Mix the essential oils with enough slippery elm powder or green clay powder to cover the affected area generously.
2. Apply the moist powder to the boil and cover with a bandage for 24 hours.

Antibacterial Oil

3 teaspoons carrier oil
20 drops tea tree essential oil
20 drops lavender essential oil
10 drops thyme essential oil

You don't want a boil to get infected; this antibacterial oil will help to protect you from that. You should, however, test it on a small area of normal skin first to make sure it's not irritating to your skin.

1. In a small bowl, combine the carrier oil with the essential oils. Mix well.
2. Hold a hot compress (above) on the boil for 10 minutes, then apply a small amount of the antibacterial oil and cover with a dressing. Repeat every few hours.

Ringworm Paste

3 teaspoons mustard seeds
water
1–2 drops sage and/or thyme essential oil

Try this antifungal paste on ringworm. If it's not better in a week, however, see a doctor.

1. Crush the mustard seeds with a mortar and pestle. Stir in enough water to make a paste, then add essential oil or oils.
2. Apply to the affected area and cover with a light bandage. Reapply once a day until the infection clears.

Dandelion Wart Treatment

freshly cut dandelion stalks or fig leaves

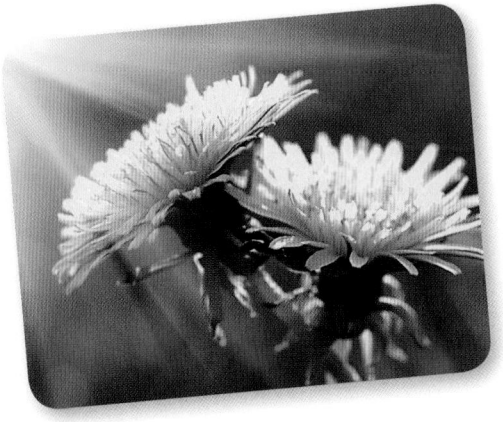

Here's an easy wart treatment straight from the backyard that won't cost you a thing. All you need are dandelion stalks or fig leaves.

1. Use the milky sap that exudes from the dandelion stalks or fig leaves and apply directly to the wart once or twice a day for several days, or until the wart pulls away from the skin. Keep the sap away from the skin around the wart and from sensitive areas such as the eyes.
2. If you are using this treatment on a child, cover the wart area with a bandage to prevent spreading the sap to sensitive skin.

Herbal Wart Treatment

1 drop tea tree, lemon, clove, thuja or thyme essential oil
1 drop almond or olive oil
1 strip bandage

Warts are mysterious—they come and go seemingly without reason. You usually don't need a dermatologist or an expensive medicine to make them disappear.

1. Soak the wart in warm water for 15 minutes. Towel dry.
2. In a small dish, combine the essential oil with the almond or olive carrier oil. Test this oil mixture on a patch of skin to make sure it isn't irritating.
3. Apply the oil mixture to the wart and cover with the strip bandage. Reapply every 24 hours.

Cuts, Bruises and Burns

First-Aid Antiseptic

2 oz (60 g) Calendula Ointment (page 292)
40 drops lavender essential oil
20 drops tea tree essential oil
10 drops chamomile essential oil
10 drops lemon essential oil

Here is a natural solution with germ-killing properties that will help soothe a minor cut or abrasion. Be sure to wash the affected area well before applying it.

1. In a small sterile jar with a tight-fitting lid, combine the calendula ointment with the essential oils, mixing thoroughly.
2. Apply a small amount to the cleaned injury. Keep the remainder in a cool, dark place for up to 2 weeks.

Calendula Ointment

3 tablespoons (15 g) fresh calendula petals
⅓ cup (80 ml) light olive oil
2 tablespoons (20 g) chopped beeswax
1 capsule vitamin E, 500 IU

Use calendula flowers (*Calendula officinalis*) for this old-fashioned therapeutic salve that has many uses.

1. Put the calendula petals in a double boiler and crush slightly with the back of a spoon. Add the olive oil and simmer for 2 hours over low heat.
2. Strain the liquid into a bowl, pressing against the strainer with the back of a spoon to extract all the oils.
3. Return the liquid to the double boiler. Over medium heat, add the chopped beeswax and stir until it melts. Remove from the double boiler and beat the mixture until it cools and becomes creamy and thick. Pierce the vitamin E capsule with a needle, squeeze in the contents and mix.
4. Spoon into a sterilized 4½-ounce jar with a tight-fitting lid, seal and keep in a cool, dark place for up to 2 weeks.

Healing Ointment

1–1½ oz (30–45 g) grated beeswax
1 cup (250 ml) olive or almond oil
2 capsules vitamin E, 500 IU
30 drops tea tree essential oil
20 drops spike lavender or French lavender essential oil
10 drops chamomile essential oil
10 drops fir essential oil

You can have this ointment on hand to treat everyday cuts and scrapes as they arise, just as you would a tube of commercial antiseptic.

1. In the top of a double boiler over low heat, melt the beeswax. Stir in the olive or almond oil. Remove from the heat. Pierce each vitamin E capsule with a needle and squeeze the contents into the mixture. Then stir in the essential oils.
2. Pour into a small sterilized jar with a tight-fitting lid and store in a cool, dark place. Use as needed on wounds. This ointment should last 1 year.

Cleansing Soap

liquid castile soap
lavender essential oil
rosemary essential oil
tea tree essential oil

Here is an antiseptic soap that will help to clean wounds properly and stave off infections. It smells good and costs very little.

1. To the bottle of castile soap, add the lavender, rosemary and tea tree essential oils (10 drops total per 2 ounces of soap). Dilute the mixture with more soap if skin is especially sensitive to any of the essential oils.
2. Use to clean cuts and abrasions.

Compress for Bruises

¼ cup (60 ml) water
¼ cup (60 ml) witch hazel or cider vinegar
2 drops lavender essential oil
2 drops rosemary essential oil
2 drops peppermint or juniper essential oil

A wet compress can relieve some of the pain of a bruise and help the healing process. This simple formula should have you feeling better in no time.

1. In a bowl, mix the water, witch hazel or vinegar and the essential oils. Soak a flannel cloth in the liquid, wring it out until nearly dry and then place over the injured area.
2. Cover with plastic wrap so the skin absorbs the essential oils, and cover the whole thing with a towel. Apply the compress for 30 minutes up to three times daily.

Anti-Bruising Oil

30 drops carrier oil
10 drops rosemary essential oil
10 drops peppermint essential oil
10 drops juniper essential oil

Use this rub very, very gently on bruises to help in the healing process.

1. In a small bowl, mix the carrier oil with the essential oils.
2. Massage the mixture gently into bruised areas every 2 hours or apply to gauze and lay over the bruises.

Two quick treatments for burns

Aloe vera gel is an effective burn salve. Pull a leaf off the plant and scoop out the clear gel. Apply directly to the burn.

Lavender essential oil also provides relief from minor burns, such as sunburn. Apply several drops of oil directly to the burn.

Oil Rub for Burned Skin

1 drop tea tree essential oil
¼ cup (60 ml) organic olive oil

This mixture gives relief to superficial burns and sunburn. You can safely use it several times a day.

1. In a small dish, dilute the essential oil with the olive oil.
2. Gently massage the mixture over the burned area.

Soothing Oil for Mild Burns

2 capsules vitamin E, 500 IU
5 drops lavender essential oil

If the burn area is large, you may need to double the ingredients for this soothing oil.

1. Pierce each vitamin E capsule with a needle and squeeze the contents into a small dish. Stir in the lavender essential oil.
2. Gently massage into the skin.

Burn Spray

1 oz (30 ml) iced water
1 oz (30 ml) aloe vera gel
25 drops (in total) lavender, chamomile, spearmint and yarrow essential oils
1 capsule vitamin E, 500 IU

Applying a spray doesn't hurt the burn the way that massaging in an oil might. This cool mixture offers relief at very little cost.

1. In a small spray bottle, mix the iced water, aloe vera and essential oils. Pierce the vitamin E capsule with a needle, squeeze its contents into the mixture and chill.
2. Shake before use and spray over burned area. Keeps in the refrigerator for several days.

Growing your own aloe vera

You can buy an aloe vera plant at any garden store or nursery. Aloes like warmth, so in colder areas, it is safer to keep the plant potted and place it near a sunny window than to plant it outdoors. (You can move the pot outdoors during the summer months.) Repot an aloe vera in a wide rather than a deep pot; it has shallow, spreading roots. Use one with a drainage hole and fill it with General Purpose Potting Mix (page 383) plus extra perlite. Don't overwater this succulent plant. Let its soil dry completely between soakings. Fertilize it yearly, in the spring, with a half-strength 10-40-10 fertilizer mixture. When you need some aloe vera gel, just cut a lower leaf off the plant and squeeze it.

Antiseptic Lotion for Burns

1 handful dried plantain leaves
½ cup (125 ml) hot water
10 drops tea tree essential oil

Nobody wants a burn to become infected. Here's a quick and inexpensive remedy with antiseptic properties.

1. In a blender, add a handful of dried plantain leaves to about ½ cup (125 ml) hot water. Begin blending, slowly adding water or plantain leaves as necessary until the mixture becomes thick, like oatmeal. Mix in the tea tree oil.
2. Spread the mixture over the affected area. You can refrigerate the remainder for several days.

Sunburn Cooler

3 tea bags or 3 tablespoons (15 g) loose tea
boiling water

For this recipe, you simply brew a pot of regular tea (any plain black leaf tea will do fine). The tannins in the tea help soothe the burning feeling.

1. In a teapot, place the tea. Pour in boiling water, cover and steep for 5 minutes. Cool.
2. Use a cloth or cotton ball to dab the sunburn with cooling tea.

Foot Care Products

Athlete's Foot Powder

½ cup (75 g) arrowroot or cornstarch
2 tablespoons (20 g) white cosmetic clay
10 drops cypress essential oil
10 drops lavender essential oil
3 drops clove essential oil
5 drops tea tree essential oil
5 drops thyme essential oil

This easy-to-make athlete's foot powder can also be used to soothe the symptoms of jock itch.

1 In a small container with a tight-fitting cover, mix the arrowroot or cornstarch with the cosmetic clay. Add the cypress, lavender and clove essential oils and mix. To make the powder antiseptic, add the tea tree and thyme essential oils.
2 Let the powder sit for a couple of days to absorb the oils, then dust on your feet once or twice a day. Keep in a dry, covered container. It should last for several weeks.

Antifungal Foot Ointment

3 tablespoons (45 ml) organic light olive oil
⅓ oz (10 g) finely chopped beeswax
50 drops of tea tree, geranium, lavender, pine, myrrh or peppermint essential oils (in any combination)

Treating a fungus with your own aromatic homemade ointment is much more pleasant than paying more for a commercial antifungal ointment. Organic, light olive oil is available in health food stores and supermarkets.

1 In the top of a double boiler, warm the oil over simmering water. Add the beeswax to the warmed oil and stir until it melts. Remove from the heat and stir until it cools. Then beat in the essential oils.
2 Spoon the ointment into a small, sterilized, widemouthed jar with a tight-fitting lid. Keep in a cool, dark place. Massage a small amount into the affected area twice a day. The ointment should keep for several weeks.

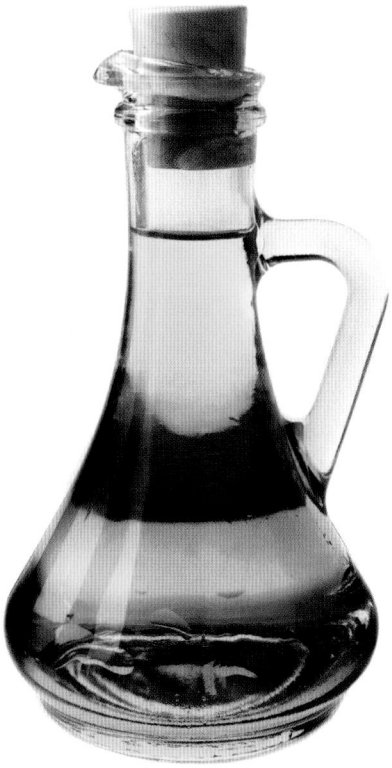

Getting an ointment to the right consistency

When making ointments, if the salve is too watery, reheat and add more beeswax. If it's too thick, reheat and add more oil.

Antifungal Solution

1–2 tablespoons (5–10 g) dried thyme
1–2 tablespoons (5–10 g) dried eucalyptus
1–2 tablespoons (5–10 g) dried lavender

Use this solution to wipe down areas affected with fungal outbreaks twice a day. It's effective and inexpensive. Before applying this solution, wash the affected area with tea tree soap (available in health food stores).

1. In a large cup, combine the herbs. Cover with 1 cup (250 ml) boiling water and steep, covered, for 10 to 15 minutes. Strain solution and cool.
2. Soak a clean cotton cloth in the solution and apply twice daily to the skin (after your shower in the morning and before bed). You can also use this solution to soak your feet.

A quick and cheap antifungal footbath

Here's a quick and easy footbath to make up in a hurry. Fill a basin with warm water and add 2 or 3 drops of mustard oil or 1 teaspoon of hot mustard powder. Soak your feet for at least half an hour. The mustard helps kill the fungus. Rinse your feet and dry thoroughly.

Corn Plaster

1 banana skin or fig skin, or pulp of a squeezed lemon
1 small dandelion leaf or garlic clove, crushed

This homemade corn plaster is very effective and costs only spare change to make.

1. Scrape the inside of the banana or fig skin until you have about 1 teaspoon of the pulp. Alternatively, you can use the flesh of a squeezed lemon.
2. In a small dish, mix the pulp with the dandelion or garlic to make a paste. Apply the paste directly to the corn, binding it in place with a small adhesive bandage.
3. When the skin is soft, gently rub the top layer of the corn away with an emery board.
4. Repeat the entire process daily until the corn disappears. For several days after the corn is gone, massage the area with a small amount of Calendula Ointment (page 292).

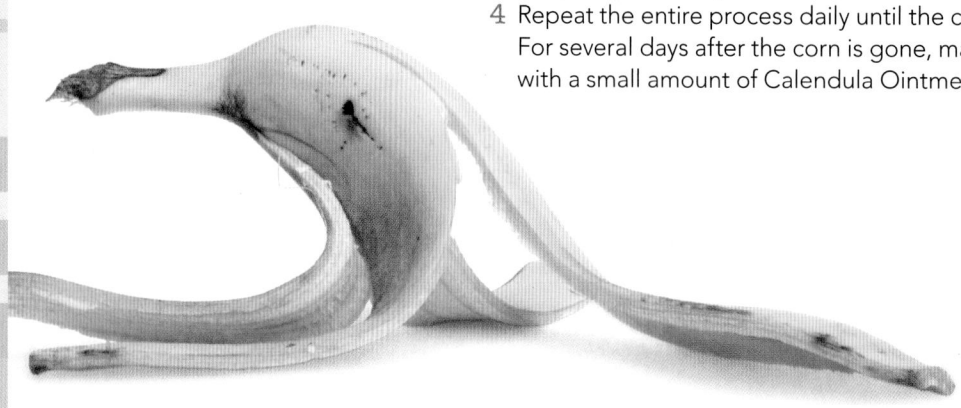

Salicylic Acid Corn Remover

5 aspirin tablets, 325 mg (adult)
½ teaspoon lemon juice
½ teaspoon water

Many commercial corn removers have salicylic acid as their main ingredient—the same active ingredient in aspirin. Here's how you can make your own salicylic acid corn remover.

1. In a small bowl, with the back of a spoon, crush the aspirin into a powder. Add the lemon juice and water and stir until the mixture forms a paste.
2. Dab the paste onto the corn and cover with plastic wrap, then place a heated towel over the wrap to help the paste penetrate more deeply. It will take several applications over several days before the corn falls off.

Lips and Mouth

Balm for Chapped Lips

¼ cup (60 ml) almond oil
3 teaspoons grated beeswax
1 teaspoon honey
1 capsule vitamin E, 500 IU
10 drops chamomile essential oil
10 drops orange essential oil
10 drops wintergreen essential oil
5 drops lavender essential oil

During winter, this homemade lip balm will keep your lips from cracking and peeling if you use it faithfully. With its lovely smell, it is a true bargain.

1. In the top of a double boiler, warm the oil, beeswax and honey over low heat until the wax melts. Remove from the heat. Pierce the vitamin E capsule with a needle and squeeze its contents into the mixture.
2. Stir in the essential oils. Store in a cool, dark place and use by dipping a finger into the balm and smoothing it on your lips.

Cold Sore Ointment

5 drops lemon balm essential oil
1 drop lavender essential oil
1 drop chamomile essential oil
1 drop bergamot or rose essential oil
10 drops jojoba oil

This is more of a liquid than an ointment, but it is just as soothing. The jojoba oil serves as a carrier oil.

1. In a small, clean jar with a tight-fitting lid, dilute the lemon balm, lavender, chamomile, bergamot or rose essential oils in the jojoba oil.
2. Smooth over the affected area several times a day.

Quickly soothe a canker sore with aloe vera

Instead of buying balm in the drugstore to coat that painful mouth sore, make your own instantly. All you need are a cotton swab and an aloe vera leaf. Dry the sore area with a cotton swab, then squeeze a bit of gel from the aloe vera leaf over the area. Repeat as often as necessary.

Mouthwash for Cold Sores

¾ cup (185 ml) water
3–4 drops clove or tea tree essential oil

This is a simple, certainly inexpensive, mouthwash that helps to soothe annoying cold sores.

1. In a clean jar with a tight-fitting lid, mix the water with the essential oil.
2. Swish the mixture in your mouth for 30 seconds, then spit it out. Cap the bottle and keep the mixture near the basin. Repeat mouthwash several times a day.

A fast cold sore preventive

The best time to prevent a cold sore outbreak is at the first tingle stage. If you feel one coming on, here's what to do. Apply 1 drop of lavender or lemon balm essential oil to the area where you feel the cold sore forming. Then hold an ice cube on top of the area for 10 minutes. This can sometimes prevent the outbreak altogether or at least reduce its severity. Repeat the whole procedure several times a day.

Cold Sore Paste

1 teaspoon finely chopped licorice root or rhizome
3 oz (90 ml) distilled water
slippery elm powder, as needed
goldenseal powder, as needed

This soothing, not-so-costly paste smothers the irritation of a cold sore and may help to heal it.

1. In a small saucepan, combine the licorice root and distilled water. Bring to a boil, then simmer for 10 minutes. Strain into a clean bowl. This makes a strong licorice decoction.
2. In a small, clean container with a tight-fitting lid, mix equal amounts of slippery elm and goldenseal powder, and moisten with the licorice decoction.
3. Apply the paste to the sore area to control pain and promote healing. Store the extra paste in the refrigerator or dilute with water and use as mouthwash.

Dental Care

Mouthwash

1 teaspoon glycerine
1 teaspoon aloe vera gel
10 drops peppermint, wintergreen or spearmint essential oil
1½ cups (375 ml) water

You don't need to spend good money on artificially flavored mouthwash that is primarily alcohol.

1 In a clean jar with a tight-fitting cap, mix the glycerine and aloe vera gel with the essential oil you have chosen. Add the water and shake well. Use as a gargle.
2 Store in a covered jar and shake well before using.

Mints

1–2 fresh leaves spearmint, peppermint, fennel or parsley
¼ teaspoon fresh or dried caraway, cardamom or fennel seeds

Instead of sugary sweets, chew on breath-freshening herbs and spices.

Chew on the herb leaves and seeds for 2 or 3 minutes. Spit out and discard.

Toothpaste

2 tablespoons baking soda
water
9 drops tea tree essential oil
9 drops peppermint essential oil

Although we can't say four out of five dentists recommend it, we do know this homemade version will cost you far less than any of the commercial brands that fill supermarket shelves. The tea tree oil provides an additional antiseptic boost to help keep gums healthy.

1 In a small bowl, mix the baking soda with just enough water to make a paste. Add the tea tree and peppermint essential oils.
2 Use the paste to brush your teeth and tongue. Cover the remaining paste and use for the next couple of days.

Gum Tonic

1 eye-dropperful of goldenseal tincture (about 20 drops)
2 drops myrrh essential oil
1 oz (30 ml) hot water

This will help treat the inflammation of bad gums without running up your grocery bill.

1 In a glass, combine the goldenseal tincture and myrrh essential oil. Dilute with the hot water.
2 Swish around your mouth and spit. Do not swallow.

Antibacterial Mouthwash

2 cups (500 ml) distilled water
2 tablespoons (10 g) green tea
2 tablespoons (10 g) dried, crumbled peppermint, spearmint or rosemary
10 drops tincture of benzoin or 1 teaspoon tincture of myrrh

When used regularly, this mouthwash can help kill many of the germs that cause gum disease.

1 In a saucepan, bring the water to a boil. In a pint jar with a tight-fitting lid, mix the green tea and peppermint, spearmint or rosemary. Pour in the boiling water, let cool, cover and steep overnight in the refrigerator.
2 Strain into a clean bottle with a tight-fitting lid. Add the tincture of benzoin or the tincture of myrrh and shake to mix.
3 Use 2 tablespoons at a time as a mouthwash for sore and/or bleeding gums. Swish and spit without swallowing.

Super Dental Floss

10 drops goldenseal tincture
3 drops myrrh essential oil
2 drops tea tree essential oil
dental floss

Save money by making your own antiseptic dental floss.

1 In a small container, combine the goldenseal tincture and the myrrh and tea tree essential oils. Cut off enough dental floss to clean between your teeth and dip it into the mixture.
2 Use the dipped floss to clean between your teeth. Make a fresh batch every time you want to floss your teeth.

Toothache-Relieving Rinse

1½ teaspoons whole cloves
1 cup (250 ml) boiling water

To quell the pain until you can get to a dentist, try this inexpensive rinse.

1 Put the cloves in a small pot. Pour in the boiling water and steep for 10 minutes. Strain into a glass.
2 Rinse your mouth with the warm infusion.

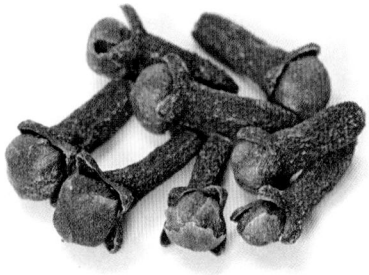

Fast toothache relief with clove oil

Until you can get to the dentist for your toothache, try this quick numbing trick. Put 1 drop of oil of cloves on a cotton swab, dip the swab in water, and then rub on the aching tooth and gum area.

Toothache-Relieving Dental Paste

2 tablespoons (20 g) ground ginger
2 tablespoons (20 g) ground cayenne pepper
water

Some people don't like cloves and need another way to relieve dental pain without using expensive pain pills with lots of side effects. Try this.

1 In a small dish, mix the ground ginger and cayenne pepper with enough water to make a paste.
2 Saturate a cotton ball with the paste and put on the painful tooth. Keep the paste off your gums because it may be irritating to them.

Joints and Muscles

Hot Pepper Rub

2 tablespoons (20 g) ground cayenne pepper
½ cup (125 ml) Green Aloe Moisturizing Lotion (page 258) or any commercial moisturizing lotion

The capsaicin in hot peppers has begun to be appreciated as a pain reliever even by commercial drug companies. Make your own for much less.

1 In a small bowl, combine the cayenne pepper with the moisturizing lotion.
2 Massage the mixture into the painful area, being careful to wash your hands afterward before touching your face or eyes.

Massage Cream

2 teaspoons grated beeswax
3 teaspoons coconut oil
¼ cup (60 ml) cayenne-infused oil
10–15 drops wintergreen essential oil
2 tablespoons (30 ml) ginger tincture
2 tablespoons (30 ml) water
2 tablespoons (30 ml) aloe vera gel
½ teaspoon borax
¼ teaspoon powdered vitamin C

This soothing massage cream will help to take care of sore muscles and your bank balance.

1 In the top of a double boiler over low heat, mix the beeswax and coconut oil and stir until the beeswax has melted. Stir in the cayenne-infused oil and the wintergreen essential oil.
2 In a separate pan, heat the ginger tincture to evaporate as much alcohol as possible, then add the water, aloe vera gel, borax and vitamin C, and bring to 160°F to 175°F on a candy thermometer. Place the ginger tincture mixture in a blender and whirl at high speed as you add the beeswax-oil mixture. Pour the resulting cream into a clean jar with a tight-fitting lid.
3 Massage the cream into sore joints as needed. Keep refrigerated for 4 to 6 weeks.

Quick-and-Dirty Muscle Rub

5 drops cayenne-based hot sauce
3–5 drops peppermint essential oil
15 drops massage oil or olive oil

Again, capsaicin comes to the rescue of tense and tired muscles that need a good massage in a hurry without costing an arm and a leg.

1 In a clean small jar, combine the hot sauce, peppermint essential oil and massage or olive oil, and mix thoroughly.
2 Rub the mixture into the affected area by hand or with a cotton ball. This may initially irritate the skin, but the irritation will disappear as the painkilling becomes more effective.
3 Clean your hands with soap and water after each application and avoid touching your eyes.

Muscle Soak

½ cup (140 g) baking soda
10–20 drops of eucalyptus, peppermint, juniper or pine essential oils
½ cup (125 g) Epsom salts
3 teaspoons juniper berries
3 teaspoons dried rosemary leaves
3 teaspoons dried chamomile flowers
3 teaspoons dried eucalyptus leaves
2 teaspoons dried lemon balm leaves
2 teaspoons dried peppermint leaves
double-layer square of cheesecloth

A luxurious hot soak with beneficial herbs is priceless for relieving tight muscles and joints. You can make your own bag of just the right herbs.

1 In a small dish, place the baking soda and add the essential oils; mix until the baking soda has absorbed the oils. In a bowl, combine the Epsom salts, herbs and the soda mixture. Place in the middle of the cheesecloth and tie up the ends to make a bag.
2 Hold beneath the running water until the tub fills, then massage your body with the bag and let it float in the tub. Soak until the water cools.

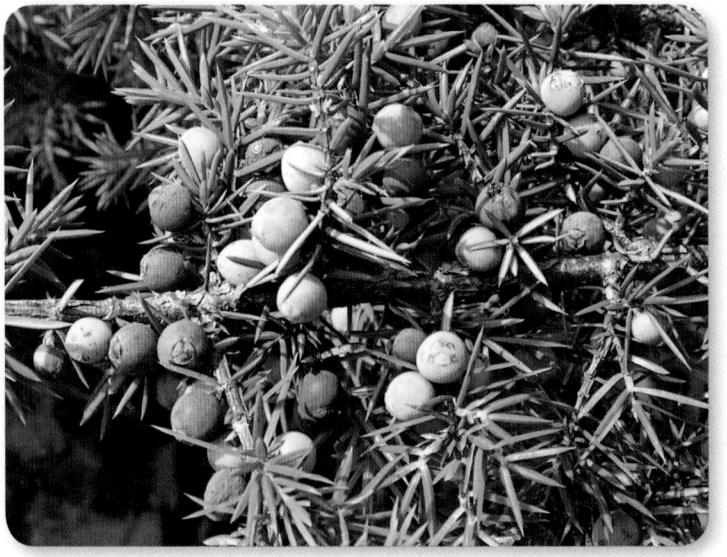

Liniment

4 teaspoons castor oil
2 tablespoons (30 ml) glycerine
2 tablespoons (30 ml) aloe vera gel
2 tablespoons (30 ml) cayenne tincture
20 drops wintergreen essential oil

This is a traditional home remedy for the athletes in your family, helping to loosen tight joints and offering relief to tired and aching limbs.

1. In a clean glass bottle with a tight-fitting stopper, combine the castor oil, glycerine, aloe vera gel, cayenne tincture and wintergreen essential oil. Shake well.
2. Massage over sore joints as needed. Refrigerate the liniment for up to 6 weeks.

Cold Pack for Strains and Sprains

3 parts water
1 part rubbing alcohol
1 plastic self-sealing freezer bag

There are all kinds of clever products on the market to use as cold packs. This one is flexible, reusable and very, very inexpensive.

1. Combine the water and rubbing alcohol in the freezer bag and freeze.
2. Wrap the frozen pack in a towel and apply to the hurting joint. The rubbing alcohol keeps the pack flexible.

Castor Oil Rub for Back Pain

5 drops ginger essential oil
5 drops peppermint or wintergreen essential oil
2 drops camphor essential oil
2 drops rosemary essential oil
1 oz (30 ml) castor oil

You don't have to pay for a special tube of rubbing cream for back pain. Instead, try this easily made rub.

1. In a small bowl, mix together the essential oils and castor oil.
2. Rub into the painful area and cover with a piece of flannel or an old T-shirt, then put a heating pad over the cloth for 15 to 20 minutes to help the rub soak in. You can double the recipe for larger areas.

Women's Problems

Muscle Relaxant for Cramps

½ teaspoon valerian tincture
½ teaspoon cramp bark tincture

Instead of taking a pill, try this less expensive, easy-to-make remedy. These tinctures are available in natural food stores or online.

Take a dose of valerian tincture and a dose of cramp bark tincture every 1 to 2 hours. These are both natural muscle relaxants.

Hot Compress for Cramps

2 tablespoons (30 ml) castor oil
10 drops ginger essential oil

You can enhance the help of a heating pad by using a touch of ginger and oil.

In a small dish, mix the castor oil and ginger essential oil. Spread the oil mixture over your abdomen, cover with a cotton or wool flannel cloth, then apply a heating pad for 20 to 30 minutes.

Anti-Cramp Tea

1 cup (250 ml) boiling water
¼ teaspoon dried raspberry leaves
¼ teaspoon dried chamomile flowers
¼ teaspoon crushed fennel seeds
¼ teaspoon dried spearmint leaves

This combination of herbs will help to relax cramps and reduce your discomfort.

1. In a large cup, pour 1 cup (250 ml) boiling water over the raspberry leaves, chamomile, crushed fennel seeds and spearmint. Steep for 10 minutes and strain into a teacup.
2. Drink for relief when the cramps hit.

Ginger Tea for Morning Sickness

1 cup (250 ml) boiling water
½ teaspoon minced fresh ginger

A simple preparation that may help to calm your stomach in the morning and reduce nausea without making you sleepy.

1. In a large cup, pour the cup of boiling water over the ginger. Steep for 10 minutes, strain into a container and refrigerate.
2. Sip in the morning when you wake.

PMS Tea

3 teaspoons chopped dried dandelion roots and/or leaves
3 teaspoons chopped dried burdock root
4 cups (1 liter) water
1 teaspoon chopped dried black cohosh rhizome or root
1 teaspoon dried cramp bark
1 teaspoon grated orange peel
1 teaspoon chopped dried licorice root

This tea is designed to help regulate hormone levels for all types of premenstrual syndrome without harming your stomach or liver.

1. In a pot, combine the dandelion roots and/or leaves and burdock root with the water. Add the black cohosh, cramp bark, orange peel and licorice root. Bring to a boil, reduce heat and simmer, uncovered, for 40 minutes. Cover and steep for 15 minutes.
2. Strain into a clean container with a tight-fitting lid.
3. Drink ½ to 1 cup (125 to 250 ml) of the tea hot or cold as needed throughout the day. Refrigerate the remainder.

Yeast Infection Cream

1 capsule acidophilus bacteria
3 tablespoons (45 g) plain organic yogurt with active cultures

You don't have to pay for expensive over-the-counter remedies for yeast infections. You can make this in no time and for very little money. Buy acidophilus bacteria capsules—the bacteria used to make yogurt—in health food stores.

1. Open the capsule and place the bacteria in a small dish. Then mix in the yogurt.
2. Apply inside the vagina with a medicine syringe at night and wear a pad to prevent leakage.

Headaches

Headache Compresses

enough chilled lavender toilet water to soak 2 washcloths
2 washcloths

To ease a tension headache after a hard day, try this cool compress.

1. In a small bowl, pour in the toilet water. Soak both washcloths in the toilet water and squeeze out the excess.
2. Lie down with a towel behind your neck. Place a wet washcloth on your forehead with the other at the base of your skull. Relax for at least 15 minutes, preferably in a darkened quiet room.

Chamomile Tea

3 teaspoons dried chamomile
1 cup (250 ml) boiling water
1 teaspoon honey (optional)

Taking a break can relieve some of the tension that causes many headaches. Inexpensive chamomile tea is particularly soothing to frazzled nerves.

1. In a small pot, place the chamomile. Pour in the boiling water and steep for 5 minutes. Strain into a teacup.
2. Sweeten with honey, if desired. Then take a few minutes to sip the hot tea slowly while sitting in a quiet spot.

Lemon Balm Tea

3 teaspoons dried lemon balm
1 cup (250 ml) boiling water
1 teaspoon honey (optional)

Lemon balm is another soothing tea herb that can relax away headaches with little fuss for small change.

1. In a small pot, place the lemon balm. Pour in the boiling water and steep for 5 minutes. Strain into a teacup.
2. Sweeten with honey, if desired. Then take a few minutes to sip the hot tea slowly while sitting in a quiet spot.

Migraine Tea

2½ cups (625 ml) water
9 teaspoons (15 g) dried lady's mantle leaves
3 teaspoons dried mint leaves

This inexpensive tea, served in a quiet, darkened room, can be very calming, but if any headache persists, seek medical advice.

1. In a saucepan, bring the water to a boil. Add the herbs and boil for 20 minutes. Remove from heat and steep for 10 minutes. Strain into a teacup.
2. Drink 1 cup (250 ml) slowly in a quiet, darkened room.

Headache Massage Oil

10 drops massage oil
3 drops peppermint essential oil
2 drops lavender essential oil
1 drop lemon, orange or lime essential oil

This fragrant aroma and gentle massage can bring a throbbing head back to health without jeopardizing your stomach or liver. If pain persists, seek medical advice.

1. In a small bowl, mix the massage oil and the essential oils.
2. Dip your fingers into the oil and then massage the oil into the temples, along the hairline, and along the base of the skull, being careful not to get any oil in the eyes.
3. Wash your hands thoroughly after each application.

Headache Oil with Vitamin E

15 drops lavender essential oil
7 drops wintergreen essential oil
1½ tablespoons (25 ml) almond or olive oil
1 capsule vitamin E, 500 IU
hot water

Here is another aromatic solution for safely massaging away a headache. Wash your hands after applying.

1. In a small dish, combine the essential oils with the almond or olive oil. Pierce the vitamin E capsule with a needle and squeeze the contents into the dish.
2. Warm the oil mixture by putting the dish in a bowl of hot water before using. Dab your fingers into the fragrant oil and gently massage your temples and the back of your neck.

Anxiety and Fatigue

Catnip Anti-Anxiety Tea

2 teaspoons dried catnip
1 cup (250 ml) boiling water

Catnip tea has a calming effect, and it may help relieve stress and combat anxiety. Sip a cup several times a day.

1. In a teapot, steep catnip in boiling water for 5 to 7 minutes.
2. Strain and drink. Serve yourself catnip tea three times a day.

Hops Anti-Anxiety Tea

2 teaspoons dried hops
1 cup (250 ml) boiling water

Your cat is casting jealous glances at your catnip tea. So try hops, the critical ingredient in beer, instead.

1. In a teapot, steep hops in boiling water for 5 to 7 minutes.
2. Strain and drink. Serve yourself hops tea three times a day.

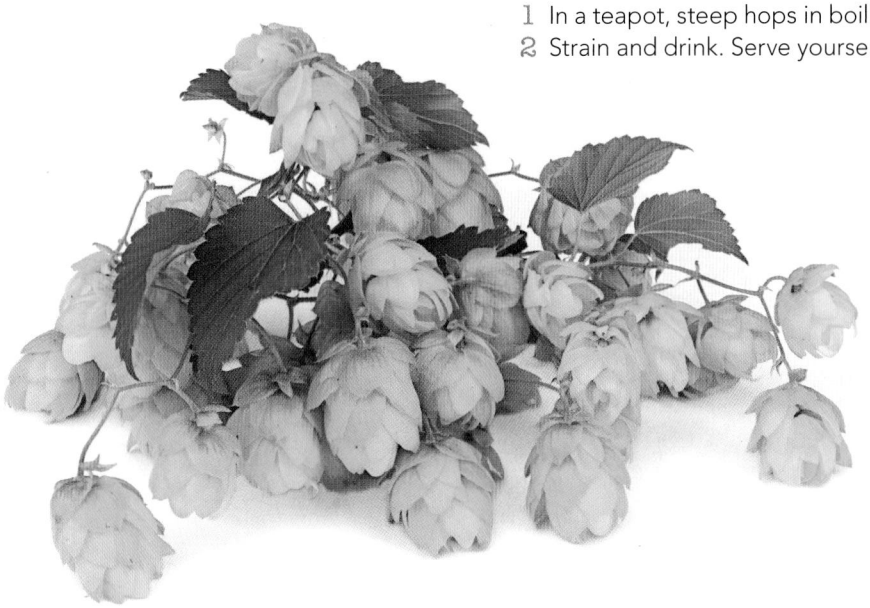

Calming Tea for Insomnia

boiling water
3 teaspoons dried chamomile or lemon balm

Many over-the-counter sleep aids may be just repackaged antihistamines. Instead, try this natural alternative.

In a small pot, pour boiling water over the chamomile or lemon balm. Steep for 10 minutes, strain and drink 1 hour before bed.

Lavender rub for insomnia

Massage a single drop of lavender essential oil into each temple before going to bed.

Sleep Pillow

4 tablespoons (20 g) sweet woodruff
2 tablespoons (10 g) lemon balm
2 tablespoons (10 g) lavender
3 teaspoons chamomile
3 teaspoons hops
3 teaspoons rosebuds
10–15 drops each chamomile, lavender, clary sage and marjoram essential oils
3 teaspoons powdered or freshly grated orris root
1 small zippered pillowcase

This aromatic small pillow will work its wonders—with no side effects—on your sleep habits.

1 In a large bowl, mix the woodruff, lemon balm, lavender, chamomile, hops and rosebuds. In a separate small bowl, mix the essential oils with the orris root. Stir this mixture into the large bowl.
2 Fill the pillowcase, zip it and add it to your bed pillows for sweet dreams.

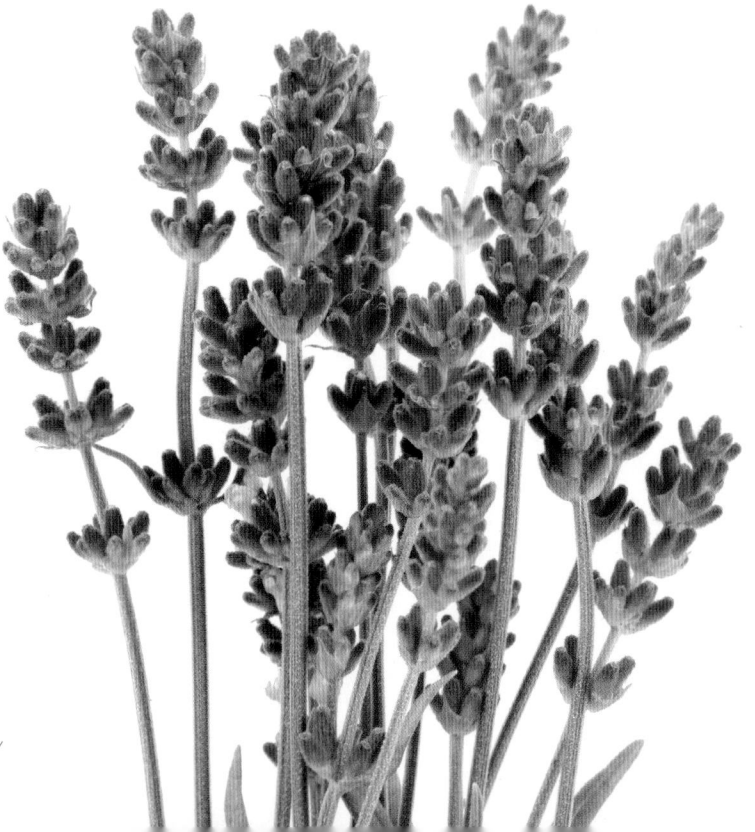

Herbal Milk Bath for Sleeplessness

½ handful lavender
½ handful chamomile
½ handful rose petals
½ handful dry powdered milk
double-layer square of cheesecloth

What is more relaxing than a nice soak in a soothing herbal bath?

1. Place the lavender, chamomile, rose petals and powdered milk on the cheesecloth and tie the corners to make a bag.
2. Place under the faucet while the water is running. Start with warm water, but allow it to cool before getting in. Cool water helps lower your body temperature, which is important for sleep.
3. Soak for 15 minutes while listening to relaxing music or a relaxation tape.

Relaxing Aromatic Bath

10 drops lavender, rose, geranium and/or bergamot essential oil

Here's another way to get sleepy or reduce stress without any pills. Keep the water relatively cool to maintain a low body temperature, important for sleep.

1. Add the essential oils to a cool bath.
2. Soak for 15 minutes while listening to relaxing music or a relaxation tape.

Invigorating Oil for Fatigue

2 parts eucalyptus essential oil
2 parts juniper essential oil
2 parts grapefruit essential oil
1 part clary sage essential oil
1 part ginger or peppermint essential oil
2 parts rosemary essential oil

These essential oils have fragrances that help to stimulate you and keep your mind alert.

1. In a clean small spray bottle, add the essential oils. Shake to mix.
2. You can use this spray in a variety of ways: spritz an entire room when you feel tired and need to keep reading. Spray a cloth, hold it up to your nose and breathe deeply. Rub into your hands. Use in a diffuser or humidifier.

Energy Tea for Fatigue

1 teacup (200 ml) boiling water
½ teaspoon dried rosemary leaves
½ teaspoon dried ginseng root
honey (optional)

This energizing tea is a real homemade pick-me-up that tastes good as well.

In a teacup, make an infusion of boiling water, dried rosemary leaves and dried ginseng root. Sweeten with a bit of honey, if you like, and drink as often as necessary.

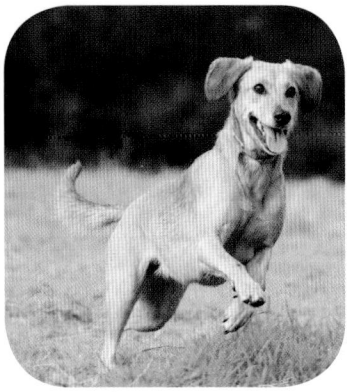

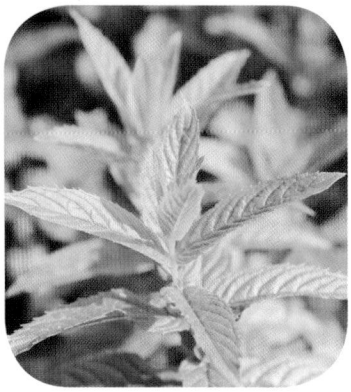

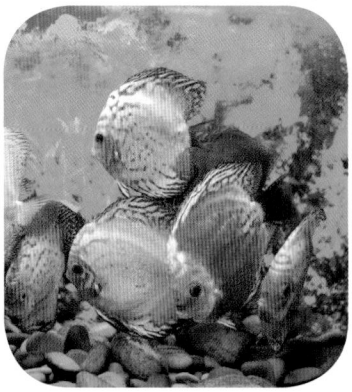

Dog Food

Calcium-Rich Dog Food ❖ Low-Fat Chicken and Rice Dog Dinner ❖ Delectable Dog Biscuits ❖ Doggie Salad ❖ Lucky Liver Treats ❖ Sweet Breath Dog Treats ❖ Doggie Birthday Cake

Dog Care Products

Brush-and-Go Dry Dog Shampoo ❖ Deodorizing Minty Dog Wash ❖ Cocktail Flea Dip ❖ Flea-Begone Bandanna ❖ Flea Powder ❖ Ear Mite Oil ❖ Firm Stool Fix

Cat Food

Wholesome Kitty Dinner ❖ Tuna Treats ❖ Catnip Crackers ❖ Quick Fish Stick Treats Sardine Balls ❖ Melon Squares ❖ Cat Grass Buffet

Cat Care Products

Baby-Fresh Litter ❖ Dry Cat Shampoo Fragrant Flea Treatment ❖ Tick Removal from Cats

Treats for Birds

Pet Bird Honey Treats ❖ Pet Bird Snacking Salad ❖ Sweet and Crunchy Bird Muffins ❖ Finch and Canary Treats ❖ Wild Bird Food ❖ Parrot Pops ❖ Premium Wild Bird Mix ❖ Healthy Hummingbird Nectar

Food for Other Pets

Guinea Pig Salad ❖ Hamster Fruit Cup ❖ Gerbil and Rabbit Salad ❖ Pet Rodent Tabbouleh ❖ Turtle and Reptile Treat ❖ Aquarium Fish Treats

Natural Pet Care Products

Our animal companions provide us not only with comfort and amusement, but also with an uncritical devotion and loyalty that is difficult to obtain elsewhere.

A loving pet provides therapy that instantly lifts its caretaker's spirits. So all of us who love pets tend to enjoy buying them expensive treats and toys. As this chapter will show you, however, you don't have to spend a fortune to keep your pet—dog, cat, bird, guinea pig, gerbil, rat, turtle or fish—well fed, healthily groomed and happily occupied.

Indulge your pets with nutritious meals that they will gobble up eagerly and healthy treats that they can enjoy without jeopardizing their health and well-being. None of these foods will strain your budget, and most are actually fun to make. And it is always reassuring to know exactly what goes into your pet's food. In the recipes that follow, you will find not only healthy everyday foods and rewards, but also special-occasion treats such as a dog's birthday cake, catnip crackers for your cat and honey treats for your pet bird.

You will also find great recipes for natural wet and dry shampoos, flea dips and breath-saving dog biscuits. For backyard bird lovers, there are recipes for inexpensive seed combinations you can mix to feed wild birds outside your window. And for young families, there are salads and treats for guinea pigs, hamsters, turtles and other childhood friends.

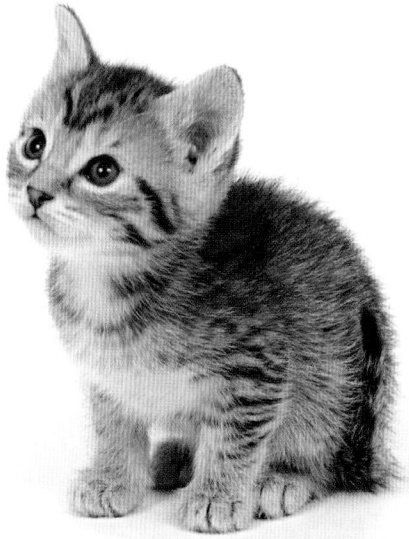

Dog Food

Calcium-Rich Dog Food

1 lb (500 g) ground chicken or beef
4 cups (about 750 g) cooked oatmeal or brown rice
½ cup (50 g) dry bread crumbs
¼ cup (60 ml) vegetable oil
3 teaspoons bonemeal (available at garden centers)
1 dog vitamin, crushed
½ cup (60 g) grated cheddar cheese

Makes 6 servings, 1 cup (about 240 g) each

This easy-to-make recipe will appeal to dogs and help to strengthen their bones. Although it is not inexpensive, it costs less than many canned dog foods, and you can vouch for the quality of its ingredients.

1. In a frying pan or skillet over medium heat, brown the meat, stirring frequently. Remove from the heat.
2. Stir in the other ingredients and enough water to keep the mixture from being crumbly.
3. Cool and store in the refrigerator for 1 week or in the freezer for up to 3 months.

Note: Feed according to the weight of your dog. Feed a 5-pound dog ½ cup daily; double the serving for every 5 pounds. Monitor your dog's weight—you may need to adjust portions to avoid obesity.

Low-Fat Chicken and Rice Dog Dinner

3 lb (1.4 kg) chicken, with skin and bone
1½ cups (280 g) cooked oatmeal or brown rice
1 dog vitamin
1 pint (500 g) fat-free cottage cheese

Makes 6 servings, 1 cup (about 360 g) each

If you want a nutritious beef-and-wheat-free diet for your pet, this combination will satisfy its appetite and may even keep its weight under control. This is also an economical dog food with fresh ingredients.

1. Poach, bake or microwave the chicken until well done. Cool and cut into cubes. Drain and reserve pan juices to use as soup stock. Discard the bones.
2. In a large bowl, mix together the cubed chicken and oatmeal or rice. Crumble the vitamin and stir it in. Drain the cottage cheese and fold it into the mixture.
3. Store in a covered container in the refrigerator for up to 1 week.

Note: Feed according to the weight of your dog. Feed a 5-pound dog ½ cup daily; double the serving for every 5 pounds. Monitor your dog's weight—you may need to adjust portions to avoid obesity.

Delectable Dog Biscuits

2 lb (900 g) Calcium-Rich Dog Food (opposite) or canned dog food
¼ cup (35 g) whole wheat flour
¾ cup (110 g) oat bran
1 cup (100 g) rolled oats
1 dog vitamin, crushed (optional)
¼ cup (25 g) grated Parmesan or cheddar cheese (optional)
½ cup (125 ml) vegetable oil

Makes 16 medium biscuits

The combination of dog food and oatmeal makes these biscuits a healthy and tasty treat for your dog. You are assured of good ingredients and a better price than commercial dog biscuits. For a nutritional boost, add a crumbled dog vitamin.

1 Preheat the oven to 250°F.
2 Mix the dog food, flour, bran, rolled oats, vitamin (if desired) and cheese (if desired for a flavor boost).
3 Add the oil slowly, mixing the dough to a consistency that can be rolled and cut with a cookie cutter.
4 Roll and cut or mold the biscuits; place on an ungreased baking sheet. Bake for 3½ hours, or until hard.
5 Cool and store in a covered canister in the refrigerator for 1 week or in a freezer for up to 1 month.

Homemade comforts for a new puppy

Puppies suffer from separation anxiety when they first leave their mother.

❖ To ease the transition, ask the breeder to put an old towel, T-shirt or other piece of clothing into the puppy's box for a few days. When you bring the puppy home, bring along the towel or clothing with the smells it recognizes and put it into the puppy's new bed.

❖ Along with this security blanket, add something that smells of you so that the pup will soon get used to its new home and associate your smell with comfort and safety.

❖ Another helpful transition aid is an old-fashioned ticking alarm clock, which emulates the mother's heartbeat.

❖ Also try filling an old sock with dried beans and microwaving it for a few seconds to create a soft, warm "body" for the puppy to snuggle up to.

Doggie Salad

1 cup (155 g) grated carrots
⅓ cup (60 g) cooked brown rice
½ cup (125 g) fat-free plain, live-culture yogurt
¼ cup (60 ml) vegetable oil

Makes 4 servings

Here's a delicious dietary supplement for your dog. Making your own costs very little and is much fresher. Dogs like carrots, which aid in digestion, freshen breath and provide vitamins. The yogurt is digestion-friendly.

1 Mix the carrots and rice in a bowl and set aside. In a second bowl, stir together the yogurt and salad oil. Pour this mixture over the carrots and rice and toss.
2 Store salad in a covered container in the refrigerator for up to 3 days. Serve ¼ cup (about 100 g) every day along with meals or as a treat.

Lucky Liver Treats

1 lb (500 g) beef or chicken livers
1 egg
1 cup (150 g) flour
¼ cup (20 g) unprocessed bran (wheat or oat)
¾ cup (110 g) cornmeal
3 teaspoons garlic powder

Makes 117 liver treats

The secret of many successful show and obedience trainers is nothing more than a little baked chewy liver nibble that dogs can't resist. Try it—your pet will jump through hoops for this homemade treat.

1. Preheat the oven to 400°F. Chop the raw livers, and then liquefy them in a blender. Add the egg, pulse to blend and then pour the mixture into a mixing bowl. Stir in the flour, bran, cornmeal and garlic powder.
2. Spread the mixture evenly into a greased 9 x 13-inch sheet-cake pan and bake for 15 minutes.
3. While still warm, cut the mixture into 1-inch squares. Turn the squares out onto a baking rack to cool and harden.
4. Store the cooled treats in a plastic self-sealing bag in the freezer to preserve freshness for up to 3 months. Serve either frozen or at room temperature.

Sweet Breath Dog Treats

3 teaspoons activated charcoal (available in fish section of pet stores)
½ cup (75 g) whole wheat flour
1 cup (150 g) white flour
¼ cup (20 g) bran cereal
½ cup (75 g) cornmeal
¼ cup (60 ml) vegetable oil
1 egg
½ cup (30 g) chopped fresh basil, wintergreen or mint
½ cup (30 g) chopped fresh rosemary or thyme
1 cup (250 ml) acidophilus milk

Makes 24 medium biscuits

Here is a specialty dog biscuit that you don't have to shell out a fortune for at a pet store. Puppies often have "puppy breath" that they naturally outgrow by the age of 6 months. If an adult dog has occasional bad breath, this tasty recipe will combat the problem. If bad breath persists, however, it may be a sign of dental or digestive problems that a vet should treat.

1. Preheat the oven to 400°F. Process the charcoal in a coffee grinder until finely ground. Mix the flours, bran, cornmeal and charcoal together in a bowl. Stir in the other ingredients.
2. Form into bite-sized patties and place on a greased cookie sheet. Bake for 20 minutes, or until dry and hard.
3. Store in a covered container in the refrigerator for 1 week or in the freezer for up to 3 months.

A quick water bowl for dog walkers

Pick up an inexpensive plastic shower cap to use as a portable pet water bowl. Stick it in your pocket when you're out walking your dog and, when needed, pull it out and fill it from a water bottle, the nearest faucet or a water fountain.

Doggie Birthday Cake

⅓ cup (50 g) flour
⅓ cup (50 g) cornmeal, bran or rolled oats
1½ teaspoons baking powder
½ teaspoon garlic powder
1 lb (500 g) ground chicken
2 tablespoons (30 ml) honey
1 large egg
¼ cup (60 g) live-culture plain yogurt
4 teaspoons vegetable oil
1 container (125 g) spreadable cream cheese
Delectable Dog Biscuits, as needed to decorate cake (page 313)

Makes 1 cake with 4 to 6 servings

People do like to make a fuss over their dogs. For a birthday or adoption anniversary, you can go to a very fancy pet store and spend a lot of money on a cake or you can make up this nutritious treat (to be meted out during the week) for much less. Here's a cake that you can feel good about offering your dog.

1. Preheat the oven to 350°F. In a medium bowl, stir together the dry ingredients. Make a well in the center and add the chicken, honey, egg, yogurt and oil. Stir just until mixed.
2. Pour into a greased cake pan and bake for 25 minutes or until the chicken is done and a toothpick inserted in the center of the cake comes out clean.
3. Turn out onto a cake rack to cool.
4. Ice the cake with cream cheese (thin cheese, if needed, with a little milk) and decorate with the dog biscuits. Refrigerate in a covered container for up to 1 week.

Dog Care Products

Brush-and-Go Dry Dog Shampoo

1 box (1 lb/500 g) baking soda

Makes 1 or more shampoos, depending on the size of dog

You can save heaps by substituting this single ingredient for a commercial dry pet shampoo. Although your pet will still need the occasional soap-and-water shampoo to remove ground-in dirt, dry shampoo will keep your dog clean and fresh smelling during cold weather or when you're traveling.

1. Test for sensitivity by rubbing a little baking soda into your dog's coat between the ears (where it can't be licked off). Wait for 5 minutes and check for reddening or other signs of irritation. If there are none, proceed.
2. Rub the baking soda into the dog's coat, working it in all the way to the skin. Be careful to avoid the eyes, nose, mouth and ears. Allow the soda to remain in the coat for a full minute to absorb oil and odor.
3. Brush the fur with a pet brush until all the baking soda and debris are removed.

Deodorizing Minty Dog Wash

1 large tube traditional-formula white toothpaste (colored or gel pastes can discolor fur)
dog shampoo
¼ cup (60 ml) cider vinegar

Makes 1 treatment

When your dog rolls in something foul-smelling—as they often do—confine it outdoors and run to the bathroom supply cabinet for help.

1 Work the toothpaste into the dog's fur from head to tail, nose to toe. Allow the toothpaste to air-dry for 20 minutes.
2 Wet the dog and apply dog shampoo, working up a full lather.
3 In a large bucket, combine the vinegar with 1 gallon of warm water. Rinse the dog with this solution (double it for a big dog) and dry as usual.
4 Repeat treatment as needed.

Cocktail Flea Dip

2 tablespoons (30 ml) vodka or dry vermouth
1¾ pints (825 ml) water

Makes 1 treatment

To check for fleas, comb your pet over a sheet of white paper: if black specks (flea dirt) drop onto the paper, treat the animal at once with this dip (double recipe for large pets). There are many expensive flea dips around, but this one does not contain harsh chemicals. To get rid of flea eggs—and future infestations—wash the animal's bedding and vacuum your house thoroughly.

1 In a large saucepan, stir alcohol into water and bring to a boil.
2 Remove from the heat, cover the pan, and allow the solution to steep for 2 hours.
3 Rub the cooled solution into your pet's fur, rinse and comb out.

Flea-Begone Bandanna

1 cotton bandanna (color and pattern of your choice)
1 small vial rose geranium essential oil
1 small vial lavender essential oil

Here's a safe, renewable, flea-repelling bandanna to make for your dog. The active ingredients are essential herb oils, which smell good to us, but fleas and mosquitoes can't stand them. (Note that this is not a tick deterrent. It should also not be considered adequate protection against mosquitoes in heartworm areas.)

1 Sprinkle several drops of each oil on the bandanna.
2 Roll the bandanna and tie it loosely around your dog's neck.
3 Launder the bandanna; retreat with oil when the scent fades.

Note: If your dog won't wear a bandanna, dab oil between its shoulder blades where it can't be licked off. Don't get oil near a dog's eyes, nose or mouth.

Natural ways to make fleas flee

Consider aromatic leaves, wood shavings and soap your first defense in your arsenal of flea repellents.

❖ Fill small drawstring bags (available at cooking supply and natural foods stores) with fresh or dried chamomile leaves, walnut leaves or cedar shavings, and tuck them into your dog's bedding (where they can't be chewed) to repel fleas.

❖ Sprinkle garlic powder or mix a crushed garlic clove into your dog's food to ward off fleabites. Both garlic and chamomile are attractive flowering perennials, so for a free supply, try growing these herbs in your flower or vegetable beds.

❖ A sprinkle of brewer's yeast (buy from health food stores) on your pets' food daily is also thought to help them repel fleas.

❖ Soap kills fleas on contact. When bathing your dog, begin by lathering the neck area and then work your way toward the tail, because fleas tend to congregate around the neck.

❖ After rinsing, rub apple cider vinegar through the fur to help repel fleas, and add a teaspoon of cider vinegar to the dog's drinking water.

Flea Powder

1 box (1 lb/500 g) baking soda
10 drops in total peppermint, lavender, rosemary, cedar, eucalyptus or rose geranium essential oils

Makes 1 treatment

This inexpensive powder will leave your dog fresh smelling and help to repel fleas. It is safe to apply as often as needed. Mix and match the oils according to your own scent preference.

1. In a mixing bowl, empty the box of baking soda, sprinkle with your personal blend of oils and stir to blend.
2. Work the treated baking soda into your dog's fur, beginning at the neck (where fleas congregate) and working toward the tail. Keep the powder away from nose, mouth, eyes and ears.
3. Allow the powder to remain on the dog for 10 minutes, then comb or brush it out along with dirt and fleas.

Note: If you have a large dog, you may need to make two or more recipes' worth.

Easy way to remove burrs and gum from fur

Burrs and chewing gum can be nearly impossible to comb or shampoo out of a pet's tangled fur. To make burrs easier to comb out, coat them with vegetable or mineral oil. Allow the oil to soften the burr for a few minutes, and then comb it out. To remove chewing gum, work creamy-style peanut butter into the gum until it dissolves, then comb out.

Ear Mite Oil

1 vitamin E capsule, 500 IU
¼ cup (60 ml) mineral oil

Makes ¼ cup (60 ml)

Ear mites can lead to serious infections and problems, including hearing loss in dogs. You can help to head off problems—and expensive vet bills—with this simple treatment. If you are too late and the problem persists, consult a veterinarian. It could be a yeast infection and not mites at all.

1. Pierce a vitamin E capsule with a needle and squeeze the contents into a small dropper bottle. Add the oil and shake. Store at room temperature.
2. To apply, hold the bottle in your hand for a few minutes to warm the oil. Put 2 or 3 drops of warm oil into the dog's ear canal and massage gently for a count of 10. Allow the dog to shake its head, then carefully swab oil and dirt from the ear. Repeat in the other ear.
3. Apply every other day for a full week.

Free pooper scoopers

❖ Save used self-sealing plastic sandwich and food storage bags to recycle as puppy toilet bags. To use a bag, turn it inside out and reach inside the clean side of the bag to grab the stool. Then pull the bag right-side-out, zip it closed and toss it in an outside bin.

❖ If you don't like the hands-on approach, you can relegate a cheap or decommissioned pair of scissors-style salad tongs to the status of pooper scooper—they work better than the real thing, and you can still make deposits into the self-sealing bags.

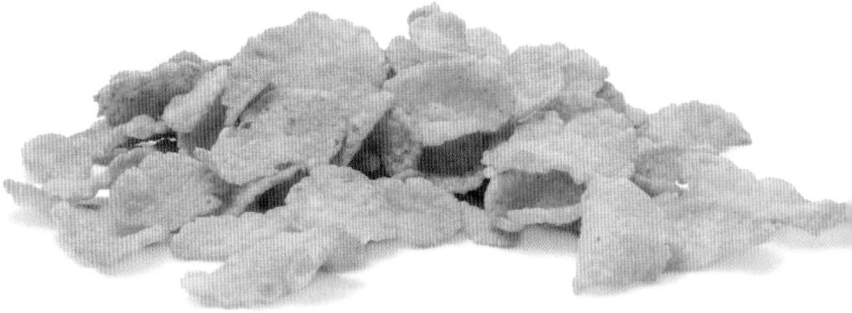

Firm Stool Fix

2 teaspoons mashed pumpkin
3 teaspoons cream cheese
¼ cup (7 g) cornflakes

Makes 1 treatment

If your pup or dog suffers occasionally from loose or runny stools, try this cheap and easy high-fiber remedy. If the problem persists, it could indicate internal parasites and you should consult a vet.

1. In a bowl, mix the pumpkin and cheese; roll the mixture into a ball and coat with the cornflakes.
2. Serve as a treat.

Cat Food

Wholesome Kitty Dinner

⅔ cup (180 g) ground chicken or beef
1 jar mixed vegetable baby food
1 cat vitamin, crumbled (optional)
⅓ cup (35 g) plain dry bread crumbs

Makes 2 or 3 servings

This nutritious meat and vegetable meal will be a welcome change of pace for your cat. You know exactly what is in it, and it's budget-friendly, too.

1. In a small saucepan over medium heat, poach the ground meat in a small amount of water until medium-rare. Remove from heat and allow to cool.
2. Stir together the meat, meat juices, vegetables and vitamin, if using. Form into bite-sized balls and roll in bread crumbs.
3. Serve as much as your cat will eat in one sitting. Store the rest in a covered container in the refrigerator for up to 3 days.

Tuna Treats

1 can oil-packed tuna
¼ cup (35 g) cornmeal
¼ cup (20 g) bran cereal
1½ cups (225 g) whole wheat flour

Makes 24 or more depending on size of treat

Cats are famous for loving tuna, and yours will jump for joy when you whip up these healthy treats that use a can of "people" tuna and a few pantry staples. As a bonus, the oil-packed tuna may help prevent hairballs. You won't find fresh treats like this at any pet store.

1. Preheat the oven to 350°F. In a large bowl, mix all the ingredients together.
2. Press the dough out on a floured board and cut into small cookies with a cookie cutter or pizza roller.
3. Place the treats on a greased cookie sheet and bake for 20 minutes or until light brown. Turn out onto a cake rack to cool. Store treats in a covered container in the refrigerator for up to 1 week or in the freezer for up to 1 month.

Trick your cat into taking medicine

Cats are choosy about what they eat, and often turn up their noses at the taste of medicine. If you have trouble getting yours to take its medicine, try smearing the medication on the back of a front paw—the cat will lick it off. If it is in pill form, crush and mix the pill with a little cream cheese to make it adhere to the paw.

Catnip Crackers

¾ cup (110 g) flour
½ cup (75 g) whole wheat flour
2 tablespoons (10 g) dried catnip (available at pet stores and in the pet aisle of some supermarkets)
½ cup (125 g) yogurt
1 egg
3 teaspoons honey
3 tablespoons (45 ml) vegetable oil

Makes 24 or more depending on the size of crackers

Cats will go bonkers for these catnip crackers, so save them for rainy-day treats and special occasions.

1. Preheat the oven to 350°F. In a medium bowl, mix the flours and catnip together. Stir in the yogurt, egg, honey and vegetable oil.
2. Press out the dough on a floured surface and cut into tiny treats using a cookie cutter or pizza wheel. Place on a greased cookie sheet and bake for 15 minutes or until golden brown.
3. Store in a covered container in the refrigerator for 1 week or in the freezer for up to 3 months.

Quick Fish Stick Treats

1 box frozen breaded fish sticks
½ teaspoon garlic powder

Makes approximately 36 treats

Cats and their human companions alike will love these instant treats made from inexpensive frozen fish sticks. Adding a sprinkle of garlic powder will help your cat repel fleas.

1. Empty the box of frozen fish sticks onto a cutting board. Sprinkle with garlic powder and cut the frozen sticks into 1-inch squares.
2. Store the squares in a self-sealing plastic bag (along with the cooking instructions from the package) in the freezer for up to 3 months.
3. To serve, remove a square and microwave it according to package directions, cool, then serve at room temperature.

Sardine Balls

1 can (6½ oz/185 g) sardines, packed in oil
¾ cup (75 g) plain bread crumbs

Makes 6 or 8 treats

Cats will meow for the fishy flavor of these wholesome little fish balls. They're easy to make, kind on the budget, and the oily fish may help keep hairballs from forming.

1. Empty the can of sardines into a mixing bowl. Mix in ½ cup (50 g) bread crumbs. Roll the mixture into bite-sized balls. When all balls are made, roll them in the remaining bread crumbs to coat.
2. Store in a sealed container or self-sealing plastic bag in the freezer for up to 3 months.
3. To serve, thaw a ball to room temperature and place in your cat's food bowl.

Make your own cat toys

Cats love toys and are especially fond of small, light, flexible and sparkly items. Avoid a costly trip to the pet store by offering these found toys to your pet.

❖ Save the foil wrappers from chewing gum and other snacks and roll them into little balls for your cat to bat around.

❖ Twist a foil wrapper into a little "bow tie" and fasten it on the end of a piece of string, then dangle it for your cat to play with.

❖ Tie these string foil-wrapper toys to doorknobs throughout the house. Your cat will love hiding behind the door and reaching around to pounce and bat at them.

❖ Create little rolling noise-makers by filling film canisters with nontoxic items, such as pieces of breakfast cereal and chopped nuts. Your cat will spend many happy hours rolling and chasing these toys.

Melon Squares

½ orange-fleshed melon
½ green-fleshed melon

Some cats love the flavor of melon. If yours is among them, keep some of these mixed melon treats on hand.

1. Peel and cube the melon flesh as you would for a salad.
2. Store melon cubes in a sealed container in the refrigerator for up to 1 week.
3. Serve 1 or 2 cubes as a treat daily.

Cat Grass Buffet

1 cup (180 g) whole oat berries
½ cup (90 g) wheat berries
½ cup (90 g) barley seeds
¼ cup (45 g) alfalfa seeds
¼ cup (45 g) rye grass seeds

Makes 4 flowerpots of grass

House cats like green "grass" to nibble on, and this recipe offers your cat long-lasting variety for little money. You can buy untreated sprouting grains inexpensively at health food stores or even cheaper at feed mills. Keep grains in sealed plastic containers in the refrigerator. Save an empty Parmesan cheese shaker to fill with seed mix: It makes sowing easier.

1. Put the grains into a sealed plastic container and shake to mix. Fill shallow, tip-resistant pots with potting soil and moisten with tepid water.
2. Sprinkle the grains thickly over the top of the soil and cover grains with a sprinkling of soil. Set the pots in a sunny window and water them as needed to keep the soil as moist as a wrung-out sponge. When the grass is about 1 inch tall, set a pot beside your cat's dinner dish and watch the fun.
3. For an ongoing supply, start a fresh pot of cat grass every other week.

Cat Care Products

Baby-Fresh Litter

cat litter to cover bottom of litter box
⅓ cup (60 g) baby powder

Makes filler for 1 litter box

The most effective way to prevent cat litter odor is also a money saver: Instead of throwing money away by filling the litter box to the top, just pour in a shallow layer. Use only 2 to 3 inches so that the litter can air-dry rapidly. Between litter changes, you can keep even the cheapest brand of litter smelling fresh with this simple, baby-safe recipe.

1. Pour the litter into a litter box to a depth of 3 inches.
2. Sprinkle the baby powder over the top of litter and stir to blend. For best results, change the litter at least once a week.

Dry Cat Shampoo

⅓ cup (25 g) unprocessed bran
⅓ cup (50 g) cornmeal
⅓ cup (35 g) rolled oats

Makes 1 shampoo

Take the stress out of bathtime for your cat by bathing it with this soothing, dry shampoo. As an added bonus, you'll save some pocket change because it's made from common pantry staples.

1. Pour the grains into a microwave-safe plastic container, seal and shake to combine. Warm in the microwave set on low for 10 seconds.
2. Rub the warm grains into your pet's fur. When finished, brush the grains out along with oil, dirt and dander.

Clever cat litter storage

If you keep your litter box in the laundry, bathroom or a walk-in closet, try storing new kitty litter in an open bag at the bottom of your clothes hamper, the corner of a closet or near the washing machine. Not only will the kitty litter absorb odors and help keep these rooms smelling fresh, but you'll also be reminded to change the litter every time you change clothes.

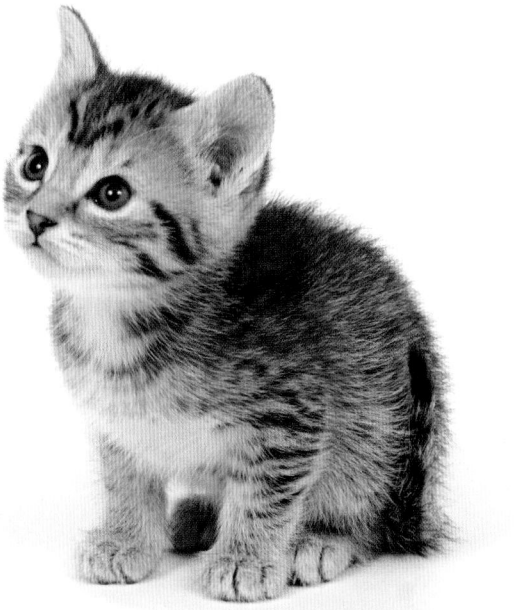

Fragrant Flea Treatment

6 drops lavender essential oil
3 teaspoons mineral oil or baby oil

Makes 1 treatment

Cats can be sensitive to any flea treatment, particularly toxic commercial flea powders. So try this mixture on a small patch of skin on the cat's stomach and wait for a day to see if there is a reaction. You must also wash the cat's bedding and vacuum the house thoroughly to get rid of flea eggs.

1. Drop the lavender essential oil and the mineral or baby oil into a small bottle and shake to combine.
2. Warm oil by holding the bottle in your hands for a few minutes.
3. Massage the warm oil into the neck area and the base of the tail where fleas congregate, then all parts of the cat, being careful to avoid contact with the cat's ears, eyes, nose and mouth. Repeat treatment when the scent is no longer detectable.

Free disposable cat litter boxes

Why clean a smelly plastic litter box when you can get biofriendly ones for free and toss them out, dirty litter and all? Make a habit of stopping by your local convenience store or beverage store and asking for their empty plastic-wrapped, shallow boxes—the kind that hold a dozen cans of soft drink. Keep the plastic on the box while in use, then pull it off and toss in the recycle bin before dumping the litter-filled box into the trash. They also make convenient toss-and-go litter boxes for traveling with your cat.

Tick Removal from Cats

petroleum jelly
hydrogen peroxide

Makes 1 treatment

Cats are sensitive to many kinds of medications and herbal treatments, including tick repellents, which are safe to use on dogs. Your best bet is to watch for ticks, especially around the face, ears and neck, and remove them according to the following recipe. However, if your cat is showing any signs at all of tick poisoning, seek veterinary advice immediately.

1. Coat the tick and surrounding skin with petroleum jelly applied with a cotton swab.
2. After the tick smothers, gently pull it, with the head intact, from the cat's skin.
3. Swab the area with hydrogen peroxide to disinfect it.

Treats for Birds

Pet Bird Honey Treats

⅓ cup (50 g) cornmeal
½ cuttlebone, finely ground (in coffee grinder or with mortar and pestle)
¼ teaspoon fine bird grit
¼ cup (40 g) mixed parakeet, finch or canary seeds
1 piece millet spray, crumbled
2 tablespoons (30 ml) honey
¼ cup (25 g) wheat germ
1 egg

Makes approximately 12 treats

Parakeets and songbirds like sweets. This calcium-rich, sweet treat is an inexpensive, wholesome snack. Most of the ingredients are already in your kitchen. You can find cuttlebone and bird grit at most pet stores or in the pet aisle of your supermarket.

1. Preheat the oven to 350°F. Place all the ingredients into a bowl and mix well. If the mixture is too thick to mold, add a little water. Press with your hands into small logs onto a greased and floured cookie sheet.
2. Bake for 30 minutes or until lightly browned.
3. Remove from the oven and turn logs out onto a cake rack to cool. Store, covered, in the freezer for up to 3 months.
4. To serve, thaw a log and fasten to cage bars with a treat clip. Renew when well nibbled.

Pet Bird Snacking Salad

3 leaves leaf lettuce, chopped, or ½ cup (20 g) chopped fresh spinach
½ cup (30 g) fresh or frozen, thawed, broccoli florets
½ cup (75 g) frozen and thawed whole kernel corn
½ apple, diced
½ segmented orange, diced
¼ cup (35 g) dried currants
½ cup (80 g) unsalted peanuts (for large birds only)

Makes about 6 servings

For optimum health, offer your bird fresh or thawed frozen fruits and vegetables daily. Forget expensive dried treats from a pet store—they can't compare in freshness, flavor or vitamins. This salad appeals to all bird species and is easy to put together by saving a little here and there from your meal preparations. Modify it as needed: You will learn quickly which ingredients your bird devours and which ingredients it leaves uneaten.

1. Toss all the ingredients in a covered bowl and store in the refrigerator for up to 5 days.
2. To serve, put a handful of salad in a shallow bowl or pottery flowerpot saucer in the cage. Offer daily and make new salad as needed.

The easy way to trap bird ticks

If your bird has ticks, hang a disposable white cloth (or a paper towel) on one side of its cage. The ticks are attracted to the bright object. After the ticks congregate on the cloth, remove and dispose in a sealed plastic bag.

Sweet and Crunchy Bird Muffins

1 small package of commercial corn, bran or oatmeal muffin mix
⅓ cup (80 ml) milk
1 egg
¼ cup (65 g) applesauce
½ cup (95 g) mixed dried fruits, unsweetened
½ cup (80 g) birdseed mix (appropriate to the species of bird)
1 bird vitamin, crumbled (optional)

Makes 6 muffins

Small-quantity corn, bran and oatmeal muffin mixes are sold cheaply in supermarkets—using them as a basis for these yummy bird treats lets you whip up treats faster than you could make them from scratch—but you can substitute your favorite muffin recipe (omit salt, which can harm birds). Plus, this all-in-one treat takes the place of several pricey commercial single-ingredient treats. For variety's sake, make all three flavors at the same time and alternate the flavors you offer your bird each day.

1. Preheat the oven to 375°F. Prepare the muffin mix according to package directions, substituting the applesauce for oil. Stir in the dried fruit, seed and bird vitamin, if using.
2. Pour the batter into greased muffin tins and bake according to package directions for 20 minutes, or until golden brown.
3. Store in a sealed container in the freezer for up to 3 months.
4. To serve, thaw a muffin and place part or all of it in the bird's cage. You can refrigerate unused portions for up to 1 week.

Finch and Canary Treats

¼ cup (60 g) crunchy Peanut Butter (page 33) or crunchy, unsweetened, low-salt commercial peanut butter
½ cup (80 g) high-quality finch seed mix
¼ cup (25 g) wheat germ

Makes 8 treats

Here's a bite-sized nutritious treat that's easy to make for small songbirds, such as finches and canaries. It is fresher and far less expensive than store-bought treats.

1. In a medium bowl, mix the peanut butter and seeds together, adding more seeds if needed to make a stiff batter.
2. Pour the wheat germ into a shallow saucer. Form the peanut butter mix into small balls and roll the balls in wheat germ to coat.
3. Serve 1 ball as a treat in a bird-proof bowl. Store leftovers in a covered container in the refrigerator for up to 1 month or freeze for up to 3 months.

Wild Bird Food

½ cup (60 g) sunflower seeds
½ cup (60 g) cracked corn
½ cup (60 g) raisins
½ cup (125 g) crunchy Peanut Butter (page 33)

Makes 2 cups

Watching backyard birds brings hours of enjoyment to adults and teaches children valuable nature lessons. This easy and inexpensive recipe—better than a bought package of birdseed—will help to attract a wide variety of colorful and interesting birds to your garden.

1. Mix all the ingredients together in a bowl. Press the mixture into an empty bird feeder or small string bag.
2. Hang the feeder in a tree.

Homemade toys for parakeets and parrots

Parrots love toys, but they can be pricey and the bigger birds can destroy them quickly. Try these time-tested and inexpensive homemade toys.

❖ Parakeets love to preen in a mirror. So, instead of paying for a fancy bird mirror, just remove the hinge from an old compact and fasten the mirror securely to the cage bars near a perch.

❖ Parrots love to climb. Satisfy this urge by tying knots along a sturdy cotton rope and hanging it from the top of the cage.

❖ Parrots also love to bite and chew, and a dog-chew toy is often less expensive and just as long lasting as a parrot chew toy. Try a rawhide "bone" or one made from nylon.

❖ Both parakeets and parrots like colorful toys, so string big wooden beads onto cotton rope and hang it for them to bat around and chew.

Parrot Pops

1 cup (125 g) high-quality mixed commercial parrot treats
½ cup (20 g) round oat cereal pieces
1 cup (185 g) dried mixed fruit, unsweetened
1 cup (160 g) unsalted peanuts
½ banana, mashed
1 egg white
6 craft sticks or lollipop handles (available at craft or kitchen supply stores)
½ cup (175 ml) honey

Makes 6 treats

These chewy sweet treats will keep your parrot happily occupied for hours. Whip them up inexpensively, then sit back and watch the fun.

1. Preheat the oven to 100°F. In a medium bowl, mix together the parrot treats, oat cereal, dried fruit and peanuts. Add the banana and egg white and stir to coat.
2. Spray muffin pan with nonstick spray, fill with mixture, insert a stick in each and press to compress. Bake for 2 hours, or until very hard. Remove pops from pan, coat each pop with honey, place on a greased baking sheet, return to oven and bake for another 10 minutes or until honey is dry.
3. Serve one treat at a time. Remove and discard uneaten parts after 4 hours. Store in a sealed container in the refrigerator for up to 1 month or in the freezer for up to 3 months.

Premium Wild Bird Mix

1 lb (500 g) striped sunflower seeds, hulls on
1 lb (500 g) black-oil sunflower seeds, hulls on
1 lb (500 g) raw peanuts
1 lb (500 g) raisins, dried blueberries, apples or other dried fruits, chopped
1 lb (500 g) cracked corn
1 small carton live mealworms

Makes 5 lb (2.5 kg)

Avoid high-priced, and often inferior, wild birdseed blends. Individual seeds are available at feed, health food and pet stores. Adding live mealworms to your mix will entice insect-eating birds to your garden.

1. In a rodent-proof metal container with a tight lid, mix together the striped sunflower seeds, black-oil sunflower seeds, peanuts, fruit and cracked corn and store in a cool area, such as the cellar or garage. Store mealworms in the refrigerator according to package directions.
2. Spread 1 or 2 scoops of the seed mixture onto a tray-type feeder and sprinkle with mealworms.

Healthy Hummingbird Nectar

2 cups (500 ml) water
½ cup (110 g) white sugar

Makes 2½ cups (625 ml)

Why buy expensive hummingbird nectar when you can make your own for next to nothing? This nectar will attract hummingbirds and orioles. Choose a feeder with a red base to attract the birds, so there's no need to use potentially harmful red food coloring. To prevent fermentation in hot weather, empty your feeder every 3 days and sterilize it by rinsing with boiling water.

1. In a small saucepan over medium heat, bring the water to a boil and then stir in the sugar until it dissolves. Return the solution to a boil. Remove from heat and cool, uncovered.
2. Store the nectar in a clean, tightly capped jar in the refrigerator for up to 1 month.
3. Sterilize the feeder by rinsing it with boiling water. Fill with fresh nectar and hang in the shade at eye level.

Food for Other Pets

Guinea Pig Salad

½ cup (25 g) chopped fresh spinach
¼ cup (40 g) grated carrot
½ cup (90 g) chopped strawberries
¼ cup (60 ml) orange juice

Makes 2 servings

Fresh vegetables and fruits should be essential parts of a guinea pig's diet. The dried treats sold in pet stores are good in a pinch, but they're expensive and a poor substitute for fresh treats. This is a vitamin-rich fresh salad that's easy to make and good enough to share with your guinea pig.

1. In a bowl, toss the spinach, carrots and strawberries with the orange juice.
2. Serve in a feeding bowl. Remove and discard uneaten salad after 4 hours. Store leftovers in a sealed container in the refrigerator for 1 day.

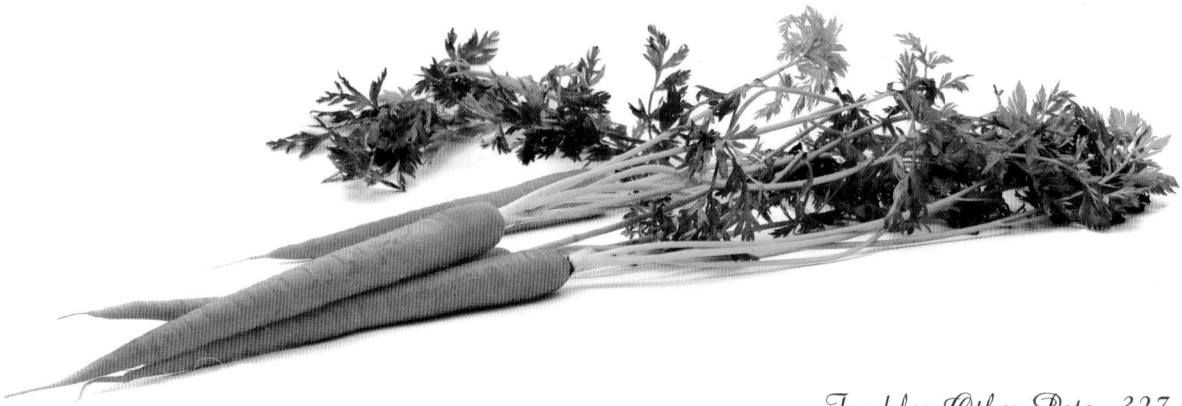

Hamster Fruit Cup

½ banana
¼ cup (40 g) grated carrot
lemon juice
3 teaspoons raisins
1 teaspoon honey

Makes 2 servings

Experts agree that dried hamster pellets and treats do not provide a complete diet and pet stores don't include a salad bar, but your hamster can scurry to its bowl for this budget-friendly sweet treat that you can whip up in no time using fresh fruits and vegetables.

1. Slice the banana and toss with the grated carrot in a bowl, adding a sprinkling of lemon juice to keep them from discoloring. Drain the juice from the bowl; add the raisins and honey and mash with a fork.
2. Serve half in a treat bowl and store the remainder in a covered container in the refrigerator for 1 day. Remove and discard uneaten treats after 4 hours.

Gerbil and Rabbit Salad

¼ cup (15 g) finely chopped spinach or leaf lettuce
¼ cup (40 g) grated carrot
1 teaspoon sunflower or pumpkin seeds, unsalted

Makes ½ cup (about 60 g)

It's important to offer pet rodents vitamin-rich fresh fruits and vegetables, and your gerbils and bunnies will welcome this healthy salad. For budget-boosting ingredients, ask for discarded outer leaves (which are more vitamin rich than inner leaves) at your produce counter, farmers' market or a restaurant salad bar. For variety, alternate seed toppings.

1. Toss the vegetables together in a bowl, top with the seeds and serve in a small treat bowl. Store leftovers in a sealed container in the refrigerator for 1 day.
2. Remove and dispose of uneaten fresh foods after 4 hours.

Pet Rodent Tabbouleh

1 cup (175 g) bulgur, uncooked
1 oz (30 ml) boiling water
¼ cup (45 g) brown rice, cooked
¼ cup (25 g) rolled oats, cooked
¼ cup (30 g) parrot seed mix
¼ cup (90 g) dark molasses
1 rodent vitamin, crushed (optional)
¼ cup (25 g) wheat germ

You just can't substitute dried pellets or grains from the pet store for fresh foods when it comes to feeding a balanced diet to rodents. This is a nutritious treat recipe for pet mice and rats. You can make it easy by saving plain, leftover grains from the family table.

1. Put the bulgur in a bowl, add boiling water and allow to stand for 5 minutes. Stir in the remaining ingredients, except wheat germ, to make a thick, crumbly mixture.
2. Form into small balls and roll in a saucer of wheat germ to coat.
3. Serve one ball daily as a treat. Discard uneaten treats after 4 hours. Store extra treats in a sealed container in the refrigerator for up to 1 week or in the freezer for up to 1 month.

Quick free playthings for pet rodents

Rodents have a never-ending need to chew, and they can rapidly demolish expensive store-bought toys. Save your wallet by collecting household "chew toys" for mice, rats, guinea pigs and bunnies, such as empty cardboard egg cartons, rolls from paper towels, food wrap and toilet paper, as well as small blocks of wood left over from woodworking projects.

Turtle and Reptile Treat

½ cup (80 g) grated carrot
½ cup (25 g) chopped lettuce or spinach
1 stalk celery, chopped
1 calcium tablet, crushed
1 teaspoon alfalfa sprouts (available at pet or health food stores)
¼ cup (35 g) chopped melon or strawberries

Makes 2 servings

To give your pet turtle a calcium boost, try this fortified daily vegetable medley. And with a few additions, this treat will also benefit lizards and other cold-blooded vegetarian pets. Reptiles have very specific dietary needs and must be housed at the proper temperature to induce an appetite.

1. For a turtle snack, place the vegetables into a bowl, sprinkle with calcium and toss. For lizards and other reptiles, add the alfalfa and fruit.
2. Serve half in a chew-proof bowl. Store the remainder in a covered container in the refrigerator for 1 day.

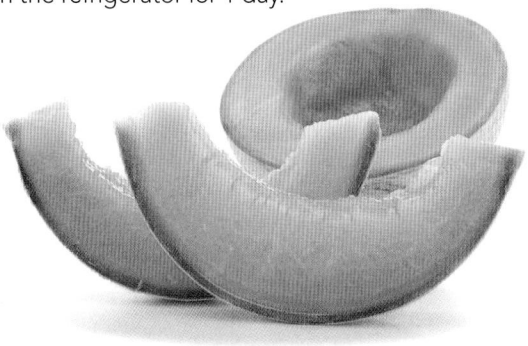

Aquarium Fish Treats

¼ cup (15 g) pureed spinach
1 earthworm, finely chopped
6 crickets
6 mealworms
6 bloodworms
¼ cup (25 g) raw beef liver, blended
1 raw shrimp, blended

The best food for your aquarium fish is a high-quality commercial fish food formulated for the species of fish, but, for variety, they enjoy fresh or fresh-frozen live food and fresh vegetables. Experiment with the treats listed here. Crickets, mealworms and bloodworms are sold at pet stores.

1. Mix the spinach plus any two other ingredients. Store a week's worth of the mix in a sealed container in the refrigerator. Freeze the rest for up to 1 month.
2. To serve, drop a piece of the mix the size of a pencil eraser into the aquarium. Continue until fish stop feeding. After 5 minutes, remove uneaten food from the bottom of the aquarium using a siphon or cooking bulb baster.

Part 3

Around the House

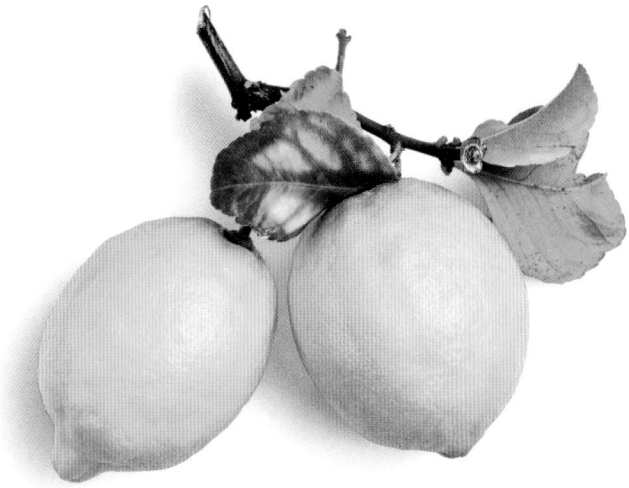

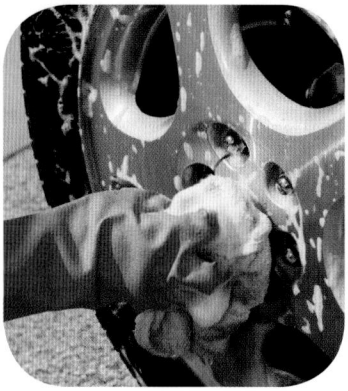

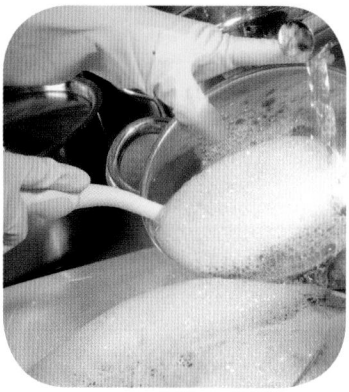

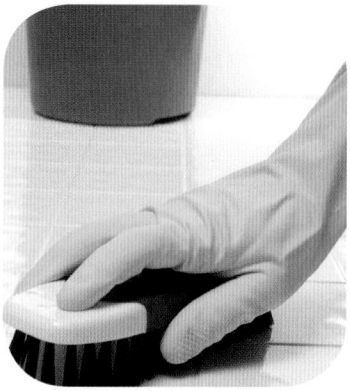

General Housecleaning

Basic Window and Glass Cleaner ❖ Super Window and Glass Cleaner ❖ Citrus Disinfectant ❖ Tough Multipurpose Cleaner ❖ Fresh-Smelling Multipurpose Cleaner ❖ Wall and Cabinet Cleaner ❖ Interior Wall Cleaner ❖ Herbal Carpet Freshener ❖ Pine Floor Cleaner ❖ Spicy Carpet Freshener

Air Fresheners

Room Freshener Spray ❖ Spicy Room Freshener

Furniture Polishes

Lemon Oil Furniture Polish ❖ No-Fuss Furniture Polish ❖ Cabinet Polish

Mold and Mildew Removers

Spot Mold and Mildew Remover ❖ Paint and Tile Mold and Mildew Remover ❖ Mold Remover for Leather and Luggage

Metal Polishes

Brass and Copper Paste Polish ❖ Cut-Lemon Brass and Copper Polish ❖ Ketchup Copper Polish ❖ Chrome and Stainless Steel Polish ❖ Quick and Easy Silver Shine

In the Kitchen

Automatic Dishwasher Detergent ❖ Dishwashing Liquid ❖ Microwave Oven Cleaner ❖ Basic Oven Cleaner ❖ Lazy Person's Oven Cleaner ❖ Oven Floor Cleaner ❖ White Goods Cleaner ❖ Scouring Powder ❖ Homemade Scrub Powder ❖ Steel Wool Soap Pads

In the Laundry

Fabric Softener ❖ Laundry Soap ❖ Stain Remover

In the Bathroom

Multipurpose Disinfectant Cleaner ❖ Easy Scrub ❖ Eucalyptus Tile Cleaner ❖ Nontoxic Bathroom Cleaner ❖ Showerhead Cleaner ❖ Nontoxic Rust Remover ❖ Nontoxic Toilet Bowl Cleaner ❖ Tougher Toilet Bowl Cleaner ❖ Drain Opener ❖ Septic Tank Activator

Cleaning the Car

Basic Car Wash ❖ Upholstery Shampoo ❖ Windshield Cleaner ❖ Vinyl and Leather Interior Cleaner

Clever Solutions Cleaning Products

Advertisements for "new and better" cleaning supplies fill home magazines, and there is a vast and competitive industry dedicated to making you think you can't exist without the latest product.

Many of these highly touted products do have seemingly miraculous ingredients that can make dirt vanish, but many actually contain traditional cleaning compounds that you can make yourself. As the recipes here show, there are lots of safe ways to clean everything in your house, using simple mixtures of inexpensive, everyday staples that you probably already have in your pantry or store cupboard.

Homemade cleaning solutions not only get the job done easily and inexpensively, but they do it without harming you or your possessions—because you know exactly what is in them. Most of these products have a long and honorable history—your grandmother probably used many of them. As you might expect, you'll see recipes that use many traditional ingredients, such as baking soda, vinegar and lemon juice. But you may be surprised to learn that you can still buy borax and washing soda at your local supermarket and even more surprised to find that tomato ketchup is a fine copper polish.

These homemade cleaning products are all very economical. White vinegar and baking soda, for example, are much cheaper than commercial fabric softeners for keeping lint off your clothes and stopping static electricity. Old newspapers are cheaper than paper kitchen towels for cleaning windows. And dried spices refresh your house far more inexpensively than any commercial room deodorizer.

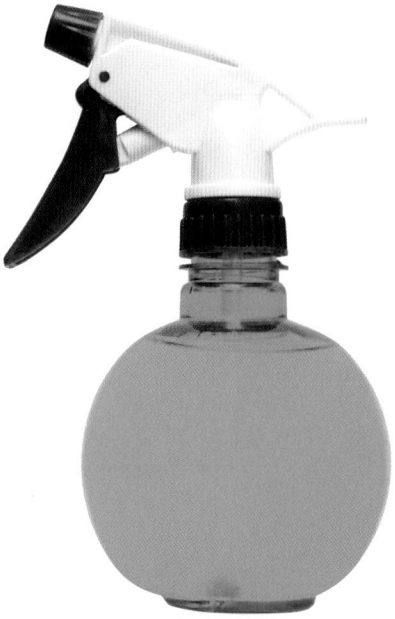

General Housecleaning

Basic Window and Glass Cleaner

½ cup (125 ml) white vinegar
10 cups (2.5 liters) water
1 clean gallon (4 liter) container
1 clean 32 oz (1 liter) spray bottle
old newspapers

Forget about all of those store-bought window cleaners. Your windows can get a professional shine for next to nothing. This recipe will clean a lot of windows. You can make a smaller batch in a quart spray bottle by mixing ¼ cup (60 ml) vinegar with enough water to fill the container.

1 Mix the ingredients in the gallon container.
2 Fill the spray bottle and spray on windows and glass items as needed. (Save the remaining cleaner for another day.)
3 Dry the glass with crumpled newspaper for added brightness.

Super Window and Glass Cleaner

⅓ cup (80 ml) white vinegar
¼ cup (60 ml) rubbing alcohol
3¼ cups (810 ml) water
1 clean 32 oz (1 liter) spray bottle
old newspapers

The alcohol in this formula helps prevent streaking.

1 Mix all the ingredients in the spray bottle. Shake the bottle well before using.
2 Spray on a dirty windowpane or other glass surface.
3 Dry with crumpled newspaper.

Citrus Disinfectant

zest from 1 orange, grapefruit, lemon or lime
3 cups (750 ml) white vinegar
1 clean quart (1 liter) container with lid
1 clean 32 oz (1 liter) spray bottle

If you like commercial orange cleaners, you'll love this fresh citrus-scented vinegar spray that is easy to make and costs very little. You can also deodorize a room by setting out a small bowl of citrus vinegar.

1 Combine the citrus zest and vinegar in the quart container. Fasten the lid on the container and store the mixture in a cupboard for 2 weeks, giving it an occasional shake.
2 Remove the zest from the container, then strain the vinegar and return it to the container.
3 To use as a spray cleaner, pour 1 cup (250 ml) of citrus vinegar into the spray bottle and fill with water.
4 To clean linoleum floors, add 1 cup (250 ml) citrus vinegar to 2 gallons (8 liters) water.

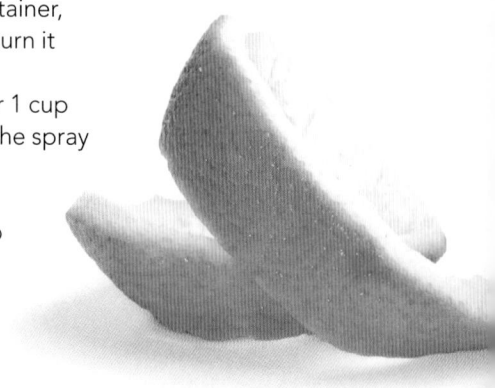

Tough Multipurpose Cleaner

3 cups (750 ml) water
⅓ cup (80 ml) rubbing alcohol
1 teaspoon clear household ammonia
1 teaspoon mild dishwashing liquid
½ teaspoon lemon juice
1 clean 32 oz (1 liter) spray bottle

When it comes to cleaning non-wood surfaces around your home, this cleaner is tough to beat. And it costs almost nothing.

1 Combine the ingredients in the spray bottle and shake well before each use.
2 Spray on countertops, kitchen appliances and fixtures, and tile or painted surfaces.
3 Wipe down with a clean cloth or damp sponge.

Fresh-Smelling Multipurpose Cleaner

3½ cups (875 ml) hot water
½ cup (125 ml) white or apple cider vinegar
1 teaspoon borax
1 teaspoon washing soda
1 teaspoon liquid castile soap
1 clean 32 oz (1 liter) spray bottle

This formula has a clean smell and works hard, despite its inexpensive ingredients. You can buy liquid castile soap at health food stores.

1 Fill spray bottle first with hot water; then add vinegar, borax, washing soda and liquid castile soap. Shake well before using.
2 Spray on countertops, kitchen appliances and fixtures, and tile or painted surfaces.
3 Wipe down with a clean cloth or damp sponge.

Wall and Cabinet Cleaner

1 cup (250 ml) clear household ammonia
1 cup (250 ml) white vinegar
¼ cup (70 g) baking soda
1 gallon (4 liters) warm water

If you have dingy cupboards, this cleaning solution will deodorize them as well as wiping up the dust and dirt.

1 Combine the ammonia, vinegar and baking soda in a large bucket, add water and give it a few stirs.
2 Use a sponge or cloth rag to wash walls, ceilings, floors or cabinets with the cleaner.
3 Wipe up the excess liquid with a clean cloth and allow to dry thoroughly before replacing contents.

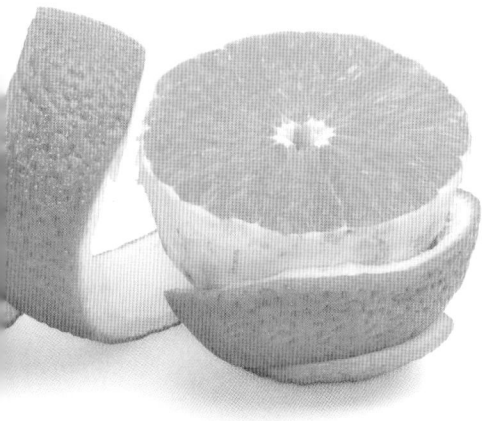

Use bread to spot-clean wallpaper

Cut the crusts off a slice of white bread and roll it up into a ball. Once the bread starts to feel slightly doughy, roll it over the bad spots on the wallpaper to lift off the dirt or fingerprints. Test the bread ball first on an inconspicuous corner.

Interior Wall Cleaner

½ cup (120 g) borax
1 tablespoon clear household ammonia
¼ cup (60 ml) white vinegar
1 gallon (4 liters) warm water

Those scuff marks and stains on your painted walls seem to appear out of nowhere. This potent cleaner will remove them without harming your paint job.

1 In a large bucket, mix all the ingredients.
2 Apply the solution to the wall with a clean sponge. Use a second clean sponge to rinse the wall with plain water.
3 To minimize streaking, start at the bottom of the wall and work up.

Herbal Carpet Freshener

large handful fresh lavender flowers
1 cup (280 g) baking soda

Many commercial air and carpet deodorizers simply mask odors. To truly freshen carpets around your home, try this inexpensive natural formula instead. (If you don't like the smell of lavender, you can also freshen up carpets with plain baking soda.)

1 In a large bowl, crush the lavender flowers to release scent.
2 Add the baking soda and mix well. Pour the mixture into a cheese shaker or a can with holes punched in the lid.
3 Sprinkle liberally on the carpet. Wait 30 minutes, then vacuum.

Pine Floor Cleaner

½ cup (50 g) pure soap flakes
¼ cup (70 g) washing soda
1 cup (225 g) salt
2 cups (500 ml) water
2 teaspoons pine oil
1 clean 16 oz (500 ml) plastic bottle with a tight-fitting lid
1 cup (250 ml) white vinegar

You shouldn't have to spend a small fortune to give your no-wax floors a pine-fresh smell. This excellent cleaner will do the job for only small change. If you can't find pure soap flakes, you can make your own by grating a bar of soap.

1 If you are making your own soap flakes, grate the soap on a coarse kitchen grater.
2 In a saucepan over low heat, combine the soap, washing soda, salt and water and stir until soap, soda and salt have dissolved.
3 Remove from the heat and allow the mixture to cool until it is lukewarm. Add the pine oil. Stir well, pour into the plastic bottle, and secure the top.
4 To use, pour 2 or 3 tablespoons of the cleaner into a half-bucket of hot water, stirring well. For large areas, you may need to double the amount.
5 After cleaning, add the vinegar to a half-bucket of clean water and rinse the floor.

Spicy Carpet Freshener

1 cup (280 g) baking soda or cornstarch
7–10 drops essential oil in your favorite scent (eucalyptus or rosewood, for example)

Add a nice smell to your rooms while you freshen the carpets with this simple mixture.

1 In a large bowl, combine the baking soda or cornstarch with the essential oil. Break up any clumps with a fork and stir well. Pour the mixture into a Parmesan cheese shaker or a can with holes punched in the lid.
2 Sprinkle liberally on the carpet. Wait 30 minutes, then vacuum.

Air Fresheners

Room Freshener Spray

1 clean 12 oz (375 ml) spray bottle
¼ cup (60 ml) rubbing alcohol
25 drops bergamot essential oil
8 drops clove essential oil
5 drops lemon essential oil
1 cup (250 ml) distilled water

Why waste your money on commercial air fresheners when it's so easy to make your own favorite scents? Use this spray judiciously, however. A room should have a hint of the spicy scent, not an overpowering perfume. You can combine up to three different essential oils to create a fragrance that suits you. Other choices include eucalyptus, lavender, geranium, grapefruit, orange, peppermint, pine, juniper, rose and spearmint.

1 In the spray bottle, combine the rubbing alcohol and the essential oils and shake well to disperse the oil. Add the water and shake for a minute or two more to blend all the ingredients thoroughly.
2 Let the mixture sit for a few days before using to allow the fragrance to blend and mature. A quick spritz is all that's needed to freshen a room.

Spicy Room Freshener

3 cups (750 ml) water
6 cloves
1 cinnamon stick
6 pieces dried orange peel

This fragrant mixture makes you think an apple pie is in the oven; real estate agents sometimes suggest putting this mixture on the stove before prospective buyers come to see the house.

In a small saucepan, combine all the ingredients and bring to a boil over medium heat. Reduce the heat and simmer, uncovered, until your home is filled with a fresh, spicy scent. (Don't let the water boil away.)

Furniture Polishes

Lemon Oil Furniture Polish

1 cup (250 ml) olive oil
⅓ cup (80 ml) lemon juice
1 clean 16 oz (500 ml) spray bottle

Shine up your wood furniture, panelling and knickknacks with this natural polish that will take you only a minute to prepare and costs very little. Discard any leftovers and make up a fresh batch each time you want to polish your wood treasures.

1 Combine the oil and lemon juice in the spray bottle. Shake well before using.
2 Apply a small amount of the mixture to a soft flannel cloth or chamois and apply it evenly over the wood surface.
3 Use a clean, dry flannel cloth to buff and polish.

No-Fuss Furniture Polish

¼ cup (60 ml) boiled linseed oil
⅛ cup (30 ml) vinegar
⅛ cup (30 ml) whisky
1 clean 16 oz (500 ml) spray bottle

How would you like a furniture polish that you can just wipe on and forget? Well, your prayers have been answered—and for a lot less than you might expect!

1 Combine all the ingredients in the bottle. Shake well.
2 Apply a small amount of polish to a clean, soft cloth and wipe on. No need to buff; the dullness evaporates along with the alcohol.

Cabinet Polish

1 teaspoon lemon juice
1 teaspoon olive oil
2 cups (500 ml) warm water

Why burn through your household budget on furniture polish for those large wood kitchen cabinets, bookshelves or wardrobes around your home? This is the perfect polish to use on big jobs—and it costs almost nothing to make. Be sure to mix up a fresh batch for each use.

1 Combine the ingredients in a bowl or container.
2 Dip a soft flannel cloth into the solution and wring it out. Wipe over the wood.
3 Buff and polish with a soft, dry cloth.

Mold and Mildew Removers

Spot Mold and Mildew Remover

½ cup (125 ml) white vinegar
3 teaspoons borax
2 cups (500 ml) hot water
1 clean 32 oz (1 liter) spray bottle

Mix up a batch of this powerful but benign-smelling disinfectant to get rid of small patches of mold and mildew that breed in bathroom medicine cabinets, windowsills and other surfaces around your home.

1 Combine the ingredients in the spray bottle. Shake well.
2 Spray on surfaces where mold or mildew is forming. Wipe off mildew, but leave the cleaning solution residue to keep mildew from returning.

Paint and Tile Mold and Mildew Remover

¼ cup (60 ml) chlorine bleach
3 teaspoons borax
1½ cups (375 ml) water
1 clean 16 oz (500 ml) spray bottle

This formula will take mold and mildew off painted and tile surfaces for the cost of your small change. Be sure the room is well ventilated as you work.

1 Combine the ingredients in the spray bottle and shake to mix.
2 Spray the painted or tile surface and wipe off mildew and mold with a clean cloth. Rinse the surface with clean water and dry with clean cloths.

Mold Remover for Leather and Luggage

½ cup (125 ml) rubbing alcohol
¼ cup (60 ml) water
1 clean 8 oz (250 ml) spray bottle

If you discover mold on your expensive luggage, handbag or leather jacket, don't just race to the dry cleaners. Instead, remove the offending growth with this simple, inexpensive mold-removal recipe. Test on a small area first.

1 Combine the ingredients in the spray bottle and shake well to mix.
2 Spray affected area. Let the solution sit for 10 to 20 minutes, then wipe off mold with a clean rag and allow the item to thoroughly air-dry.

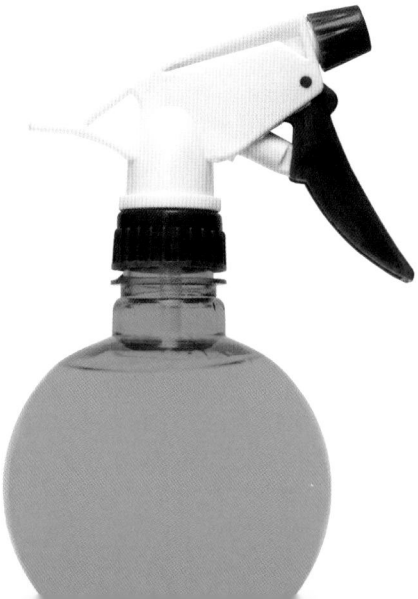

Metal Polishes

Brass and Copper Paste Polish

¼ cup (35 g) flour
¼ cup (55 g) salt
¼ cup (60 ml) vinegar
¼ cup (60 ml) hot water
1 teaspoon lemon juice

Use this simple, nontoxic—and very inexpensive—polish to brighten up all your tarnished unlacquered brass and copperware. (Lacquered items only need dusting.)

1 In a small bowl, combine all the ingredients to form a paste.
2 Using a soft cloth, rub the mixture onto the metal surface.
3 Rinse the object thoroughly in warm water (remember that salt is corrosive).
4 Dry with soft, clean cloths and then buff to a shine with a soft flannel cloth or chamois.

Cut-Lemon Brass and Copper Polish

½ cup (125 ml) white vinegar
2 tablespoons salt
½ lemon

Here's an even easier way to shine up unlacquered brass or copper objects—and a useful way to use up leftover half lemons.

1 In a saucepan over medium heat, heat the vinegar for 5 minutes, then pour it into a small bowl and stir in the salt.
2 Dip the lemon into the mixture and rub it over the object, concentrating on the most heavily tarnished areas.
3 Thoroughly rinse the object in warm water and dry with soft, clean cloths. Buff to a shine with a soft cloth.

Ketchup Copper Polish

½–1 cup (125–250 ml) tomato ketchup
¼–1 lemon, juiced

This simple polish can be a bit messy, but it works like a charm on unlacquered copper—and it's completely nontoxic. Can your old copper polish say that?

1 In a small bowl, combine the ketchup and lemon juice and stir to mix. How much you need of each ingredient depends on the size of the object you want to polish, but keep the ratio of ketchup to lemon juice about 8:1.
2 Spread out some old newspapers on your work surface. Rub the mixture over the copper piece's surface. Let it sit for 5 to 10 minutes.
3 Thoroughly rinse the copper piece in warm water and dry with soft, clean cloths. Buff to a shine with a soft cloth.

Chrome and Stainless Steel Polish

¼ teaspoon baby oil
½ cup (125 ml) club soda

Baby the chrome and stainless steel finishes around your home with this simple one-two set of cleaners. They remove stains as well as dirt and fingerprints cheaply and quickly.

1 Apply a few drops of baby oil to a soft cloth or piece of flannel and wipe down the chrome or stainless steel surface. Moisten the second soft cloth with club soda, and rinse off the oil.
2 Dry and buff with a soft, dry cloth.

Quick and Easy Silver Shine

4 cups (1 liter) hot water
3 teaspoons baking soda or washing soda
3 teaspoons salt
1 sheet aluminum foil

Want a really easy, inexpensive and amazingly effective way to polish your silver without any smelly chemicals or commercial products? This is easier than using a silver dipping cleaner.

1 Fill the kitchen sink with about 4 cups (1 liter) hot water.
2 Dissolve the baking soda or washing soda and salt in the water, then place the sheet of aluminum foil at the bottom of the sink.
3 Rest the tarnished silver on the foil for 10 seconds. Remove and dry with a soft flannel cloth.

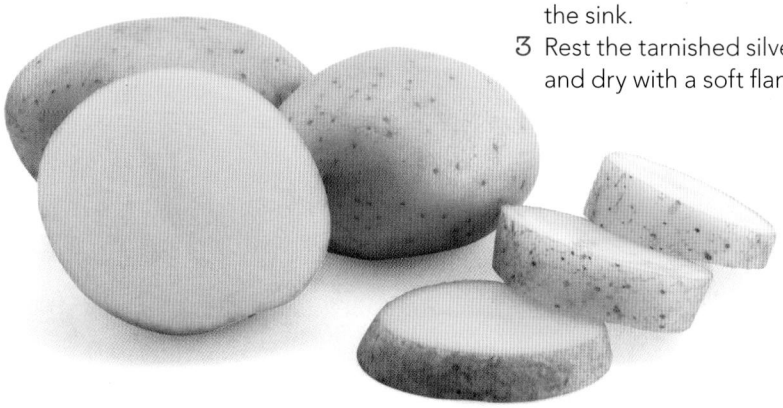

Potato rust remover for tin pans

Tin pie plates and other kitchen utensils are subject to rust if they are not dried carefully after each washing. Here, for little more than the price of a potato, is a way to restore your tinware without harsh chemicals. Peel a potato and cut it into easy-to-handle pieces. Put some baking soda or salt in a saucer. Then dip a cut piece of potato in the soda or salt, and rub it over the rust spots. Rinse the tin utensil and dry thoroughly.

In the Kitchen

Automatic Dishwasher Detergent

2 cups (480 g) borax
2 cups (560 g) washing soda
1 clean 32 oz (1 kg) plastic container with cover

Even if you live in a hard-water area, this simple, inexpensive detergent recipe will help keep your dishes shiny and spotless.

1 Combine the borax and washing soda in the container and seal it tightly for storage.
2 For each load of dishes, put 2 tablespoons of the mixture in the dishwasher soap dispenser.

Fast, cheap rinsing agent for your dishwasher

Here's an easy way to get those dishes sparkling in your automatic dishwasher without using any chemical rinsing agents. Just stop the dishwasher during its rinse cycle and add 1 to 1½ cups (250 to 375 ml) white vinegar. Or pour the vinegar into the rinse compartment beforehand (being careful not to overfill). Then wash the dishes as usual.

Dishwashing Liquid

¼ cup (25 g) pure soap flakes (or a bar of pure soap, for grating)
1½ cups (375 ml) hot water
¼ cup (60 ml) glycerine
½ teaspoon lemon oil
1 clean 16 oz (500 ml) squirt bottle

This dishwashing soap for washing dishes by hand is inexpensive and really gets your dishes clean. It's mild on your hands, too.

1 If you are unable to find pure soap flakes, lightly grate a bar of pure soap on a coarse kitchen grater.
2 In a medium jug, pour the soap flakes into the hot water and stir with a fork until most of the soap has dissolved. Let the solution cool for 5 minutes.
3 Stir in the glycerine and lemon oil. A loose gel will form as it cools. Use the fork to break up any congealed parts and pour the liquid into the squirt bottle. Use 2 to 3 teaspoons per sink or dishpan of hot water to clean dishes.

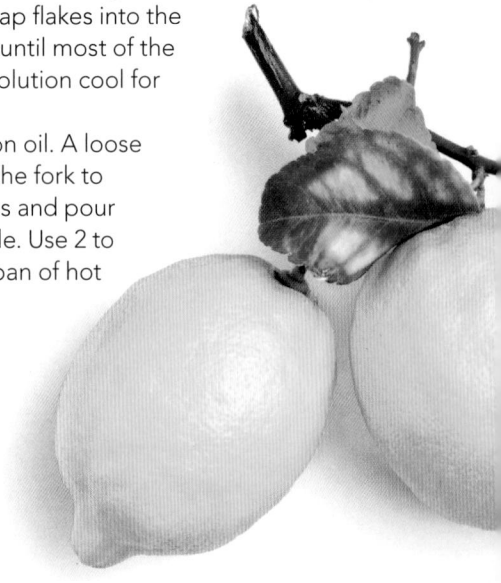

Microwave Oven Cleaner

1½ cups (375 ml) water
3 tablespoons lemon juice, 3 tablespoons baking soda or 2 cups (500 ml) white vinegar

You don't need harsh cleansers and lots of elbow grease to clean your microwave. For the price of a lemon, some baking soda or some white vinegar, you can just wipe away the splatters and stains inside.

1. In a microwave-safe bowl, combine the water and lemon juice or baking soda, or just pour the vinegar. Place the uncovered bowl inside the oven, and run the microwave on high for 3 to 5 minutes, allowing the liquid to condense on its inside walls and ceiling.
2. Carefully remove the bowl with a towel or pot holder (it will be very hot!), and wipe the interior of the oven with a dishcloth or paper towel.

Basic Oven Cleaner

2 tablespoons (30 ml) liquid soap
2 teaspoons borax
1 clean 16 oz (500 ml) spray bottle
2 cups (500 ml) warm water
½ cup (140 g) baking soda in an open bowl

Try this odorless recipe the next time you need to clean your oven, and leave those caustic chemical-based oven cleaners where they belong—on the store shelf.

1. Pour the soap and borax into the spray bottle and add the warm water. Shake well to dissolve the borax.
2. Spray the solution on the oven's surfaces, giving special attention to dried, cooked-on spills.
3. Let the mixture sit for 30 minutes to 1 hour, then scrub the oven surfaces with a damp scrub pad dipped in the baking soda. Rinse with clean water.

Lazy Person's Oven Cleaner

¾ cup (185 ml) clear household ammonia
1 cup (280 g) baking soda in a widemouthed dish

Here is the recipe for a cheap, almost effortless oven cleaner that is still very effective.

1. Pour the ammonia into a small bowl and leave it overnight in a closed, cool oven.
2. The next day, remove and discard the ammonia and wipe down the oven's interior surfaces with moistened paper towels or damp sponges dipped in baking soda.

Oven Floor Cleaner

½ cup (125 ml) water
1–2 cups (280–560 g) baking soda
1 teaspoon liquid detergent

This recipe is for cleaning up the oven floor after a sticky sweet pie or a too-full casserole has spilled over and caused a real mess. You don't need expensive, caustic commercial oven cleaners to deal with it. You probably already have everything you need on hand.

1 Sprinkle water along the bottom of the oven.
2 Spread enough baking soda over the surface to coat it entirely, and sprinkle more water on top of it.
3 Let the paste sit overnight. The next morning, the grease and grime will be loosened enough for you to wipe it up with damp paper towels or dishcloths.
4 Once you've wiped up the core of the mess, use the liquid detergent on a damp sponge to remove any remaining residue. Rinse with water and let dry.
5 Repeat if necessary.

White Goods Cleaner

8 teaspoons (40 ml) dishwashing liquid
1 oz (20 g) cornstarch
1 cup (250 ml) water
1 cup (250 ml) white vinegar
a few drops herbal essential oil

Regular wiping with this solution will remove grubby finger marks and leave the surfaces of freezers, refrigerators and washing machines looking like new without scratching them.

1 Put all the ingredients in a plastic spray bottle and shake gently to combine.
2 Spray a fine mist of the mixture over the grubby surface and wipe clean with a soft cloth.

Scouring Powder

1 cup (280 g) baking soda
1 cup (240 g) borax
1 cup (225 g) salt
1 clean 32 oz (1 kg) plastic container with cover

You don't need chlorine bleach to clean stains off the nonporous surfaces in your kitchen and bathroom. This scouring powder is very effective, a lot safer to use and far more economical.

1 Combine the ingredients in the container and mix well. Close the container tightly to store.
2 To clean a stained surface, sprinkle some of the powder onto a damp sponge or directly onto the surface to be cleaned. Scour, rinse and dry.

Homemade Scrub Powder

2½ cups (700 g) baking soda
1½ cups (335 g) salt
2 tablespoons (30 g) cream of tartar
1 clean 32 oz (1.5 kg) plastic container with lid

Use this mixture to scrub off grease and grime from your stainless steel and enameled cookware. (If you use baking soda on aluminum cookware, it may cause darkening.)

1 Mix all the ingredients well, and store in a tightly sealed plastic container.
2 To use, pour 2 to 3 tablespoons of powder onto cookware and scrub with a brush or nylon scrubber that's been slightly moistened with water. Rinse well and dry with a soft cloth.

Steel Wool Soap Pads

1 bag steel wool pads (available at hardware stores)
3 tablespoons (60 g) Homemade Scrub Powder (above)

Those popular prepackaged steel wool soap pads are great for getting tough stains and cooked-on foods off your pots and pans, but they can be rough on your hands. These homemade steel wool pads work just as well and are easier on both your wallet and your skin.

1 If you've purchased large pads, use sharp scissors or shears and carefully cut them into rectangles approximately 3 inches long by 2 inches high.
2 Spread a layer of scrub powder over the cooking surface, moisten the steel wool pad with warm water and scrub away stains. Rinse well with water. Dry with a soft, absorbent towel.
3 To make your pads last longer, squeeze out remaining water and keep them in a bowl lined with aluminum foil.

In the Laundry

Fabric Softener

¼ cup (70 g) baking soda
½ cup (125 ml) white vinegar

Here's a simple recipe for keeping your fabrics soft and fluffy. It's gentle on your clothes and much easier on your wallet than commercial fabric softeners.

1 Fill the washing machine with water.
2 Add the baking soda and then the clothing.
3 During the final rinse cycle, add the vinegar (pouring it into the softener dispenser if your washing machine has one).

Laundry Soap

½ cup (50 g) pure soap flakes (or a bar of pure soap)
½ cup (140 g) baking soda
¼ cup (70 g) washing soda
¼ cup (60 g) borax
1 clean 16 oz (500 g) plastic container with lid

This basic laundry soap gets clothes just as clean as commercial cleaners; it just costs a lot less.

1. If you cannot find soap flakes, lightly grate a bar of pure soap on a coarse kitchen grater.
2. In a large bowl, mix all the ingredients together. Store in a tightly sealed plastic container.
3. Use about ½ cup (110 g) of the mixture instead of detergent in each load of laundry.

Stain Remover

⅓ cup (80 ml) clear household ammonia
½ cup (125 ml) white vinegar
¼ cup (70 g) baking soda
2 tablespoons (30 ml) liquid castile soap
6 cups (1.5 liters) water
1 clean half-gallon (2 liter) recycled plastic container
1 clean 16 oz (500 ml) spray bottle

Stains are always easier to get out if you treat them before they set (club soda is effective for lifting many stains before they dry). You can use other ingredients found around your home to remove many common types of stains (see Removing Common Stains, below).

1. Mix all the ingredients in the ½-gallon container. Pour some of the solution into the spray bottle. Shake well before each use.
2. Spray liquid onto the stain and leave for 3 to 5 minutes. Launder as usual.

Removing common stains

❖ **Automotive Oil and Grease Stain Remover**
4 cups (1 liter) cola soft drink
For severe stains, soak garment in cola overnight. Rinse and launder the next morning.

❖ **Grass and Bloodstain Remover**
1 teaspoon 3% hydrogen peroxide
¼ teaspoon clear household ammonia
Mix the ingredients in a small bowl. Rub the mixture on the stain. As soon as the stain fades, rinse and launder.

❖ **Perspiration Stain Remover**
1 cup (250 ml) white vinegar
¼ cup (55 g) salt
8 cups (2 liters) warm water
Mix the ingredients in a bucket and soak the garment for 1 hour before washing.

❖ **Red Wine Remover**
3 teaspoons borax
2 cups (500 ml) warm water
Mix the ingredients together in a small bowl. Dip the garment in the solution, let it soak for 1 minute, then launder.

❖ **Tomato Sauce Remover**
½ cup (125 ml) 3% hydrogen peroxide
3 cups (750 ml) water
Mix the ingredients in a dishpan or bucket. Soak the garment in the solution for 30 minutes before laundering.

❖ **Whitening Yellowed Whites**
½ cup (125 ml) white vinegar
6 cups (1.5 liters) warm water
Mix ingredients in a dishpan or bucket. Soak clothes in the solution overnight and launder the next morning.

Vinegar: fabric softener plus

Who would have guessed that a single cup of an everyday staple—white vinegar, which costs almost nothing—could do everything that many people use a fabric softener, a color setter, a disinfectant and a bleach to do? Just add 1 cup (250 ml) distilled white vinegar to your washing machine's rinse cycle, and it will help to kill any bacteria in the wash, set the color of newly dyed fabrics, keep clothes lint- and static-free, brighten small loads of white clothes and eliminate the need for fabric softeners.

In the Bathroom

Multipurpose Disinfectant Cleaner

2 teaspoons borax
½ teaspoon washing soda
2 tablespoons (30 ml) lemon juice
¼ cup (60 ml) white vinegar
3 cups (750 ml) very hot water
1 clean 24 oz (1 liter) spray bottle

Here's a good all-purpose disinfectant that is easy to use and is much cheaper than commercial bathroom cleaners.

1. Combine the borax, washing soda, lemon juice and vinegar in the spray bottle.
2. Slowly add the hot water, then vigorously shake the bottle until the powdered ingredients have dissolved. Shake the bottle before each use.
3. Spray on tile and ceramic surfaces and wipe with a damp, clean cloth.

Easy Scrub

¼ cup (60 g) borax
½ teaspoon vegetable-oil-based liquid soap, such as castile
½ teaspoon lemon juice

You don't need to buy special cleaners for your vulnerable kitchen and bathroom surfaces. This homemade soft scrub gets out tough stains on surfaces that are easily scratched, including ceramic sinks and countertops, and costs very little per cleaning job.

1. In a small bowl, combine the borax and liquid soap to make a smooth paste.
2. Stir in the lemon juice and mix well.
3. Place a small amount of the paste onto a clean, damp sponge, apply to the surface, then rinse off and dry the surface with a clean cloth.

Eucalyptus Tile Cleaner

½ cup (50 g) pure soap flakes (or a bar of pure soap)
1 cup (125 g) chalk or diatomaceous earth
1 cup (280 g) baking soda
1 teaspoon eucalyptus essential oil
1 clean recycled 16 oz (500 g) jar with metal top

This fresh, tangy powder will leave your kitchen and bathroom tiles shiny and clean for a fraction of the price of commercial cleaners.

1 If you cannot find soap flakes, lightly grate a bar of pure soap on a coarse kitchen grater. Then, in a small bowl, crush the soap flakes with the back of a spoon until powdered (or grind them in a blender).
2 Mix in the chalk or diatomaceous earth and the baking soda, breaking up any lumps.
3 Sprinkle the essential oil over the surface of the powdered mixture and stir it with the spoon. Stir for several minutes to disperse oil throughout the mixture, then spoon the mixture into a screw-top jar or can with some holes punched in the lid.
4 Cover the holes with masking tape to keep the powder dry between uses. Let the mixture sit for 1 week before using to be sure the essential oil has been thoroughly absorbed. Sprinkle surface with powder, scrub with a damp sponge and rinse with clear water. Dry with a soft towel.

Nontoxic Bathroom Cleaner

1⅔ cups (450 g) baking soda
½ cup (125 ml) liquid soap
½ cup (125 ml) water
2 tablespoons (30 ml) white vinegar
1 clean 16 oz (500 ml) squirt bottle with lid

This is a terrific deep-cleaning cleanser for any bathroom surface. It cuts through soap scum and mildew and costs very little to produce.

1 Mix the baking soda and liquid soap in a bowl. Dilute with the water and add the vinegar. Stir the mixture with a fork until any lumps have been dissolved. Pour the liquid into the bottle. Shake well before using.
2 Squirt on area to be cleaned. Scrub with a nylon-backed sponge. Rinse off with water. Keep lid on between uses.

Showerhead Cleaner

¼ cup (70 g) baking soda
1 cup (250 ml) vinegar
1 plastic sandwich bag
adhesive tape or a large bag tie

Use this "explosive" mix to blast away mineral deposits blocking up your showerhead. You don't need a plumber to clean your showerhead when you can do it yourself.

1 Pour the baking soda and vinegar into the bag over a sink. Wait a minute or two for the foaming to stop and then place the opened end of the bag over the showerhead, which should be submerged in the solution.
2 Secure the bag to the showerhead stem with the tape or bag tie. Let the showerhead soak in the solution 1 to 1½ hours. Wipe off the showerhead with a soft cloth.

Nontoxic Rust Remover

1 lime (a second one may be needed for some jobs)
¼ cup (55 g) salt

Commercial rust removers are among the most toxic compounds found around the home. But here's a completely safe and surprisingly effective way to give rust stains on bathtubs and sinks the brush-off.

1. Squeeze the lime over the rust spots, then cover the moistened area with salt.
2. Let the mixture sit for 3 to 4 hours.
3. Use a nylon scrubber to scrub the mixture off. The rust should be gone. Repeat for really stubborn stains.

Nontoxic Toilet Bowl Cleaner

1 cup (240 g) borax
½ cup (125 ml) white vinegar

Clean and sanitize your toilet bowl without harmful chlorine! For no-scrub convenience, simply pour in this mixture and leave overnight.

1. Flush the toilet to wet the sides of the bowl.
2. Sprinkle the borax around the toilet bowl, then liberally drizzle some vinegar on top. Let the toilet sit undisturbed for 3 to 4 hours before scrubbing with a toilet brush.

Tougher Toilet Bowl Cleaner

⅔ cup (160 g) borax
⅓ cup (80 ml) lemon juice

For tougher jobs, try this potent paste that still has no chlorine and costs much less than commercial toilet bowl cleaners.

1. In a small bowl, combine the ingredients to form a paste.
2. Apply the paste to the toilet bowl using a sponge or rag. Let the paste sit for 2 hours, then scrub off. Flush the toilet.

Drain Opener

½ cup (140 g) baking soda
1 cup (250 ml) vinegar
1 teapot boiling water

Don't bother with those caustic commercial cleaners; try this simple, inexpensive and safe way to unclog drains instead.

1. Pack the drain with baking soda, then pour in vinegar.
2. Keep the drain covered for 10 minutes, then flush it out with boiling water.

Fast and easy drain freshener

Here's an easy way to eliminate drain odors while maintaining the proper pH and health of your septic system. Run warm tap water for several seconds, then pour 1 cup (280 g) baking soda into the drain. Wait an hour and flush with a teapot of boiling water. For best results, repeat once every 2 weeks.

Septic Tank Activator

2 cups (440 g) sugar
4 cups (1 liter) simmering water
2 cups (300 g) cornmeal
2 packages (7 g each) dry yeast

If you detect a persistent unpleasant odor from your septic tank, it's probably due to a "die-off" of sewage-digesting bacteria. Before you call in your local septic tank specialist, try using this simple recipe to give the little beasties a boost.

1 Dissolve the sugar in a saucepan of simmering water and cool to lukewarm. Mix in the cornmeal and the yeast.
2 Once the solution has been mixed, flush it down the toilet (flush twice, if necessary). For best results, do this before turning in for the night or when there will be no activity in the bathroom for several hours.

Cleaning the Car

Basic Car Wash

½ cup (125 ml) mild dishwashing liquid
½ cup (140 g) baking soda
about 1 gallon (4 liters) warm water

Taking your car to a commercial car wash can be a costly habit to maintain—and the results aren't as satisfying as when you do it yourself. This soap is tough on grime but gentle on your car's finish and your wallet.

1 Mix the ingredients in a clean gallon container. Shake until all the baking soda is dissolved.
2 To use, mix 1 cup (250 ml) solution in a bucket of warm water.

Upholstery Shampoo

6 tablespoons (30 g) pure soap flakes (or a bar of pure soap)
2 tablespoons (20 g) borax
2 cups (500 ml) boiling water

Use this shampoo on a regular basis to freshen up fabric interiors that get a lot of use. It's much cheaper than commercial upholstery cleaners and does the job just as well.

1. If you cannot find soap flakes, lightly grate a bar of pure soap on a coarse kitchen grater.
2. In a large bowl, mix the soap flakes and borax together. Slowly add the boiling water, stirring well to thoroughly dissolve the dry ingredients.
3. Let the mixture cool, then whip into a foamy consistency with an eggbeater.
4. Brush dry suds onto the upholstery, concentrating on soiled areas. Quickly wipe off with a damp sponge.

Windshield Cleaner

3 cups (750 ml) glycerine
1 cup (250 ml) rubbing alcohol
2 cups (500 ml) water
1 clean 32 oz (1.5 liter) spray bottle

You shouldn't have to buy commercial windshield cleaner. Keep a spray bottle of this solution in your trunk (along with some old newspaper to wipe off the grime). Be sure to wipe off any solution that gets on rubber or plastic gaskets or wipers with a damp cloth because prolonged contact with alcohol may damage them.

Combine the liquid ingredients in the spray bottle and shake well before using.

Vinyl and Leather Interior Cleaner

2 tablespoons (30 ml) vegetable-oil-based soap, such as castile
¼ cup (60 ml) olive oil
1 teaspoon lemon essential oil

Put the life back into your car's vinyl or leather interior with this fresh-scented polish without paying auto-parts-store prices.

1. Mix the ingredients well in a small bowl. Apply with a sponge.
2. Wipe off with a soft cloth.

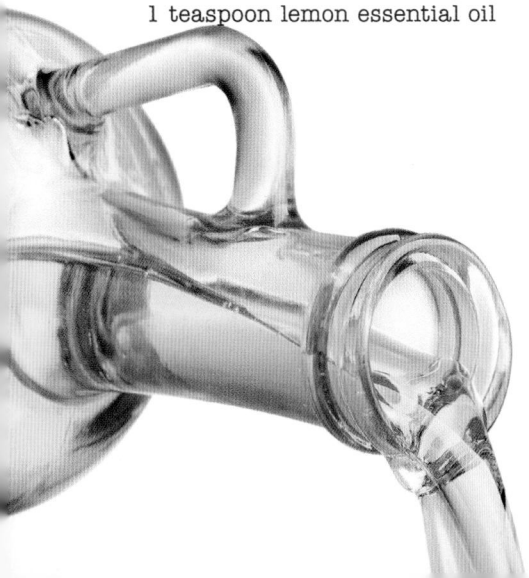

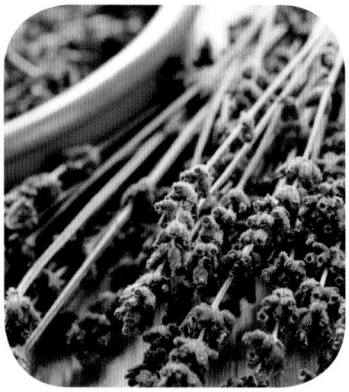

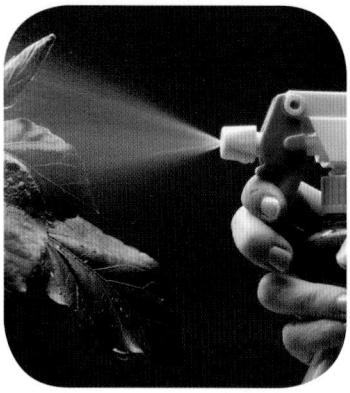

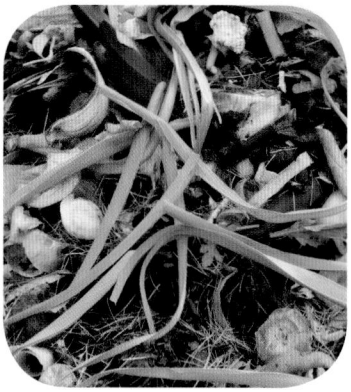

Household Compounds

Fabric Paste ❖ Wallpaper Stripper ❖ Oil-Paint Stain ❖ Varnish-Based Stain ❖ Nontoxic Stain for Children's Wood Projects ❖ Furniture Finish Test ❖ Leaking Toilet Test

Craft-Making Supplies

Craft Paste ❖ Pottery Glue ❖ Paper Glue ❖ Homemade Art Chalk ❖ Play Bubbles ❖ Vegetable Easter Egg Dyes ❖ Homemade Play Clay ❖ Simple Play Dough ❖ Finger Paints ❖ Basic Flower Drying ❖ Drying Medium for Preserving Flowers ❖ Potpourri Mixes ❖ Lemon-Scented Potpourri ❖ Rolled Beeswax Candles

Household Pest Repellents

Homemade Flypaper ❖ Moth Repellent Cedar Sachets ❖ Cockroach Bait ❖ Citronella Mosquito Candles ❖ Pungent Moth-Repelling Bundles ❖ Aromatic Moth-Repelling Sachets ❖ Ant Traps ❖ Carpet Flea Remover

Garden Helpers

Spot Weed Killer ❖ Red Clay Stain Remover ❖ Rust Remover ❖ Fire Starters ❖ Whitewash ❖ Water Repellent for Exposed Wood

Garden Soil Care

Compost ❖ Green Manure Soil Conditioner ❖ Seaweed Soil Conditioner ❖ Wood-Ash Potassium Boost ❖ Coffee Grounds Fertilizer

Garden Pest Deterrents

Blood and Bone Rabbit and Possum Repellent ❖ Repellent for Four-Footed Pests ❖ Garlic Possum Repellent ❖ Soap Repellent ❖ Easy Earwig Trap ❖ Slug and Snail Trap ❖ Alcohol Insect Treatment ❖ Homemade Insecticide ❖ Aspirin Systemic Insecticide ❖ Antifungal Compost Tea ❖ Baking Soda Fungal Fix ❖ Bug Blaster Soap Spray ❖ Fruit Fly Trap ❖ Rhubarb Insect Solution ❖ Ammonia Plant Conditioning Spray ❖ Oil Spray Insecticide Concentrate ❖ Insect Repellent

Houseplants

Sterile Seed-Starting Mix ❖ Lightweight Seed Mix ❖ Flowerpot Sterilizer ❖ General-Purpose Potting Mix ❖ Booster for Early Spring Flowers ❖ Repellent for Houseplant Pests ❖ Houseplant Food

Useful House and Garden Products

Running a household is a challenge. These days, just keeping a house operating smoothly takes money and ingenuity. But you can lessen the drain and strain with some of the easy-to-make products in this chapter.

Here you will find time-honored recipes for wallpaper pastes and strippers, furniture stains and other useful household compounds. There are safe, natural ways to help keep your home pest-free, along with ideas for providing fun for children—and adults—with busy hands. And you can make them all with a minimum of money and a maximum of good results.

Keeping your outdoor space beautiful and productive without spending a fortune or using a lot of chemical compounds is also a concern of most householders. Here are recipes and formulas for helping to keep your garden weed-free without using expensive manufactured herbicides and for making your own organic compost and natural soil conditioners and fertilizers. The many recipes for homemade garden pest deterrents will provide you with a choice of effective solutions to classic garden problems that neither cost very much nor taint the atmosphere. Simply by using ingredients that you already have in your kitchen, you can help to foil everything from black spot on your roses to slugs in the flower beds—and keep rabbits and possums out of your vegetable patch or shrubs. You will also discover some useful seed and potting mixes and other natural products that you can make to give your indoor plants a boost.

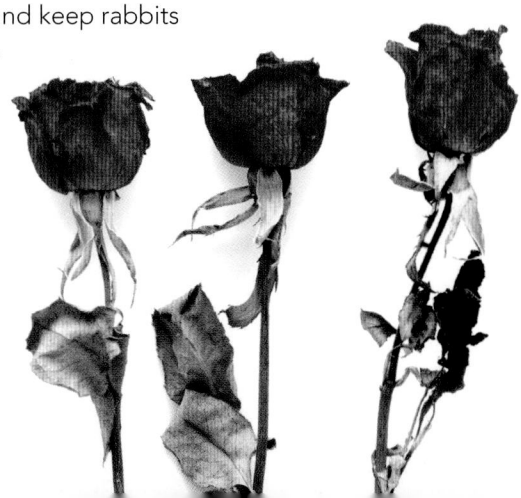

Household Compounds

Fabric Paste

fabric to cover the area
bottled liquid starch

Covering a less than perfect wall with attractive fabric is an old decorating trick that you probably already know. Using liquid starch as your glue may surprise you. It's now cheap and easy to add some color to a wall, under the wainscoting or inside an alcove.

1 Select a fabric that is medium to light weight. Cut the fabric to the lengths needed and soak the cut pieces, one at a time, in a tub filled with liquid fabric starch. Press the fabric to the wall as you would if wallpapering, smoothing out wrinkles, and allow it to dry.
2 When you want to remove the fabric, simply pull it away from the wall and rinse away any starch that remains on the wall with a sponge or wet towel.

Wallpaper Stripper

wallpaper scoring wheel or wire-bristle brush
1⅓ cups (330 ml) very hot water
⅔ cup (170 ml) liquid fabric softener
sponge
paint roller
wallpaper scraper or putty knife

Removing old wallpaper is never fun, but you can make it easier by heating up your own homemade stripper. For a large room, make up batches of the stripper so that it always goes on hot.

1 Score the wallpaper lightly with a scoring tool or wire-bristle brush so that the stripper solution will be absorbed beneath the paper's water-resistant surface.
2 In a bucket, mix the hot water and fabric softener. Apply this stripper to small areas with a sponge. You can cover larger areas with a paint roller soaked in the hot solution.
3 Allow the stripper to soak into the wallpaper for 20 minutes, then scrape the paper off the wall with a wallpaper scraper or putty knife, being careful not to gouge any of the plasterboard or plaster underneath.
4 Reapply the stripper solution to stubborn spots or if stripping multiple layers of paper. When the paper is removed, rinse the wall with a sponge and clean water, and allow it to dry before priming to paint or applying new paper.

Oil-Paint Stain

artist's oil paints in tubes (one or more colors, as needed)
gum turpentine

This stain is perfect for coloring wooden picture frames because you can use the exact colors of a painting to make the artwork coordinate with the frame, thinning the pigment to allow the natural wood grain to show. If you want traditional wood colors, choose raw umber (equivalent to walnut), burnt umber (mahogany) and yellow ochre (golden oak).

1. Mix equal parts oil paint and turpentine in a clean, widemouthed jar. Test the hue and opacity of the stain on a scrap of wood. This flexible stain can be easily modified. If it is too opaque, add turpentine; if it is too transparent, add more oil paint. If you want a unique shade, mix paints as needed. Be sure to mix enough stain for the entire project, as it is hard to duplicate a custom stain if you run short.
2. Brush the stain on the wood and allow it to dry to the touch before varnishing. If you want more grain to show, wipe the freshly stained wood with a clean, lint-free cotton cloth (such as an old T-shirt) moistened with turpentine.

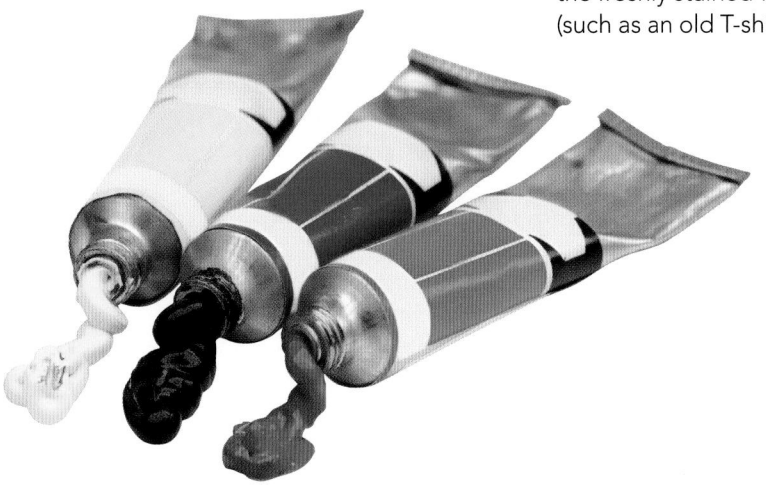

Fast fix for furniture scratches

You don't have to refinish a piece of wooden furniture, trim or floor just because it has a few scratches. (In the case of an antique, refinishing can actually reduce its value.) Here is an easy, inexpensive way to disguise a scratch. Get a children's crayon in a color that closely matches the wood's finish. Burnt sienna, sienna and yellow ochre are among the most useful colors. Then just rub the sharpened crayon over the scratch and buff to blend it in. If you want permanent coverage and the piece is less valuable, use a felt-tip marker instead; then apply some paste wax as directed to add sheen.

Varnish-Based Stain

varnish
paint thinner
stain
1 varnish-quality natural- or nylon-bristle brush
extra-fine sandpaper
tack cloth (available from hardware stores)

Some wood species, such as maple, are so hard that they don't absorb stain satisfactorily. If you find that this is the case, you can still "stain" a piece of furniture by tinting the sealer and varnish with the wood stain of your choice. This custom-tinted varnish recipe solves the problem and is a little less than a commercial product.

1 Stir together 2 parts varnish, 2 parts paint thinner and 1 part stain in a widemouthed jar to create a tinted sealer coat. Stir slowly to avoid bubbling. Brush onto a smoothly sanded piece of wood and allow to dry overnight before varnishing.
2 Sand the sealed piece of furniture lightly and wipe down with a tack cloth. To deepen the stain color, add stain, as desired, to tint the varnish in the can. When mixing color, remember that the color will deepen with each coat of varnish. Test the color on a scrap of wood or inconspicuous part of the project before proceeding. When the color is right (it should be transparent enough to allow wood grain to show through), brush the varnish onto the entire piece, taking care to avoid drips or streaks. Allow the varnish to dry overnight.
3 If a second coat of varnish is needed, repeat Step 2. Allow the varnished piece to dry for 2 days before using.

Nontoxic Stain for Children's Wood Projects

⅓ cup (60 g) powdered tempera paint
1 cup (250 ml) water
widemouthed 1 quart (1 liter) jar
paintbrush
nontoxic spray or brush-on, water-based varnish

If you have a child who is old enough for simple woodworking projects or for painting precut blocks and plaques, you'll want to try this recipe. It gives you brightly colored, safe stains that cost very little compared to the name-brand counterparts.

1 Pour the powdered paint into the jar. Add the water, screw on the lid and shake to mix.
2 Apply to wood with a paintbrush and allow the project to dry overnight.
3 Paint details and allow to dry overnight. Varnish the project with a water-based, nontoxic varnish, according to package directions, to preserve the color and add an attractive glossy surface. Dry as directed before using.

Four unexpected uses for vinegar

Shock Cure

If you have static electricity around the house in winter, try this simple, cheap vinegar cure.

1 Mix 1 cup (250 ml) white vinegar with 1 cup (250 ml) water in a 16 oz (500 ml) or larger spray bottle.
2 Spritz a dust cloth with the solution and wipe plastic tabletops, venetian blinds and upholstery to remove dust and discourage it from returning on static currents.

Glue Begone

You don't need to buy small bottles of expensive glue removers—you can wipe stubborn adhesive tags from store-bought products with a little household staple.

1 Dip a clean cloth into white vinegar and rub it over glue spot until it loosens. Remove glue with a dry corner of the cloth. Use a plastic spatula to lift any stubborn spots.
2 Rinse the spot with a clean, damp cloth, and then polish with a dry cloth.

Hand Deodorizer

There is nothing more irritating than a strong fish, onion or garlic smell that sticks to your hands. Here's the cheap and easy answer.

1 Wash your hands with soap and water as usual, then pour vinegar over your clean hands and rub in for a few seconds.
2 Rinse and dry hands as usual.

Mineral Deposit Remover

If you live in an area with hard water, sooner or later you'll notice that your coffee maker takes longer to brew and the coffee doesn't taste as good, your carpet steamer doesn't work as well as it did, and your steam iron may stop steaming. Here's how to make them all like new again.

1 To clean coffee makers, steam-cleaning machines and steam irons, pour ½ cup (125 ml) white vinegar into the water reservoir (or more as needed to fill the reservoir), turn the machine on and allow it to run until all of the vinegar passes through.
2 Then fill the reservoir with clean water and run the entire reservoir of clean water through the machine to rinse out the vinegar residue. With coffee makers, repeat rinsing stage, if needed.

Furniture Finish Test

nail-polish remover
cotton balls

With this simple process, you'll be able to determine the kind of finish used on a piece of furniture and the type of stripper you'll need to buy, saving both time and money. When working with chemical finish removers, use eye protection, wear rubber gloves that are designed for this use, and work in a well-ventilated place, such as a garage with opened doors.

1 Saturate a cotton ball in nail-polish remover and hold it briefly against an inconspicuous part of furniture, such as the bottom of a chair runner, side of a drawer or back of a table leg.
2 If the furniture finish becomes sticky or begins to dissolve, it is a lacquer-based finish, such as shellac or oil-based varnish, and you should buy a liquid furniture refinisher or rubbing alcohol to remove the finish.
3 If the finish is unaffected by the nail-polish remover, it is a plastic-based varnish, such as polyurethane, and you should strip it with paint remover.

Leaking Toilet Test

10 drops food coloring

Toilets can leak undetected, leading to an expensive waste of water and, sometimes, ruined floors. You don't need a plumber to find out. Here's how to test a toilet for leaks yourself.

1. Add food coloring to the cistern on the back of the toilet and leave it for 1 hour.
2. When the hour is up, examine the water in the toilet bowl. If colored water has leaked into it, you need to replace the toilet-cistern ball. Buy a replacement at a hardware store and, following directions on the package, put in the new ball.
3. If any colored water has leaked onto the floor, you need to call a plumber.

Craft-Making Supplies

Craft Paste

4 cups (1 liter) water
¼ cup (55 g) salt
1½ cups (225 g) white flour (more or less as needed)

Flour paste is a time-honored favorite for paper crafts, like decoration making and papier-mâché. It is easy and cheap to make at home.

1. In a saucepan, bring the water to a boil, and then remove from heat.
2. Stir in the salt and add the flour a little at a time, stirring constantly to prevent lumping, until the mixture reaches the consistency of very thick gravy. Cool and use.
3. Store leftover paste in a sealed container in the refrigerator for up to 5 days. Discard paste if mold forms or if it smells spoiled.

Pottery Glue

1½ teaspoons glycerine
4½ teaspoons gum arabic
¼ teaspoon water
rubber bands (optional)
duct tape (optional)

Use this traditional homemade recipe to make durable glue for repairing broken pieces of crockery or china.

1. In a small bowl, mix the glycerine, gum arabic and water thoroughly and store in a small, sealed bottle.
2. Coat both sides of the surfaces to be glued with the mixture and clamp them together with strong rubber bands or duct tape until the glue dries (about 1 hour).
3. Wash mended objects carefully by hand; do not place them in a dishwasher or on the stove. Do not use for hot liquids.

Paper Glue

1 cup (125 g) cornstarch
3 cups (750 ml) water
¼ cup (60 g) light corn syrup or glucose syrup
2 teaspoons white vinegar

This inexpensive homemade glue is more transparent than flour paste and is good for gluing pieces of paper together where looks count, such as scrapbooking or making greeting cards.

1 Mix and cook ½ cup (60 g) cornstarch, 1½ cups (375 ml) water and all the corn syrup and vinegar over medium heat until thickened. Remove from heat.
2 In a separate bowl, stir together the remaining ½ cup (60 g) cornstarch and ½ cup (125 ml) water. Blend into heated mixture. Store in a sealed container in the refrigerator for up to 2 months.

Homemade Art Chalk

cardboard toilet-paper tubes or plastic taper candle molds (available at craft stores)
masking tape
parchment paper
disposable milk or ice-cream carton
1½ cups (225 g) plaster of Paris
¾ cup (185 ml) water
paint stirring stick
8 teaspoons powdered tempera paint color (or mix 4 teaspoons colored paint and 4 teaspoons white paint for pastel colors)

Whether you need an ongoing supply of chalk for the family blackboard or simply want to supply budding artists with an endless supply of pavement chalk, here is an easy and inexpensive way to make your own.

1 Cover one end of each mold (toilet-paper tubes for fat pavement chalk and taper candle molds for blackboard-sized chalk) with masking tape to prevent leaks. Line the molds with parchment paper so that the finished chalk will release easily.
2 In a disposable container, stir the plaster of Paris and water together slowly with a paint stirring stick. Divide the solution into two or three containers if you are making more than one color of chalk. Add the paint powder to each container and stir to distribute the color evenly.
3 Sit the baking-paper-lined molds upright on a flat surface, fill with the chalk mix and tap the sides of the mold to release any air bubbles. Allow the chalk to air-dry for 3 days before unmolding. The chalk should slide out of the cardboard tubes or candle molds.
4 Make up new batches as needed until all desired colors are made.

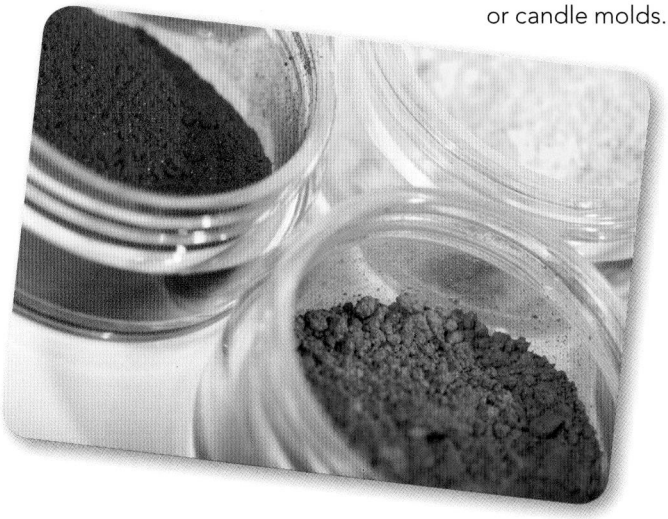

Play Bubbles

½ cup (125 ml) dishwashing detergent
1½ cups (375 ml) water
2 teaspoons sugar
1 teaspoon glycerine

Bubbles are a great party starter for kids of all ages, and this easy recipe makes lots of bubbles. Use your imagination—you can create bubble blowers out of open-ended cookie cutters and empty juice cans with both ends cut out. Instead of blowing bubbles, you can hold these blowers and whisk them through the air to release streams of bubbles.

1 In a medium bowl, slowly mix the ingredients, using a spoon or whisk to avoid foaming.
2 Pour the mixture into shallow bowls, dip blowers into the bowls, and wave them through the air to make big bubbles.

Vegetable Easter Egg Dyes

peels of 2 or more onions
½ cup (100 g) frozen spinach, thawed
1 fresh beet

You can make your own colorful natural Easter egg dyes very cheaply from vegetable juices. To make patterns on the already hard-boiled eggs, draw the design with a nontoxic wax pencil or crayon and then dip the eggs into hot dye long enough to color the egg without melting the wax. For a lacy pattern, soak a piece of fabric lace in melted paraffin and wrap around an egg while the wax is still soft. Put the wrapped egg in a spoon and dip into hot dye just long enough to color it. Remove the egg, and peel off the fabric to reveal a lacy colored pattern.

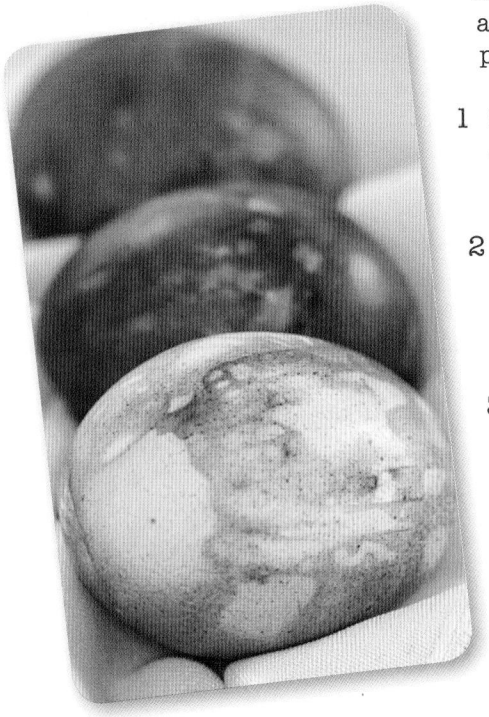

1 For yellow eggshells: In a saucepan of water, boil the onion peels for 20 minutes or until the water turns yellow. Remove onion peels, add eggs and boil for 5 minutes. Remove eggs and set aside to cool.
2 For green eggshells: In a saucepan of water, boil the spinach for 20 minutes or until the water turns green. Strain out spinach and return green water to saucepan, add eggs and boil for 5 minutes. Remove eggs and set aside to cool.
3 For red eggshells: Cut the beet into small pieces and put in a saucepan of water, boil for 20 minutes or until the water turns red. Remove beet pieces, add eggs and boil for 5 minutes. Remove eggs and set aside to cool.

Homemade Play Clay

4 cups (600 g) plain flour
1 cup (225 g) salt
1½ cups (375 ml) water
food coloring kit

This simple, money-saving recipe is great for making children happy on a rainy afternoon, but it is also the basis of Christmas tree ornaments, beads and other sophisticated crafts. The recipe makes doughlike "clay" that bakes hard in the oven and can be painted and coated with a craft varnish for a permanent and professional finish.

1 Preheat the oven to 350°F. Mix ingredients together and knead for 5 minutes. You can divide the dough into portions and add drops of food coloring at this point, or model the white "clay" and paint the finished piece. Put unused clay into sealed plastic bags and use within 4 hours of mixing.
2 Place finished pieces on a baking sheet and bake for 1 hour, or until hard.

Simple Play Dough

2 cups (300 g) plain flour
1 cup (225 g) salt
8 teaspoons (40 ml) vegetable oil
4 teaspoons cream of tartar
2 cups (500 ml) water
food coloring or nontoxic powder paint

A perennial favorite, this inexpensive dough can be played with, then returned to the fridge and stored for another day. Why buy commercial play dough when it's cheap to make?

1 Combine all the ingredients, except food coloring or powder paint, in a saucepan and stir over medium heat for about 3 to 5 minutes until a stiff dough forms.
2 Cool, then divide into portions and add a different food coloring to each portion. Work the coloring thoroughly through the dough. Store in self-sealing bags in the fridge.

Finger Paints

½ cup (60 g) cornstarch
2 cups (500 ml) cold water
6 small plastic containers with snap-on lids
food coloring kit

You can feel good about giving little artists finger paints that you make yourself from kitchen pantry staples that you know are safe—and washable.

1 In a small saucepan, combine the cornstarch and water. Bring to a boil over high heat, stirring constantly until thickened. Remove from heat and let cool to room temperature.
2 Divide the cornstarch mixture evenly among the containers. Put several drops of food coloring into each container and stir to distribute colors evenly.

Basic Flower Drying

selection of flowers, such as roses, hydrangeas, everlasting daisies, Queen Anne's lace or baby's breath
rubber bands
string

Dried flowers can make a very natural-looking floral arrangement that will last you a long time. And if you do the drying yourself, the cost is minimal. Some candidates can come from your own garden and others you can find elsewhere. If you like roses, for example, you can often get wilted ones from a florist at no cost. (They won't look wilted when they are dried.) Try to get a dozen or more flowers with stems.

1 Remove the leaves from the stems. Then bundle the stems together in groups of six with a rubber band. Hang the bundles upside down by string from a rod or a clothesline in a dry, warm place, such as a cupboard or the attic. The stems are hung upside down so that the flowers don't flop over during drying.
2 Leave bundles for a week or two or until the flowers are dry to the touch.

Drying Medium for Preserving Flowers

1 lb (500 g) borax
1 lb (500 g) cornmeal
1½ teaspoons salt
flowers and flower buds
artist's brush with pointed tip

Many flowers dry better in a drying medium, which you can make yourself much more economically than if you buy it. Most flowers dry best and last longest when they are picked fresh and are just beginning to open. This drying medium will dry many kinds and colors of flowers and buds, although you must recreate their stems with floral wire and floral tape. To preserve their color, display dried flowers out of direct sunlight.

1 Preheat the oven to 200°F. In an open casserole, mix the borax, cornmeal and salt. Bake uncovered for 30 minutes, stirring occasionally, to dry the contents completely.
2 Pour half of the drying mixture into a shoebox or plastic storage container. Set aside the remainder of the drying mixture.
3 Make a shallow well in the center of the mix. Trim the stem of a bud or flower to 1 inch long. Hold the flower and trickle cornmeal mix between its petals to fill the blossom. Place the flower into the well in the container of mix, stem end down. Repeat with as many flowers as will fit in the container.
4 Pour the remainder of the mix over all flowers until they are buried. Set the container in a warm, dry, dark place, such as a closet, for 2 weeks.
5 After drying, remove the flowers carefully from the cornmeal mix and brush the mix from the petals with an artist's brush. Fasten the flowers and buds for arrangements onto floral wire stems with floral tape. You can hot-glue the short stems to wreaths and gift packages.

Potpourri Mixes

3 cups dried flower petals, herb leaves and small pine cones (optional)
3 tablespoons (30 g) dried orris root or orris root powder (available at craft or herb stores)
10 drops essential oil (one type or a blend of your choosing)

A bowl of fragrant, flowery potpourri can fill a room with the essence of summer—even in the middle of winter. Make potpourri to perfume your own home—or as homemade gifts. If you don't have a garden, ask your florist for past-their-peak flowers, such as lavender, statice and roses, and lemon leaves that you can dry (see Drying Medium for Preserving Flowers, opposite).

1 In a large bowl, mix together flower petals, herb leaves, small pine cones, if using, and orris root.
2 Sprinkle essential oils over the dry ingredients and stir to distribute the fragrance.
3 Display in an open bowl out of direct sunlight and add a couple drops of oil, as needed, to refresh the fragrance.
4 Store, or give as a gift, in a sealed glass or plastic container.

Lemon-Scented Potpourri

1 cup (15 g) dried calendula flowers
1 cup (20 g) dried chamomile flowers
½ cup (10 g) dried lemon balm
½ cup (10 g) dried lemon verbena
½ cup (15 g) dried lemon thyme
½ cup (10 g) dried basil
½ cup (80 g) finely diced dried lemon peel
3 tablespoons (30 g) orris root powder
½ teaspoon lemon verbena essential oil
6 drops chamomile essential oil

If you like a citrus scent, you'll love the fresh perfume of this colorful mixture. If you have other lemon-scented leaves, such as lemon-scented geranium or lemon-scented tea tree, feel free to add them.

1 Combine all the ingredients and mix well. Put in a sealed container and leave for a few weeks to mature.
2 To use, transfer potpourri to open bowls and stir gently to release the scent.

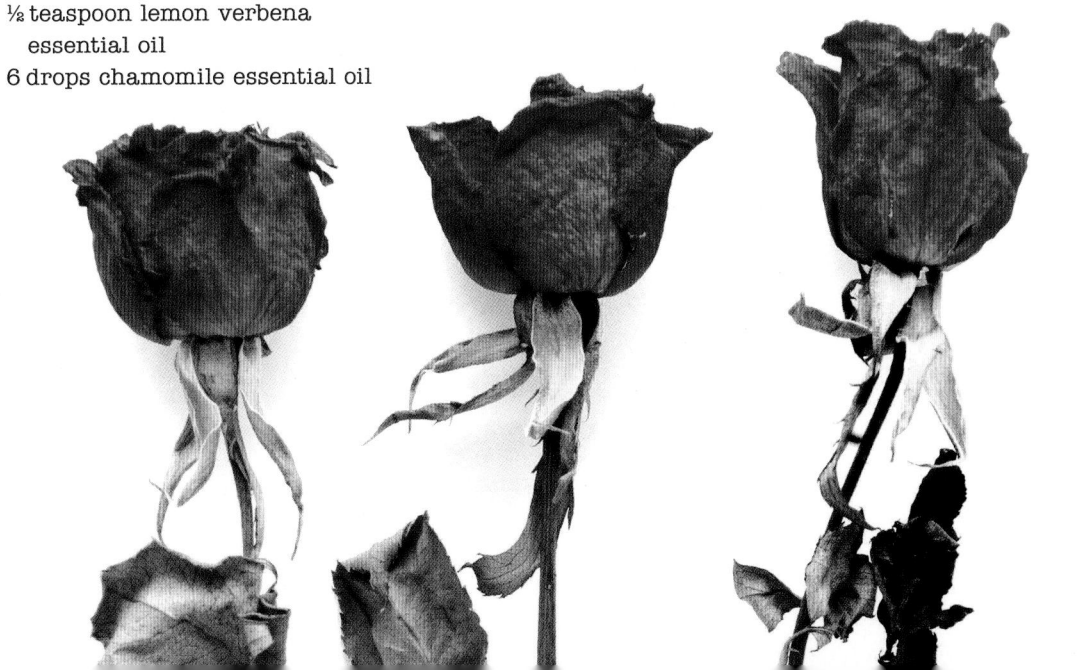

Rolled Beeswax Candles

sheets of beeswax (as many as the number of candles desired)
wicking

Candles rolled from sheets of beeswax are simple to make and long-burning. They make elegant gifts.

1 Cut wicking 3 inches longer than the sheets of beeswax.
2 Melt a small amount of beeswax in a double boiler over low heat. Soak the wicks to saturate in wax, remove and stretch out straight on a sheet of parchment paper to cool.
3 Warm the beeswax sheets until malleable with an electric hair dryer set to its lowest setting. Lay a prepared wick on the edge of a sheet, placed on a flat surface. Roll the sheet tightly and evenly around the wick until it is as thick as desired.
4 Trim excess beeswax with a utility knife, and seal candle seam with a heated butter knife. Repeat steps for remaining candles.

Household Pest Repellents

Homemade Flypaper

½ cup (110 g) corn syrup or glucose syrup
3 teaspoons brown sugar
3 teaspoons white sugar
6 strips brown paper (cut from a paper bag)

Why buy flypaper when you can make your own? All you need is a brown paper bag, a little bit of sugar and some corn or glucose syrup.

1 Combine the syrup and sugars in a shallow bowl.
2 Poke a hole at the top of each strip of brown paper. Soak the paper in the syrup mixture overnight.
3 Scrape the paper strips across the edge of the saucer to remove excess syrup and hang the finished flypaper strips near windows and doors.
4 Replace when the strips are covered with insects.

Moth Repellent Cedar Sachets

2 pairs colorful adult or baby socks
1 bag cedar shavings (often sold at pet stores as bedding)
satin or grosgrain ribbon
clothes hanger

You can have the benefits of a moth-repellent cedar closet or cedar-lined drawers at a fraction of the cost of the real thing with these fragrant cedar sachets.

1 Fill the socks with cedar shavings—adult-sized for closets and baby-sized for drawers.
2 Tie the tops of the socks closed with coordinating ribbon.
3 Tie large sachets to clothes hangers and hang in closets to freshen air and repel moths. Tuck the little ones into lingerie and woollens drawers.

Cockroach Bait

1 metal coffee can with plastic lid
1 old-style beer-can opener (that cuts V-notches)
2 tablespoons (20 g) borax
3 teaspoons flour
3 teaspoons sugar

Cockroaches are attracted to damp areas, such as under the kitchen sink, but this inexpensive solution will kill them if they eat it. Remember to store pest treatments, such as this, in sealed and labeled bottles in a childproof cabinet.

1 Punch holes around the base of the empty coffee can, using the beer-can opener. Label the can with a sign that reads "Cockroach Killer."
2 In a small bowl, mix the ingredients together. Put the mixture in the coffee can, snap on the lid, and place it under the sink or wherever you've seen cockroaches. Lock the undersink cupboard if you have children or pets.
3 Refill the can or create additional cans as necessary.

Citronella Mosquito Candles

1 package wicking
one 10 lb (4.5 kg) block paraffin
crayons (colors of your choice), roughly chopped
citronella essential oil
molds
cooking spray
1 package mold seal

Citronella is a natural mosquito repellent that you can use indoors or out. Mold the candles in containers that you already have, such as soup cans, or use clay flower pots and leave them in the mold. Buy wicking, paraffin and mold seal at craft stores.

1 Cut wicking 4 inches longer than the mold's height. Melt some of the wax in a double boiler over very low heat and soak the wicks until saturated. Lay out straight on parchment paper to cool.
2 Lightly spray the inside of each mold with nonstick cooking spray, and seal with mold seal if it doesn't have its own.
3 Stick the wick to the bottom of the mold with a bit of mold seal. Tie the other end to a small stick or skewer, pull the wick taut and lay the stick across the mouth of the mold.
4 Melt the remaining wax in a double boiler, never letting it exceed 194°F (use a candy thermometer to check). Use oven mitts to handle hot wax to prevent burns. Lower heat, add the crayons and a few drops of citronella oil and stir to distribute evenly.
5 Pour the wax into the molds, stopping ½ inch from the top. Place the molds in a pan of cold water (use pot holders), taking care not to splash water into the mold. Let cool for 1 hour.
6 When the mold is cool, remove the candle. Trim the wick and smooth the bottom of the candle by standing it in a pot of warm water. If you used a two-part mold, trim any ragged seams with a paring knife.

Pungent Moth-Repelling Bundles

1 small bundle southernwood, camphor, tansy or sweet woodruff
1 rubber band
string
1 clothes hanger

Moths dislike the strong fragrance of certain herbs. They also avoid cupboards that are regularly aired out, so every once in a while leave your closet or chest of drawers cracked open for a day, and make an herbal repellent.

1. Bind together a small bundle of fresh herbs (either one kind or a blend) by fastening a rubber band around the stems.
2. Tie a bundle to an empty clothes hanger and hang it in the closet among woollen clothes, or tuck it under drawer-liner paper in a drawer containing woollens.

Aromatic Moth-Repelling Sachets

10 inches (25 cm) fine material, such as silk or nylon netting
dried lavender flowers
dried elder flowers

This sachet containing lavender and elder flowers makes a lovely aromatic gift and will also keep your drawers fragrant and moth-free.

1. Fold the fabric with right sides together and cut to create an 8 x 8-inch square plus a ½-inch seam allowance on all four sides. Sew three seams.
2. Turn the pouch right side out and fill with flowers. Tuck the remaining seams inside and stitch the bag closed by hand.
3. Place in drawers or chests with woollens to repel moths.

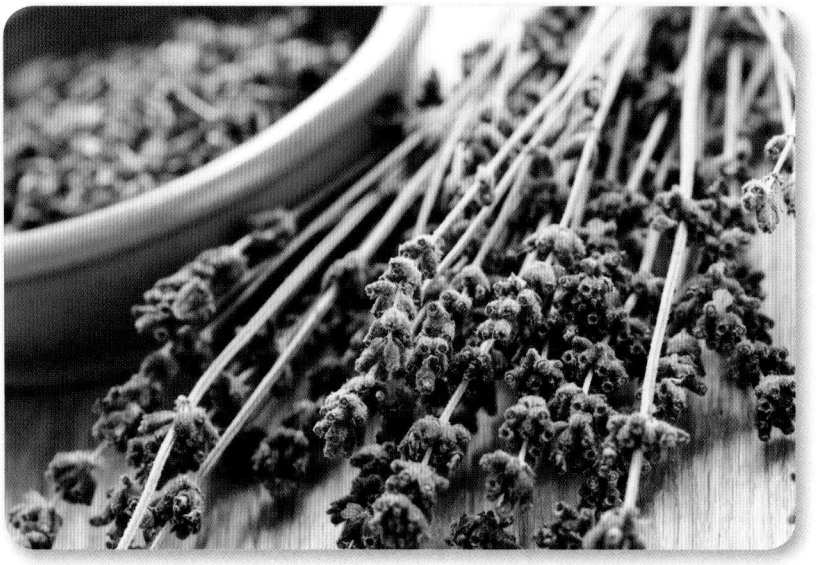

How to keep pet food ant-free

Placed on the floor, pet food bowls are like a natural magnet for ants. Here's a simple, totally nontoxic way to keep ants away. Set an empty pie plate where you usually feed your pet. Fill the pet's bowl with food and set it into the pie plate. Pour water into the pie plate, filling it to the rim. Ants and other crawling insects cannot cross this "moat" to reach the pet food.

Ant Traps

3 cups (750 ml) water
1 cup (220 g) sugar
4 teaspoons borax
3 clean 8 oz (250 g) screw-top jars
cotton balls
old-style beer-can opener (that cuts V-notches)

Here's an easy, inexpensive way to round up the ants that begin to invade your house each summer.

1. In a jug, mix the water, sugar and borax together. Loosely pack the jars half-full of cotton balls and saturate the balls with the solution.
2. Pierce jar lids with the can opener, making 2 or 3 holes just large enough to admit ants.
3. Place the baited jars where ants are active, but make sure jars are out of the reach of pets and children. Attracted by the lethal sugar and boric acid mixture, ants will crawl into the traps.

Carpet Flea Remover

3 mothballs
duct tape

If fleas hitchhiked indoors on your pet, try this simple, effective and cheap fix for freshening and debugging your carpets, using your vacuum. Wear rubber gloves when handling mothballs and be sure to keep pets and children away while you work.

1. Cut a small slit into the disposable vacuum bag liner and drop in mothballs. Seal the slit with a piece of duct tape. If you have a bagless vacuum, simply drop the balls on the floor and vacuum them up, or open the canister and drop them in.
2. Vacuum as usual. Fleas that are vacuumed up will be killed by the mothballs in the bag or canister. Drop in new mothballs when you change the disposable bag or empty the canister.

Garden Helpers

Spot Weed Killer

boiling water

Weeds that pop up between flagstones and in cracks of the footpath are hard to dig out of the small crevices. Control weeds in your terrace or walkway by dousing them with this very simple solution!

1. Boil a kettle full of water.
2. Douse weeds with the boiling water, wait 1 day and check for withering. If the weeds resist, repeat. Keep boiling water away from garden beds.

How to protect plants when spot-treating weeds

It's difficult to spot-treat weeds that sidle up to your favorite garden plants without killing the good plants. Here's how to keep the weed killer on the weed and off your prized peonies: Cut the bottom out of a large, 2 liter clear plastic soft drink bottle or 1 gallon (4 liter) container and remove the lid. To isolate a weed for treatment, set the bottomless bottle over it, stick the weed-killer spray applicator into the lid opening and spray. Be sure to label the bottomless bottle with the pesticide being used and to store it in a locked cabinet with other pesticide equipment.

Red Clay Stain Remover

table salt
vinegar

If you garden in an area with clay soil, you know all too well how its red color stains your clothes. Set aside an old pair of jeans just to garden in. When they're caked with mud, use this simple recipe to keep stains off the clothes you wash them with.

1. Drape the muddy jeans over the back of a garden chair or lay them out on a picnic table and rinse vigorously with a garden hose.
2. In a small jar, add vinegar to the salt, a little at a time, to make a paste. Rub the paste into the mud stains, allow to sit for 20 minutes, then launder as usual.

Sure and safe weed controls

In the old days, gardeners had to outsmart weeds because there were no chemical weed killers. Take a few tips from them, save a trip to the garden center, and keep your garden weed- and chemical-free.

1 Weed early and often to keep weeds from taking hold. Hold the hoe blade horizontal to the ground and scrape weed seedlings from the vegetable garden and in and around ornamentals. Avoid tilling deeply—it can bring buried seeds to the surface, where they will sprout. To save your back, use an ergonomic hoe with a gooseneck that lets you stand up straight.
2 Burn weeds that pop up in the driveway or between pavers with a small propane torch or kill them with boiling water.
3 Spread a 3-inch-deep layer of organic mulch, such as straw, wood chips or compost, around the base of plants to smother weeds and retain soil moisture.
4 Pull any weeds sprouting from potted nursery plants before planting them in your garden.
5 Apply granulated lime according to package directions to lawns in the autumn, using a fertilizer spreader. Most lawn weeds can't thrive in alkaline soil.

Rust Remover

white vinegar
paper towels
steel wool

Use vinegar as a rust remover for old hinges, screws and metal garden furniture exposed to the elements.

1 Fill a widemouthed jar half-full of vinegar, drop in small rusty parts, screw the lid on and soak for a few days until rust loosens. Remove the objects, rinse and carefully dry.
2 Soak a paper towel in vinegar and lay it over furniture surfaces to loosen rust. If the rust is stubborn, cover the saturated towel with plastic wrap to keep the towel damp. Sit the piece out of direct sunlight for a few days. Remove the wrapping, steel-wool the spot smooth, rinse and dry. Paint, if desired.

Fire Starters

1 lb (500 g) paraffin wax
scraps of kindling wood
cake cooling rack

If you use this simple recipe to make your own fire starters, you'll never have to dash to the hardware store at the last minute when you'd rather be enjoying your outdoor fireplace or charcoal barbecue.

1 Melt the paraffin in the top of a double boiler over low heat or in a slow cooker set on low heat.
2 Dip wood scraps into the melted wax to cover completely, remove and arrange on the cooling rack to harden.
3 When the wax cools, store the waxed wood scraps in an old coffee can in a cool place. To use, place one or two scraps at the bottom of your fireplace or charcoal barbecue and stack logs or charcoal over them. Use a long-handled match to light the starters, which will act as long-burning igniters for your fire.

Whitewash

1 cup (225 g) table salt
2 cups (450 g) hydrated lime
1 gallon (4 liters) water or milk

Whitewash is a wood coating that has been used for hundreds of years. In the days when paint was an expensive luxury, whitewash was popular for painting farm buildings and fences. Whitewash has no binders and will slowly wear away in rain, which is why it was routinely painted on greenhouse roofs to shade plants in summer. To finish a traditional project or to shade your greenhouse, try this simple recipe. While whitewash must still be mixed by hand, the ingredients, including color tints, are sold at concrete supply stores.

1 Stir the ingredients together slowly in a metal bucket, taking care not to splash. The ingredients will become warm as they are mixed. Add more lime or water as needed to achieve the color and consistency of milk. For a more permanent paint, substitute fresh milk for water.
2 Allow the mixture to cool before painting on wood and allow it to air-dry.

Caution: Mix whitewash outdoors; wear protective eye goggles and old clothes. Be careful not to splash the mixture on your skin when mixing and rinse it off right away if any does get on your skin. Mix whitewash in a metal bucket, because it heats up as the ingredients combine and may affect a plastic container.

Water Repellent for Exposed Wood

1 quart (1 liter) exterior varnish (spar or polyurethane)
1 clean 1-gallon (4 liter) paint can
1 cup (130 g) grated paraffin wax
1 stirring stick
mineral turpentine
paintbrush or roller

Try this recipe for a long-lasting, waterproof coating for decks, shutters and other wooden items that are exposed to the elements. If you plan to stain the wood, do so before applying the water repellent. If you want to paint or varnish, apply the water repellent first and allow it to dry before painting or varnishing.

1 Pour the varnish into the paint can. Add the wax and stir slowly until the wax dissolves.
2 Add mineral turpentine until the can is full and stir slowly to mix all the ingredients without creating air bubbles.
3 Brush or roll the treatment onto raw or stained wood and allow to dry for 4 hours before using, painting or varnishing.
4 If you want to paint the wood, prime with oil primer after the water repellent dries, allow the primer to dry as directed on package label, then paint.

Garden Soil Care

Compost

6 parts dried (brown) plant material (dry leaves, straw, sawdust or paper)
1 part fresh (green) plant material (grass clippings; vegetable scraps; coffee grounds; horse, cow or chicken manure)

Compost is the best natural soil amendment you can use. It contains valuable plant nutrients and plant disease-fighting organisms, and it also makes soil moisture-retentive and easier to till. Best of all, compost is free when you make your own. You can make your compost in a bin (3 feet square is ideal) or simply pile the ingredients on the ground. If you turn the pile periodically, it will break down faster, but even if you pile it and leave it for a year, it will break down.

1 Put a layer of brown material directly on the ground, then add a layer of green material. Continue to layer brown and green material to a height of 3 feet. Water with a hose as needed to keep the pile as moist as a wrung-out sponge.
2 To speed up decomposition, use a hay fork to puncture and turn the pile to allow air into its center. In rainy weather, cover the pile with a tarp to prevent saturating it.
3 If the pile becomes smelly, it is too wet—mix in more brown ingredients. When the pile looks like rich, crumbly black soil and has a sweet, earthy fragrance, it is ready to use in the garden or as mulch.

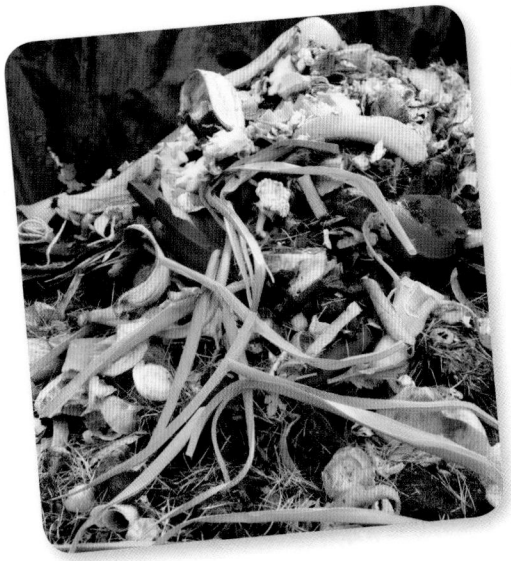

An inexpensive, very helpful soil test

A complete soil test costs much less than you'd think and is one of the best investments you can make in your garden. The test results will provide an exact prescription for fertilization, liming and adding trace elements.

Knowing what your soil needs allows you to furnish your plants with ideal conditions with no wasted effort. For testing locations and to order a kit by mail, check your phone book or do an online search.

Green Manure Soil Conditioner

mixture of "green manure" seeds (grasses and legumes)

Often called "green manures," these are annual crops that thrive in cool weather, improving the soil and protecting garden soil from erosion and weeds. Use a combination of grasses and legumes. Check with your local nursery for a list of seeds to suit your area.

1. After clearing vegetables or annual flowers from a bed in autumn, sow green manure seeds in cleared beds according to package directions.
2. In early spring, 3 to 4 weeks before planting time, dig the green manure into the soil, or harvest it at the lower stem and use it for mulch. As it decomposes, green manure adds humus to the soil and acts as fertilizer for the next crop.

Seaweed Soil Conditioner

seaweed

Seaweed is actually higher in nitrogen and potassium than most animal manures and is also a rich source of trace elements. Check with beachside municipalities if they are happy to have you haul it away.

1. To cleanse seaweed of salt, pile it where runoff will be directed to a storm drain, such as on your driveway. Allow several rains to rinse away the sea salt, then add the seaweed to your compost pile or dig it into garden beds in the autumn.
2. To make seaweed tea, steep an old pillowcase filled with seaweed in a bucket of water for 1 week. Remove and discard the bag, dilute the liquid to the color of weak tea, and water your plants with it.

Water-wise gardening techniques

You can save water and still have a beautiful garden. All it takes is noting moist and dry areas of your property and choosing the right plant for the right place.

❖ **Target practice** Think of your yard as radiating outward from your house like a bull's-eye target. The wettest areas are closest to the house—especially around outdoor faucets where water drips, and the next wettest area is within reach of a 50- to 100-foot garden hose. Beyond the reach of your hose are the driest areas.

❖ **Plant with care** Grow water lovers, like ferns and annuals, near the house, and select drought-tolerant perennials with deep roots that can reach groundwater, such as echinacea (coneflower), rudbeckia and ornamental grasses, outside the reach of your garden hose.

❖ **Consider climate** If you live in a mild-winter climate, choose water-conserving garden plants that are native to drier regions. Or select plants that are native to your specific area, which are naturally adapted to your local soil and rainfall.

Fertilizer, free for the asking

Healthy plants are naturally resistant to insects and diseases, and natural fertilizers are the best way to ensure healthy plants and a balanced garden ecosystem. No matter where you live, good sources of fertilizer may be available, free for the hauling, at farms and from neighbors who have pet rabbits or chickens. All you have to do is ask for animal manure to enrich your compost.

Wood-Ash Potassium Boost

wood ashes

Wood ashes from a fireplace or woodstove (not coal or charcoal ashes) are a free source of the plant nutrients potassium, calcium and phosphorus. They can also be used to decrease soil acidity, similarly to lime. Benefits of treating soil with ashes include improved hardiness and flavor of fruits. Be sure to apply in small amounts or compost well before applying to keep the caustic ashes from burning plants. Water-soluble nutrients can leach from ashes, so be sure to use fresh ones that have not been exposed to rain.

1. Apply 5 to 10 lb (750 g to 1.5 kg) of ashes per 100 square feet of garden in the autumn.
2. To reduce soil acidity, use wood ashes as a substitute for ground limestone: See package directions for limestone and apply up to twice as much wood ashes as it recommends. Allow ashes to weather over the winter before planting.

Coffee Grounds Fertilizer

coffee grounds

Acidic coffee grounds make an excellent soil conditioner or mulch for acid-loving plants such as conifers, azaleas and rhododendrons. You can often have as much of the used grounds as you need, free for the taking, from your local cafe.

1. Apply a 3-inch-thick mulch of coffee grounds around the base of acid-loving plants, leaving a 6-inch ring of bare soil around the trunk of the plant to discourage fungal collar-rot diseases and trunk-eating insects.
2. For a complete fertilizer, 2-4-2 analysis, mix 4 parts coffee grounds with 1 part composted wood ashes, and work into soil in autumn.

Garden Pest Deterrents

Blood and Bone Rabbit and Possum Repellent

blood and bone fertilizer

They may be cute, but when rabbits and possums munch on your prized garden produce or gnaw the bark of young trees, they wear out their welcome. Blood and bone is an organic fertilizer that is high in nitrogen, the nutrient most needed by green plants. But more importantly, the rabbits and possums associate the smell of it with predators and will avoid gardens treated with it.

1. Sprinkle the fertilizer over the soil around garden perimeters and in garden beds according to package directions.
2. Reapply after heavy rains.

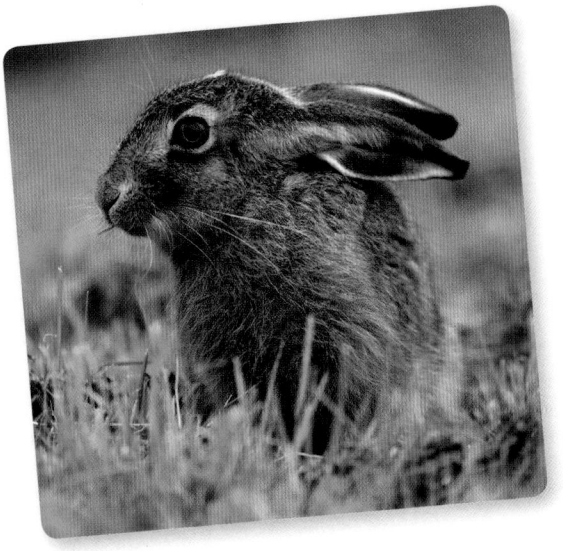

Use fencing to keep rabbits out

Use fence wire or shade cloth with holes small enough to discourage chewing and exclude the tiniest rabbit. Wrap young tree trunks with shade cloth to keep rabbits from gnawing the bark. To protect a vegetable garden, staple chicken wire that has small holes along the inside of your garden fence. For the most effective control, bury the fencing a foot deep to keep rabbits from digging under it.

Repellent for Four-Footed Pests

water
ammonia
mothballs

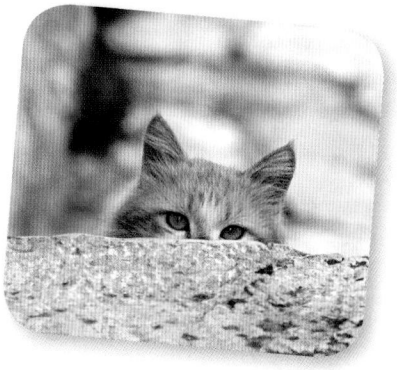

Whether it's rats, stray cats or possums treating your trash like an all-you-can-eat buffet or mice and rats looking for a holiday home in your barbecue, you can get four-footed pests to keep clear with a couple of inexpensive household products.

1. In a spray bottle, mix a solution of half water and half ammonia. Liberally spray the mixture on trash cans or other areas visited by animal pests. If trash cans sit outside, swab them out with full-strength ammonia after every emptying.
2. Place a handful of mothballs in a shallow dish or pan and set into an unused barbecue to repel mice, possums and rats. Remove mothballs when the barbecue is in use. Tuck a few mothballs into garden furniture cushions before storing them over the winter to repel nesting mice. Be sure to keep mothballs, which are toxic, out of the reach of children and pets.

Garlic Possum Repellent

8–10 cloves garlic, crushed
4 cups (1 liter) hot water

Possums can be a great nuisance in the garden, but they hate the taste of garlic. Whip up this brew and they'll soon be feeding elsewhere. You can also use ground fresh chile peppers or fish sauce in the solution instead of garlic.

1. In a bowl, mix the crushed garlic into the hot water and allow to stand overnight.
2. Strain the mixture into a spray bottle and spray foliage. Repeat every few days (or after rain) until the possums get the message.

Soap Repellent

several bars or scraps of deodorant bath soap (not floral scented)
long nail or drill with ⅛-inch bit, or old socks
string

This repellent works for some animals such as deer. Deer dislike the smell of deodorant soap. Collect soap scraps and tie them into an old sock for a long-lasting, environmentally safe protection for prized plants. Fresh bars of soap make an even stronger deterrent. One bar can protect a 9-square-foot area, so space the bars as needed to protect vulnerable plants.

1. Remove the soap from the wrapper, make a hole in one end of a bar with the nail or the drill, and run a piece of string through the hole. If using soap scraps, drop them into the toe of an old sock and tie the open end closed with string.
2. Tie the soap (or soap-filled sock) to the branch of a shrub or tree with string or attach to a stake in the garden bed. Replace when the soap is diminished by rain.

Easy Earwig Trap

several sheets of used newspaper
string

These fearsome-looking insects can be identified by the pincers at the ends of their tails. Although earwigs don't hurt people, these nocturnal feeders can nibble plants overnight. Try this nontoxic control made with recycled newspaper. This technique also works with slaters.

1. Roll several thicknesses of newspaper into a tight cylinder and secure with string. Dampen the rolled paper and place on the soil near eaten plants.
2. Check the newspaper roll each morning to see if earwigs are hiding inside. If so, dispose of them in a securely tied trash bag and set out a new roll. Continue this routine until earwigs are under control.

Slug and Snail Trap

1 teaspoon dry yeast
1 teaspoon sugar
1 cup (250 ml) tepid water
stale beer (optional)
1 or more clear plastic drinking-water bottles and caps

Slugs and snails devastate prized garden plants by chewing round holes in the leaves, leaving telltale shiny slime trails. They climb up into plants like hostas and marigolds to feed after sundown and, in the morning, crawl down to hide in mulch or garden debris. Here's a nontoxic recipe for catching them.

1. Mix the yeast, sugar and water together and allow it to rest for 5 minutes. Pour just enough yeast solution (or stale beer) into an empty drinking-water bottle, so that when you lay it on its side the liquid does not run out.
2. Lay the bottle on its side under a plant that shows slug or snail damage or place under a vulnerable plant as a preventive measure. Slugs and snails will be attracted by the yeasty odor, crawl in and drown.
3. Check the bottle daily and, when full, replace the lid, throw it away and make a new trap. Make as many as you need—these traps may not be beautiful, but they look better than the skeletal remains of a slug-eaten plant in the garden.

A quick slug and snail barrier

When you don't have time to set elaborate traps for these garden pests, make an unbroken ring of wood ashes around your favorite flowers. Snails and slugs will turn away from caustic ashes. Make sure that you reapply the ashes after it rains.

Alcohol Insect Treatment

1 cup (250 ml) rubbing alcohol
1 cup (250 ml) water

Rubbing alcohol is a tried-and-true homemade treatment for soft-bodied garden pest insects such as aphids and mealybugs. Traditionally, it was advised that you dab it onto individual insects with a cotton swab, but this is a time-consuming task. Try this speedy spritz instead.

1. Combine the alcohol and water in a spray bottle and shake to combine.
2. Before treating, spray one leaf of the infested plant as a test to make sure there are no reactions, such as browning. If not, spray the entire plant, including undersides of leaves and flower buds. Avoid spraying open flowers, which may turn brown if treated with alcohol.
3. Repeat every other day for 3 days to kill hatchlings. Monitor plants and spray again as needed. Label the bottle and store it out of the reach of children and pets.

Homemade Insecticide

10 cloves garlic
3 teaspoons vegetable or mineral oil
3 cups (750 ml) hot water
1 teaspoon dishwashing liquid (not laundry or dishwasher detergent)

When aphids, whiteflies and other insect pests become a problem in the garden or on your houseplants, don't rush to the market for an expensive spray. Make your own from these kitchen-tested ingredients. Store all garden treatments, such as this, in a sealed and labeled bottle in a childproof cabinet.

1. In a blender, puree the garlic, skin and all, and oil.
2. Strain the mixture through a sieve into a quart (1 liter) jar. Add water and dishwashing liquid. Close the jar and shake gently to mix.
3. Decant the mixture into a spray bottle (you can clean and reuse a cleaning product spray bottle). Spray infested plants, making sure to cover both sides of the leaves. Apply every 3 days for a week to control hatching insect eggs. Repeat as needed after rain or when problems arise.

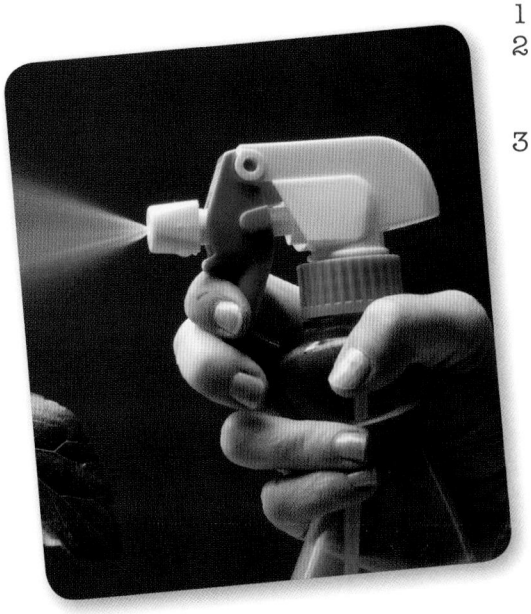

Outsmarting stinging insects

You can avoid attracting stinging insects, such as bees, wasps and mosquitoes, by being careful about what you wear or how you smell while gardening or sitting on the patio. Here are some smart suggestions:

1 Stinging insects that strike during daylight hours are attracted to flower colors—red, pink, yellow, orange and purple—so wear clothes in cool shades of blue, green, black, gray or white for yard and garden work.

2 Many stinging insects are also attracted to floral and fruity scents, so forgo perfume, scented shampoo, scented hair conditioners and fragrant body lotions.

3 Stinging insects are often repelled by herbal scents. Wear a broad-brimmed hat in the garden and tuck sprigs of rosemary, chrysanthemum or marigold flowers into the brim to repel insects. Or, if you don't want to wear a hat, put the sprigs into the pocket of a T-shirt.

Aspirin Systemic Insecticide

1½ regular-strength aspirin (450 mg in total)
5 gallons (10 liters) water

Plant experts have experimented successfully with watering plants with aspirin-water as a systemic insecticide and promoter of plant growth. Plants naturally produce some salicylic acid, which aspirin contains, as a natural protection. When watered with the aspirin solution, treated plants absorb extra salicylic acid, which helps them repel sucking insects, and they produce strong, healthy growth.

1 In a large watering can, stir the aspirin into the water until dissolved. Water plants as usual with treated water or put it in a spray bottle and use as a foliar spray.
2 Treat plants twice monthly with aspirin water.

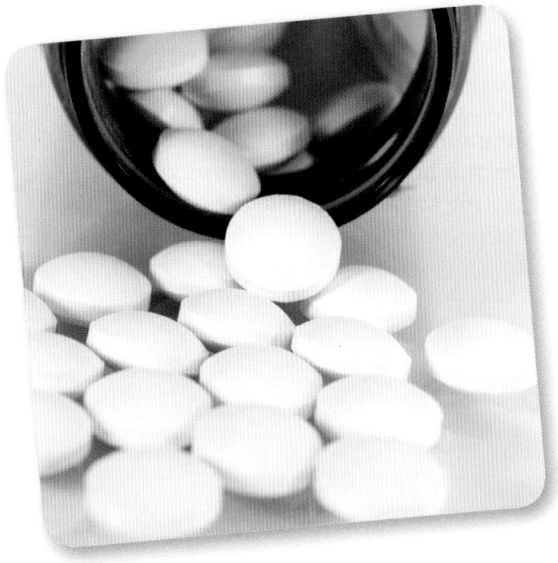

Antifungal Compost Tea

1 gallon (3–4 liter) bag compost
1 empty burlap bag or old pillowcase
string
10 liters water

Compost is not just a great soil conditioner and fertilizer. It also contains beneficial organisms that resist soil-borne fungal diseases. To discourage the formation of fungus on plants, such as brown patch, sooty mildew and powdery mildew, make a "tea" treatment using common garden compost.

1 Place compost in the bag, tie the bag shut with string and drop it into a bucket of water.
2 Set the bucket in a sunny spot, and steep the bag in the water for 2 or 3 days—until the water turns dark brown.
3 Remove the bag of compost (use the contents as mulch). Dilute the remaining solution with water to the color of weak tea. Spray it on roses, zinnias, phlox and other plants that are susceptible to fungal infections. Repeat twice monthly during the growing season to prevent outbreaks.

Baking Soda Fungal Fix

1 teaspoon baking soda
1 teaspoon dishwashing liquid (do not use laundry or dishwasher detergent)
4 cups (1 liter) warm water

When a baking soda solution is applied to fungus-prone plants, such as roses, before signs of mildew appear, it can prevent diseases such as powdery and sooty mildew and black spot. This spray is cheap and easy to make—keep it on hand and apply as needed. To further discourage fungal diseases, keep plant leaves as dry as possible by watering the soil without splashing the leaves, and mulch plants with compost.

Pour the ingredients into a large spray bottle and shake to mix. Spray both sides of leaves and stems.

Bug Blaster Soap Spray

3 teaspoons dishwashing liquid (do not use laundry or dishwasher detergent)
1 gallon (3.75 liters) water

Dishwashing liquid is harmless to the environment and is safe to use in the house. Outdoors it also makes an effective control for soft-bodied insects, such as thrips, caterpillars, aphids and mealybugs, because the soap breaks down their protective coverings, causing the pests to dehydrate.

1 Stir the dishwashing liquid into the water. Fill a spray bottle and test-spray one or two leaves of an infested plant. Wait a day, and if the leaves are not damaged, spray the entire plant. Be sure to coat the stems as well as both sides of the leaves.
2 Repeat the treatment twice a week until the pests are no longer visible. Then repeat as often as needed.

Fruit Fly Trap

1 quart (1 liter) plastic bottle with lid
bait, such as yeast spread, port wine or vanilla essence and sugar
rubbing alcohol

In many areas, fruit flies can completely ruin your home-grown crop. Instead of resorting to deadly sprays, hang a few of these simple traps in your trees to reduce the fruit-fly population.

1 Punch several ¼-inch holes in the neck of the plastic bottle.
2 Put a little of your bait substance in the bottom of the bottle along with a few drops of rubbing alcohol.
3 Hang the trap in the fruit tree, just above the lower leaves. Replace the bait at least twice a week. Start using the traps about 6 weeks before harvest time and continue until the fruit has been picked.

Rhubarb Insect Solution

3 stalks rhubarb with leaves
3½ quarts (3½ liters) water

Rhubarb is an attractive perennial plant that not only makes good pies but also makes an insecticide that is toxic to sucking insects. This recipe is for ornamental plants only. Do not spray on herbs, fruits or vegetables because rhubarb leaves are toxic to humans and animals.

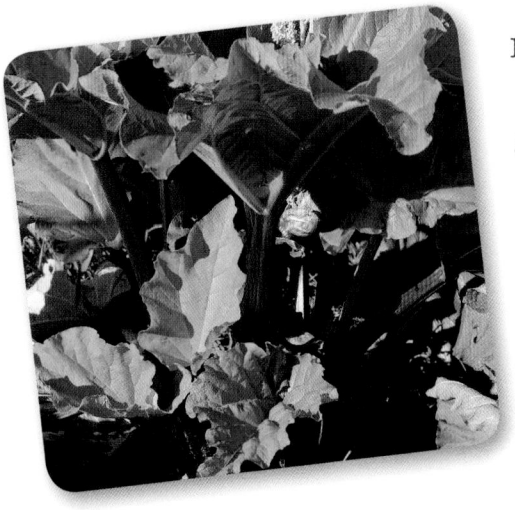

1 Chop the rhubarb leaves and stems. In a stockpot, combine the rhubarb and water. Bring to a boil, reduce the heat and simmer, uncovered, for 1 hour.
2 Cool to room temperature and strain liquid into a spray bottle through a funnel. Spray mixture on infested plants at 3-day intervals for 10 days. Repeat as necessary.

Use scented mulch to keep insects away

Trimming herbs frequently, especially removing flower stalks, helps them maintain lots of tender, flavorful new growth. Sprinkle the sprigs and flowers that you don't use in the kitchen along garden paths as aromatic and insect-repelling mulch.

Ammonia Plant Conditioning Spray

1 part household clear ammonia
1 part dishwashing liquid (do not use laundry or dishwasher detergent)
7 parts water

Ammonia is a concentrated form of nitrogen, which is the nutrient most needed by green plants. You can make an inexpensive all-purpose fertilizer and insecticidal spray using ammonia and soap. The soap helps the ammonia stick to the leaves and also kills soft-bodied insects. Mix as much as you need for garden plants and lawns. Store all garden treatments, such as this, in a sealed and labeled bottle in a childproof cabinet.

1. In a large container, combine the ingredients.
2. Fill a spray bottle and apply the mixture to stems and both sides of leaves for garden plants. Use a hose-end applicator to spray the lawn.

Oil Spray Insecticide Concentrate

3 teaspoons dishwashing liquid (do not use laundry or dishwasher detergent)
1 cup (250 ml) vegetable oil

Some plant pests and fungal infections are hard to eradicate because they have shells or waxy coatings that protect them from traditional treatments. You can, however, smother tough-shelled scale, the eggs of many insects and even mildew infections by coating them with oil. Store all garden treatments, such as this, in a sealed and labeled bottle in a childproof cabinet.

1. In a pint (500 ml) container, combine the ingredients to form a spray concentrate. Store it in a sealed, labeled container.
2. To apply, mix 1 or 2 teaspoons concentrate with 1 cup (250 ml) water in a spray bottle and apply to stems and both sides of plant leaves. Reapply after it rains.

Insect Repellent

sprigs fresh rosemary
sprigs fresh basil
sprigs fresh thyme

This fragrant, herbal smoke will help to deter flies and mosquitoes at your next barbecue. However, it is a mild solution and extra protection should be used in areas with mosquito-transmitted diseases.

1. When you remove food from the barbecue, spread out a handful of pungent culinary herbs on the top rack where they will smoke, but not burn.
2. Allow the herbs to cook and release their fragrances.

Houseplants

Sterile Seed-Starting Mix

1 part sifted garden soil
2 parts sphagnum peat moss
2 parts coarse sand
1 baking potato

Mature plants develop defenses against many kinds of insects and diseases, but fragile seedlings can be wiped out by soil-borne diseases or insects. Use this money-saving recipe to make a sterile potting medium for sprouting garden seeds and also for making potting soil to protect valued houseplants.

1 In a large container, mix the soil, peat moss and sand together.
2 To sterilize, moisten and place the mixture in a shallow baking pan with a baking potato and bake at 200°F until the potato is done. This is a smelly process, ideal for doing on an outdoor barbecue. Discard the potato.

Lightweight Seed Mix

1 part vermiculite
1 part milled sphagnum moss
1 part perlite

This mix is made of sterile materials bought at a garden center and does not need to be baked.

1 In a large container, mix all the ingredients together.
2 Moisten with warm water before using.

Flowerpot Sterilizer

1 part household bleach
10 parts water

Just because a flowerpot is used and dirty, you don't need to toss it. Whether clay, plastic or ceramic, the pot can be superficially cleaned with a strong blast from a garden hose. If the pot has white, crusty mineral deposits, scrape them off with an old knife (scraping clay pots will sharpen the knife). When the pot is free of dirt and minerals, sterilize it to kill insect eggs and plant diseases.

1 Mix the bleach and water, making enough to fill a tub that is deeper than the largest pot you want to sterilize.
2 Place the cleaned pots in the tub and allow them to soak for 20 minutes.
3 Remove sterilized pots, rinse again with clear water and set them in the sun to dry. They are now ready for new plants.

General-Purpose Potting Mix

1 part perlite
1 part finished compost
1 part topsoil

The compost in this mix contributes disease-fighting microorganisms and nutrients to help mature indoor and outdoor potted plants thrive.

1. Mix all the ingredients together and store them in a waterproof, sealed container.
2. To modify this mix to suit succulents, cacti and other plants that need sharply drained soil, increase the perlite to 2 parts, or add 1 part builder's sand to the original recipe.
3. Before filling a large pot, invert several small plastic pots on the bottom of the larger pot, then fill with soil. The air space beneath the small pots will aid drainage and lighten the overall weight of the pot.

How to overwinter herbs indoors

To preserve culinary herbs for use throughout the winter months, dig the plants from the garden toward the end of summer and transfer them to pots. Place the pots on a sunny windowsill indoors. For the best results, select vigorous but compact plants and use 6-inch clay pots.

Booster for Early Spring Flowers

1½ gallons (5½ liters) warm water (110°F to 115°F)
1 3-gallon (10 liter) bucket
1 cotton ball
cloudy ammonia
1 plastic trash bag

Get a jump on spring by forcing branches of flowering shrubs and trees to bloom early indoors. In late winter, watch for flower buds to swell on spring bloomers, such as quince and ornamental cherry trees. Prune enough branches to fill a tall vase.

1. Cut stems, crush the cut ends with a hammer and place them in the bucket of warm water.
2. Saturate a cotton ball with cloudy ammonia and drop the ball into the bucket.
3. Put the bucket of stems in a clean trash bag, tie it closed, and then leave it in a warm place indoors until the buds begin to open. Then arrange the stems in a vase of clean water and set them out in a room for a long-lasting bouquet.

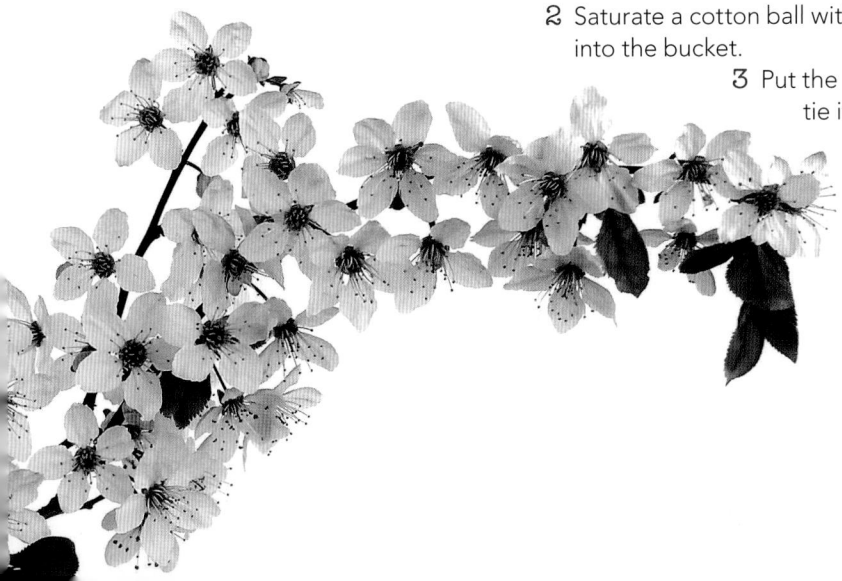

Reblooming houseplants

When you receive a special flowering plant as a gift, it can be heartbreaking to have to throw it away after it finishes blooming, but it doesn't have to end this way. With a little effort, you can keep these plants from year to year and get them to rebloom.

❖ **Hippeastrum (*Amaryllis*)** After blooming, set the plant in a sunny spot and water as usual, letting it die back naturally, as you would for any bulb. This will occur sometime between late summer and early autumn. Remove the withered foliage. Keep the plant in a cool (about 55°F), dark place over winter (such as a cellar or garage) and do not water it. At the end of winter, bring the plant out into the light and warmth. Water and fertilize it, and flowers should appear by early summer.

❖ **Poinsettia** As the length of the day increases in spring, poinsettias will stop blooming, but their foliage will remain fairly attractive. They can be placed outside in the warm months, but be sure to do a hard pruning in midsummer (cut stems back to 2 inches above the soil). During early autumn, put the plants on a strict light schedule: 14 hours of total darkness at night, 10 hours of bright light during the day. Any light at all during the dark period can disturb the cycle, which is why some people place the plants under trash cans or in a cupboard at night. Once the flower heads have formed, you can bring the plants back into normal conditions.

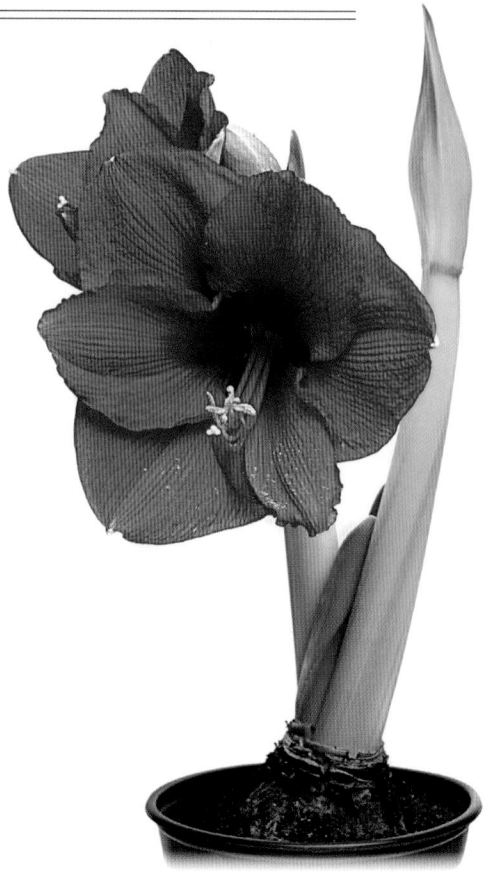

Repellent for Houseplant Pests

1 large clear plastic dry-cleaning bag
6 mothballs
1 twist tie

If you have a houseplant that is bothered by aphids, mealybugs or other insect pests, you can banish them with this simple, no-mess recipe. Use rubber gloves when handling moth balls.

1. Put the infested plant, pot, and saucer into the dry-cleaning bag. Moisten the soil, drop mothballs into the bag and tie the bag closed with a twist tie.
2. Set the bagged plant in a bright place that is out of direct sunlight for 1 week. At the end of the week, remove the plant and put it in its usual home, then dispose of the bag and mothballs. Repeat the treatment as needed until pests are gone.

Houseplant Food

2 bucketfuls fresh horse or cow manure or 1 bucketful poultry manure
1 burlap bag
rope
1 barrel or trash can
water

For an easy organic food for houseplants, try this recipe for "manure tea."

1. Dump manure into the burlap bag. Tie the bag shut with one end of a long rope and place it in an empty barrel or trash can.
2. Fill the barrel or trash can with water and leave the bag to steep for a week, using the rope occasionally to jerk it up and down and mix the liquid.
3. Thin the "tea" to the color of weak tea and apply monthly to the soil around houseplant roots. Keep reserved tea in labeled jars with tight lids, out of the way of children and pets.

How to create a lush indoor garden

If you display your houseplants all in one area, you will get a lush visual effect, and the plants will benefit from the heightened humidity gained by grouping the pots of moist soil.

Arrange the potted plants on a waterproof covering, with the shorter ones at the front and rows of successively taller ones behind. For extra protection, set water-collecting saucers under each pot. To increase the humidity of the garden, include a few vases or decorative bowls filled with pebbles and water.

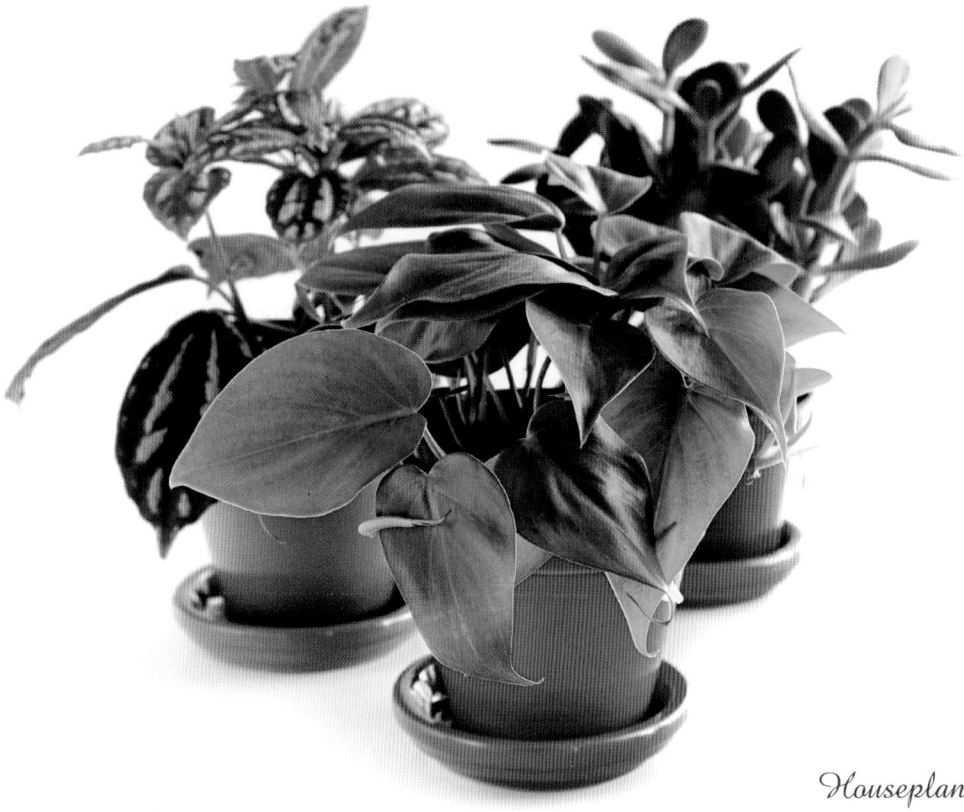

Index

A

acne remedies, 288–89
additives, 10–11
aftershave recipes, 272, 273
Aioli (garlic mayonnaise), 30
air fresheners, 337
alcohol. See rubbing alcohol; wine and spirits
almond extract, 261
almond oil, 245, 259
almonds, 247, 264
aloe vera
  growing, 294
  health and beauty uses, 258, 273
  home remedy uses, 278, 285, 293, 294, 298
aluminum foil, 321, 341
amaryllis care, 384
ammonia
  buying, 20
  cleaning uses, 335, 343
  garden uses, 375, 381, 383
  laundry use, 346
  precautions for, 21
Angel Cake, 118
angelica seed, 253
aniseed, as antacid, 276
antacids, spices as, 276
Antibacterial Drawing Paste, 290
Antibacterial Oil, 290
antifungal remedies
  for garden, 379
  medicinal, 295–96
Antipasto Platter, 143
Antiseptic Lotion for Burns, 294
Ant Traps, 367
anxiety remedies, 307
appetizers. See snacks and appetizers
apples, apple juice
  Apple and Raisin Muffins, 107
  Apple Ginger Jelly, 80
  Applesauce, 58
  Electrolyte Drink, 277
  freezing, 88
  Hot Mulled Cider, 163
  Perfect Apple Pie, 126
appliances, 13, 14
apricots
  Apricot Oat Bars, 141
  Dried-Apricot Jam, 76
  freezing, 88
Aquarium Fish Treats, 329
arnica essential oil, 273
arrowroot, as powder base, 262, 268, 295
artichokes, 147, 244
asparagus, freezing, 85
aspirin, 297, 378
athlete's foot remedies, 295–96
Automatic Dishwasher Detergent, 342
avocados, 151, 256

B

Baba Ghanoush, 150
baby powder, for cat box, 322
back pain remedy, 303
bacon, 109, 182
bagels, 111
baked goods. See specific types
baking equipment, 14
baking mixes, homemade, 61
baking powder substitute, 96
baking soda
  buying, 20
  car care use, 350
  cleaning uses, 336, 337, 341, 343, 344, 345, 348, 349, 350
  garden uses, 379
  health and beauty uses, 254, 267, 268, 299
  home remedy uses, 285, 302
  laundry uses, 345
  pet care uses, 315, 317
Balsamic Vinaigrette, 35
bananas
  Banana, Sour Cream, and Honey Face Mask, 248
  Banana Cake, 119
  Banana Nut Bread, 96
  Chocolate-Nut Frozen Bananas, 237
  Corn Plaster, 296
  Honey Banana Ice Cream, 223
  as wrinkle fighter, 249
  Youthful Skin Face Mask, 248
Barbecued Spareribs, 168
Barbecue Sauce, 52, 167
barley, 158, 187
basil
  Insect Repellent, 381
  Pasta with Classic Basil Pesto, 183
  Salsa Verde, 32
Bath Gel, 264
bath powders, 267–68
bath products, 263–68
bathroom cleaners, 347–50
bath treatments. See specific ailments
beans
  Baked Beans, 168
  Black Bean Soup, 188
  freezing, 86
  Hummus, 150
  Refried Beans, 170
  Tuscan-Style Three-Bean Salad, 201
Béarnaise Sauce, 54
beauty products
  bath products, 263–68
  body care, 257–63
  face care, 242–51
  foot care, 270–71
  hair care, 254–57
  hand and nail care, 268–69
  lips and mouth care, 251–54
  men's products, 272–73
  storage of, 260
  tips and equipment for, 15–18
beef
  Beef Barley Soup, 187
  Beef Stock, 49
  bouillon cubes, 49
  Calcium-Rich Dog Food, 312
  Chili Con Carne, 166
  Chinese Crispy Beef Stir-Fry, 169
  Lasagna, 186

Savory Meat Mix, 166
Spaghetti Bolognese, 179
Spicy Beef Pie, 177
Thai Beef Salad, 196
Wholesome Kitty Dinner, 319
beer
Beer Bread, 92
Beer Shampoo, 254
as meat tenderizer, 47
beeswax
Galen's Cold Cream, 250
in lip balms, 251–52, 297
Love Your Feet Cream, 270
Rolled Beeswax Candles, 364
beets, 85, 151
bell peppers, 73, 85
benzoin tincture, 289, 300
bergamot
Bacteria-Fighting Citrus Mouthwash, 253
Body Spray, 262
Relaxing Aromatic Bath, 309
Room Freshener Spray, 337
berries. See specific types
beverages. See cold drinks; hot drinks
bird food, 324–27
blackberries, freezing, 88
blackberry leaves, 277
black cohosh, 305
blanching technique, 85
bleach
buying, 20
garden use, 382
mold and mildew removal, 339
precautions for, 21
blondies, 130
Blood and Bone Rabbit and Possum Repellent, 374
Blood-Orange Champagne Granita, 230
bloodstains, 346
Bloody Marys, 159
blueberries
Blueberry Ice Cream, 221
Blueberry Muffins, 108
Blueberry Syrup, 58
freezing, 88
Three-Berry Jam, 79
Blue Cheese Dressing, 39
body care treatments
Almond Exfoliating Body Scrub, 261
body oils by skin type, 259
Body Powder, 262
Body Spray, 262
Cellulite Massage Oil, 260
Citrus Cologne Splash, 260
Citrus Moisturizer, 258
Cranberry Sugar Scrub, 261
Deodorant, 263
Green Aloe Moisturizing Lotion, 258
Shaving Gel for Women, 259
Simple Fragrant Body Splash, 260
Simple Sugar Scrub for Dry Skin, 261
Summer Body Splash, 259
Warm Herbal Body Treatment, 257
boil remedies, 290
borax
buying, 20
cleaning uses, 335, 336, 342, 343, 344, 347, 349, 351
craft use, 362
laundry use, 346
mold and mildew removal, 339
pest control, 365, 367
bottling (canning) techniques, 68, 72
bouillon cubes, homemade, 49
Bouquet Garni, 41
bran, 108, 322
Brandied Peaches, 217
brass polishes, 340
bread
Bread and Butter Pudding, 213
for cleaning wallpaper, 335
French toast, 139–40
muffins, 107–9
quick breads, 92–98, 141
rolls, 110–15
yeast breads, 99–106
breakfast foods
cereals, 26–27
treats, 139–42
brewer's yeast. See yeast and brewer's yeast
brioche, 103
broccoli, freezing, 86
brownies, 132
bruise remedies, 293
brussels sprouts, freezing, 86
bubble bath recipes, 263
Bubbles, Play, 360
bug bites, 284–85. See also itch relievers
Bug Blaster Soap Spray, 379
burdock root, 305
burn remedies, 293–94
butter, clarifying, 57
Butter Cake, 118
buttermilk substitute, 94
Butter Pecan Ice Cream, 227
Butterscotch (candy), 205
Butterscotch Sauce, 60

C

cabbage, 195
Cabinet Cleaner, 335
Cabinet Polish, 338
Caesar Salad, 198
Caffe Latte, 160
Cajun Seasoning Mix, 43
cakes and icings
Angel Cake, 118
Banana Cake, 119
Basic Cake Mix, 61
Butter Cake, 118
Cheesecake with Strawberry Glaze, 120
Chocolate Buttercream Icing, 122
Chocolate Cake, 117
Chocolate Ganache Icing, 121
Cream Cheese Icing, 122
Cupcakes, 121
Devil's Food Cake, 117
Orange Cake, 119
Simple Glaze Icing, 122
Spice Cake, 116
Vanilla Icing, 121
Calcium-Rich Dog Food, 312
calendula
Calendula Ointment, 292
First-Aid Antiseptic, 291
Healing Calendula Lotion, 286
camphor, 366
candles, making, 364

candy
Butterscotch, 205
Candied Citrus Peels, 211
Caramels, 206
Fudge, 206
Gumdrops, 204
Lollipops, 205
Marshmallows, 210
Pastel Mint Patties, 207
Peanut Brittle, 208
Peanut Butter Cups, 209
Pralines, 207
Rocky Road, 209
Toffee Bars, 208
candy thermometers, 204
canning (bottling) techniques, 68, 72
Caper-Dill Eggs, 146
cappuccino. See coffee
Caramel Cappuccino, Frosty, 155
Caramels, 206
Caramel Sauce, 60
caraway seed, 276, 299
car cleaners, 350–51
cardamom seeds, 299
Caribbean Spicy Meat Rub, 45
carpet care
Carpet Flea Remover, 367
fresheners for, 336, 337
carrot essential oil, 259
carrot oil, 260
carrots
Carrot Bread, 97
Doggie Salad, 313
freezing, 86
Cassis Sorbet, 233
castile soap, buying, 20
castor oil, 278, 303
cat care, 319, 321, 322–23
cat food, 319–21
cat litter boxes, 322, 323
catnip, 307, 320
cauliflower, 69, 86
cayenne pepper
Cajun Seasoning Mix, 43
Hot Pepper Rub, 301
Liniment, 303
Massage Cream, 301
Quick-and-Dirty Muscle Rub, 302
for sore throat, 281
Toothache-Relieving Dental Paste, 301
cedar
for flea control, 317
Moth Repellent Cedar Sachets, 364
cedarwood essential oil, 285
Cellulite Massage Oil, 260
cereal recipes, 26–27
Chai, 162
Chalk, Homemade, 359
Challah, 102
chamomile
Anti-Cramp Tea, 304
Basic Skin Toner, 244
in body oil, 259
Calming Tea for Insomnia, 308
Chamomile Shampoo, 256
Chamomile Tea, 306
Delicately Scented Bath Powder, 268
for flea control, 317
in hair rinses, 255
Herbal Milk Bath for Sleeplessness, 309
in itch relievers, 285
Rich Neck Moisturizer, 243
Salve for Eczema or Dermatitis, 287
Sleep Pillow, 308
Soothing Tea for Heartburn, 276
Stomach-Calming Tea, 276
Warm Herbal Body Treatment, 257
Chapped Lips, Balm for, 297
cheese. See also cream cheese
Blue Cheese Dressing, 39
Cheese and Parsley Bread, 93
Cheese Sauce, 56
Cranberry Cheddar Muffins, 109
Light Blue Cheese Dressing, 39
Marinated Goat Cheese, 147
Penne with Four-Cheese Sauce, 181
Quesadillas, 149
Spinach-Feta Phyllo Triangles, 148
Chermoula, 44
cherries, freezing, 88
Chest Compress, 279
Chest Rub, 279
chewing gum, removing from dog fur, 317
chicken
Calcium-Rich Dog Food, 312
Chicken Liver Paté, 144
Chicken Noodle Soup, 189
Chicken Nuggets, 139
Chicken Seasonings Mix, 42
Chicken Stock, 50
Classic Chicken Pie, 176
Creamy Chicken Salad, 198
Curried Chicken Salad, 199
Doggie Birthday Cake, 315
Low-Fat Chicken and Rice Dog Dinner, 312
Tandoori Chicken, 175
Thai Green Chicken Curry, 171
Wholesome Kitty Dinner, 319
chickpeas, 150
chile peppers
Chili Jam, 67
Sweet Chili Sauce, 33
chili powder
Chili Con Carne, 166
Chili Eggs, 146
recipe for, 43
Chinese Crispy Beef Stir-Fry, 169
Chinese Fried Rice, 174
chocolate
Brownies, 132
Chocolate Buttercream Icing, 122
Chocolate Cake, 117
Chocolate Chip Cookies, 128
Chocolate Chip Lip Balm, 252
Chocolate Chip Muffins, 107
Chocolate Chocolate Chip Ice Cream, 225
Chocolate-Dipped Strawberries, 219
Chocolate Ganache Icing, 121
Chocolate Mousse, 216
Chocolate-Nut Frozen Bananas, 237
Chocolate Pops, 236
Chocolate Pudding, 211
Chocolate Sauce, 60
Cocoa, 161
Cocoa Lip Balm, 252
Devil's Food Cake, 117
Fudge, 206
Hiccup Reliever, 277
Hot Chocolate Viennese, 161

Mint Chocolate Chip Ice Cream, 226
Rich Chocolate Ice Cream, 225
Rocky Road candy, 209
Rocky Road Ice Cream, 224
substitute for, 132
Chrome and Stainless Steel Polish, 341
chutneys, 74–75
Cider, Hot Mulled, 163
cinnamon
Cinnamon Oatmeal Milk Bath, 266
Cinnamon-Raisin Swirl Bread, 104
Cinnamon Rolls, 113
Cinnamon Soap, 265
Spicy, Minty Mouthwash, 253
Spicy Room Freshener, 337
citronella essential oil, 284, 365
citrus. See also specific fruits
Bacteria-Fighting Citrus Mouthwash, 253
Candied Citrus Peels, 211
Citrus Cologne Splash, 260
Citrus Disinfectant, 334
Citrus Marmalade, 84
Citrus Moisturizing Treatment, 258
Citrus Sorbet, 233
Zingy Citrus Bath Salts, 267
clarifying process
butter, 57
cooking stocks, 51
clay. See cosmetic clay; green clay; Play Clay, Homemade
cleaning products
air fresheners, 337
bathroom cleaners, 347–50
car cleaners, 350–51
furniture polishes, 338
general housecleaning, 334–37
kitchen cleaners, 342–45
laundry products, 345–47
metal polishes, 340–41
mold and mildew removers, 339
Cleansing Liquid for Acne, 289
Cleansing Soap, 292
clove
Mouthwash for Cold Sores, 298
Spicy, Minty Mouthwash, 253
Spicy Room Freshener, 337
for toothache, 300
Cobb Salad, 200
Cockroach Bait, 365
Cocktail Flea Dip, 316
Cocktail Sauce, Seafood, 28
cocoa. See chocolate
coconut, 129, 224
coffee
Caffe Latte, 160
Cappuccino Granita, 231
Cappuccino Mix, 161
Coffee Grounds Fertilizer, 373
Frosty Caramel Cappuccino, 155
Iced Coffee Slush, 155
cold and cough remedies
Chest Compress, 279
Chest Rub, 279
Cough Drops, 281
Cough Suppressant, 280
Cough Suppressant Tea, 280
Decongestant Salve, 282
Drops for Earache, 283
Gargle Solution, 281
Herbal Inhalant, 283
Humidifier Booster, 283
Mustard Powder Plaster, 280
Mustard Seed Plaster, 279
Saline Spray for Sinuses, 283
Slippery Elm Tea, 281
Sore-Throat Lozenges, 282
Steam Cough Relief, 280
Steam Treatment, 282
Cold Cream, Galen's, 250
cold drinks
Bloody Marys, 159
Classic Iced Tea, 154
Cranberry Iced Tea, 154
Frosty Caramel Cappuccino, 155
Fruit Juice Spritzer, 159
Ginger Beer, 156
Iced Coffee Slush, 155
Lemonade Syrup, 156
Lemon Barley Water, 158
Lemon Squash, 157
Orange Blossom, 157
Sangria, 160
Sparkling Fruit Bowl, 158
sweetener for, 155
Traditional Lemonade, 157
Cold Pack for Strains and Sprains, 303
cold sore remedies, 297–98
Coleslaw, Classic, 195
comfrey, for hair care, 255
compost, 371
Compost Tea, Antifungal, 379
compresses
Chest Compress, 279
Compress for Bruises, 293
eye compresses, 243
Headache Compresses, 305
Hot Compress for Cramps, 304
condiments and spreads, 28–33
conditioners. See hair care products
congestion. See cold and cough remedies
constipation remedies, 278
cookies, slices and brownies, 128–33
cooking stocks, 49–51
cookware, 12, 14
copper polishes, 340
corn, freezing, 87
cornichons (Pickled Gherkins), 67
cornmeal
Corn Bread, 93
Cornmeal Hand Scrub, 269
craft use, 362
Dry Cat Shampoo, 322
corn remedies, 296–97
cornstarch
cleaning uses, 337, 344
craft use, 359
health and beauty uses, 256, 267, 268, 295
corn syrup, 210, 364
cosmetic clay, 289
cough remedies. See cold and cough remedies
Country Pork Sausages, 145
craft-making supplies
Basic Flower Drying, 362
Craft Paste, 358
Drying-Medium for Preserving Flowers, 362
Finger Paints, 361
Homemade Art Chalk, 359
Homemade Play Clay, 361
Paper Glue, 359
Play Bubbles, 360

Potpourri, 363
Pottery Glue, 358
Simple Play Dough, 361
Vegetable Easter Egg Dyes, 360
cramp bark, 304, 305
cranberries
Cranberry Cheddar Muffins, 109
Cranberry Iced Tea, 154
Cranberry Sugar Scrub, 261
crayons, for furniture scratches, 355
cream
Fettuccine Alfredo, 181
Peachy Complexion Cream, 244
substitution for, 178
cream cheese, 120, 122
crème anglaise (Custard), 59
Crème Brûlée, 214
Crème Caramel, 215
Crescent Rolls, 112
croutons, homemade, 36
cucumbers
Cucumber Astringent, 245
Dill Pickles, 66
Pickled Gherkins (cornichons), 67
Pickle Relish, 68
Sweet Pickles, 66
Tzatziki, 153
cupcakes, 121
currants, freezing, 89
curry pastes, 46, 171
curry powder
Curried Chicken Salad, 199
Curried Eggs, 146
Curry Puffs, 149
Curry with Rice, 170
recipe for, 45
Custard Pie, 125
custards, 59, 214–15
customization, of homemade products, 11
Cuticle Cream, 269
cuts and scrapes, 291–93
cypress essential oil, 295

D

dandelion
Corn Plaster, 296
Dandelion Wart Remover, 291
PMS Tea, 305
Dandruff Treatment, 254
deli-style dishes
Baked Beans, 168
Barbecued Spareribs, 168
Barbecue Sauce, 167
Basic Rice Pilaf, 175
Chili Con Carne, 166
Chinese Crispy Beef Stir-Fry, 169
Chinese Fried Rice, 174
Curry with Rice, 170
Pad Thai Noodles with Shrimp, 172
Pork Korma with Potatoes and Spinach, 171
Refried Beans, 170
Savory Meat Mix, 166
Singapore Noodles, 173
Stir-Fried Vegetables, 169
Tandoori Chicken, 175
Thai Green Chicken Curry, 171
Tomato Herb Tarts, 167
dental care, 252–54, 299–301
Dental Floss, Super, 300
Deodorant, 263
Deodorizing Minty Dog Wash, 316
dermatitis remedies, 286–87
desserts and sweets
cakes and frostings, 116–22
candy, 204–11
cookies, slices and brownies, 128–33
custards, 214–15
frozen pops, 235–37
frozen yogurt, 228–29
fruit, 217–19
granitas, 230–32
ice cream, 220–27
ices, 230
meringues, 127
mousses, 216–17
pies, 123–26
puddings, 211–13
sherbets, 232–33
sorbets, 233–35
dessert sauces, 58–60
Deviled Eggs, 146
Devil's Food Cake, 117
diarrhea remedies, 277
digestive distress remedies, 276–78
dill
as antacid, 276
Caper-Dill Eggs, 146
Dill Pickles, 66
dips, 150–53
Dishwasher Detergent, 342
Dishwashing Liquid, 342
disinfectant cleaners, 334, 347
Dog Biscuits, Delectable, 313
dog care, 314, 315–18
dog food, 312–15
drain cleaners, 349, 350
dried fruit. See fruit (fresh and dried); specific fruits
drying techniques
herbs, 41
Oven-Dried Tomatoes, 73
dry mixes, 61
dry shampoo
for people, 256
for pets, 315, 322
dry skin, 243, 259
dyes, vegetable, 360

E

earache remedy, 283
Ear Mite Oil, 318
Earwig Trap, Easy, 376
Easter Egg Dyes, 360
Easy Scrub, 347
economics, of homemade products, 10
eczema remedies, 286–87
eggplant, 150
eggs
Deviled Eggs, 146
Egg Salad, 197
Egg-White Toner, 245
Nourishing Conditioner, 257
Quiche Lorraine, 178
safe use of, 13, 30
elderberries, for hair care, 255
elder flower, 242, 366
Electrolyte Drink, 277
Energy Tea for Fatigue, 309
environmental benefits, of homemade products, 11
epsom salts, 267, 302
equipment
food products, 12–14
health and beauty products, 16–17
household and gardening products, 21
Essential Oil Itch Soother, 285
essential oils. See also specific types

for body oil by skin type, 259
buying, 20
versus fixed, 16, 245
precautions for, 17–18
eucalyptus
Antifungal Solution, 296
Chest Rub, 279
Cough Drops, 281
Decongestant Salve, 282
Eucalyptus Foot Lotion, 271
Eucalyptus Tile Cleaner, 348
Flea Powder, 317
Herbal Inhalant, 283
Humidifier Booster, 283
Insect Repellent, 284
Invigorating Oil for Fatigue, 309
Muscle Soak, 302
Soothing Gel for Insect Bites, 285
Steam Cough Relief, 280
eyes, beauty products for, 242–43

F

Fabric Paste, 354
fabric softener
recipe for, 345
vinegar as, 347
in Wallpaper Stripper, 354
face care products. See also skin outbreaks
Almond Mayonnaise Scrub, 247
Anti-Wrinkle Eye Cream, 242
applying masks, 250
Artichoke Facial, 244
Banana, Sour Cream, and Honey Face Mask, 248
banana wrinkle fighter, 249
Basic Skin Toner, 244
Cucumber Astringent, 245
Deep-Cleansing Facial, 247
Egg-White Toner, 245
eye compresses, 243
Facial Cleansing Mask, 246
Galen's Cold Cream, 250
grape cleanser, 246
Green Clay Purifying Face Mask, 246
Honey Mask, 247
Lemon Skin Toner, 245
Mask for Oily Skin, 249
Oatmeal Exfoliant, 249
Peachy Complexion Cream, 244
Rich Neck Moisturizer, 243
Simple Eye Makeup Remover, 242
skin type and, 243
Strawberry Yogurt Mask, 251
Tired Eye Remedy, 242
Youthful Skin Face Mask, 248
fast foods, 136–39. See also snacks and appetizers
fatigue remedies, 309
fences, for repelling rabbits, 374
fennel, 299, 304
fertilizers, 371–73, 381
Fettuccine Alfredo, 181
fever remedies, 284
Fig Jam, Lemony, 77
film canisters, as cat toys, 321
Fines Herbes, 41
Finger Paints, 361
Fire Starters, 369
Firm Stool Fix (for dogs), 318
First-Aid Antiseptic, 291
fish and seafood
cat food, 319, 320
Fish Stock, 50
New England Clam Chowder, 189
Pad Thai Noodles with Shrimp, 172
Pasta with Seafood, 182
Quick Shrimp Laksa, 190
Salad Niçoise, 201
Shrimp Salad, 200
Taramasalata, 152
Tuna Salad, 199
fish food, 329
fixed oils, versus essential oils, 16, 245
flatulence remedy, 278
flea control products
for carpet, 367
for pets, 15, 316–17, 323
floor cleaner, 336
Flowerpot Sterilizer, 382
flowers
amaryllis and poinsettia, 384
Booster for Early Spring Flowers, 383
drying, 362
potpourri, 363
Flypaper, Homemade, 364
Focaccia, 101
food coloring, 358, 361
food preservation
bottling (canning), 68, 72
drying, 41
freezing, 13, 43, 85–89
food safety, 13, 30
foot care products, 270–71, 295–97
freezers, 13
freezing techniques, 85–89
French Bread, 99
French Dressing, 40
French Fries, Oven-Baked, 137
French Onion Soup, 193
French toast, 139–40
French Vanilla Ice Cream, 220
frozen foods
frozen pops, 235–37
fruit, 88–89
ice cream, 220–27
vegetables, 85–87
fruit (fresh and dried). See also specific fruits
bird and pet food, 325–27
bottling (canning), 68
desserts, 59, 217–19, 235, 237
Dried Fruit Compote, 218
freezing, 88–89
Fruit and Nut Cereal, 26
Sparkling Fruit Bowl (punch), 158
Fruit Fly Trap, 380
Fruit Juice Spritzer, 159
Fudge, 206
fungal diseases, in plants, 379
fungal infections, in people, 295–96
Furniture Finish Test, 357
furniture polishes, 338
furniture scratches, 355

G

Gardener's Hand Cream, 268
gardening products
disease control, 379
fire starters, 369
pest control, 374–81
rust and stain removers, 368, 369
soil care, 371–73
tips and equipment for, 19–21
water conservation, 372

weed control, 368, 369
wood protection, 370
Gargle Solution, 281
garlic
Aioli (garlic mayonnaise), 30
Corn Plaster, 296
Cough Suppressant, 280
Drops for Earache, 283
for flea control, 317
Garlic Possum Repellent, 375
Garlic Vinaigrette, 35
Homemade Insecticide, 377
Gazpacho, 194
Gel Soap, 264
geranium essential oil
Antifungal Foot Ointment, 295
in body oil, 259
Cellulite Massage Oil, 260
Healing Oil Bath, 286
Relaxing Aromatic Bath, 309
Gerbil and Rabbit Salad, 328
gift baskets, 102
ginger
Apple Ginger Jelly, 80
Cough Suppressant, 280
Ginger Beer, 156
Gingersnaps, 130
Ginger Tea for Morning Sickness, 304
Hot Compress for Cramps, 304
Melon Ginger Jam, 78
for motion sickness, 277
Orange Ginger Marinade, 48
Soothing Tea for Heartburn, 276
Toothache-Relieving Dental Paste, 301
ginseng root, 309
glass cleaners, 334
Globe Artichokes in Olive Oil, 147
glues
recipes for, 354, 358–59
removal of, 357
glycerin, 20, 351
goldenseal, 299, 300
Graham Crackers, 133
granitas, 230–32
Granola, 27
Granola Bars, 140
grapefruit, 84, 334
grapefruit essential oil, 309
grapes
as facial cleanser, 246
Grape Jelly, 81
grass stains, 346
Gravy, 52
grease stains, 346
Greek Salad, 195
green beans, freezing, 86
green clay
Acne Facial Scrub, 288
Antibacterial Drawing Paste, 290
Green Clay Purifying Face Mask, 246
Poison Ivy Lotion, 285
Skin Rash Drying Paste, 286
Green Curry Paste, 46
Green Manure Soil Conditioner, 372
Green Tomato Chutney, 75
Guacamole, 151
Guinea Pig Salad, 327
Gumbo, 192
Gumdrops, 204
Gum Tonic, 299

H

hair care products, 254–57
Hamster Fruit Cup, 328
hand and nail care products, 268–69, 357
hard water deposits, 357
headache remedies, 305–7
Head Lice Treatment, Natural, 257
Healing Ointment, 292
health and beauty products. See beauty products; home remedies; specific ailments
health benefits, of homemade products, 10–11, 19
Heartburn, Soothing Tea for, 276
Hemorrhoid Pads, 278
herbs. See also specific herbs
Bouquet Garni, 41
Chicken Seasoning Mix, 42
drying, 41
Fever Tea, 284
Fines Herbes, 41
freezing, 43
as gifts, 42
growing, 383
for hair care, 255
Herbal Bath Bag, 265
Herbal Carpet Freshener, 336
Herbal Inhalant, 283
Herbal Milk Bath for Sleeplessness, 309
Herbal Tea for Flatulence, 278
Herbal Wart Remover, 291
Herb and Bacon Muffins, 109
Herb Dressing, 38
Herb Dressing Mix, 37
Herbes de Provence, 42
Herb Vinaigrette, 34
infusions, 277
as insect-repelling mulch, 380
Italian Herb Blend, 42
Lemon Herb Marinade, 48
oils flavored with, 35
potpourri, 363
precautions for, 17–18
Steam Treatment, 282
Tomato Herb Tarts, 167
vinegar flavored with, 37
Hiccup Reliever, 277
Highlight Rinse, 255
hives remedies, 287
Hollandaise Sauce, 55
homemade product benefits, 7–8
home remedies. See also specific ailments
storage of, 260
tips and equipment for, 15–18
honey
Banana, Sour Cream, and Honey Face Mask, 248
Cough Suppressant, 280
Honey Banana Ice Cream, 223
Honey Lip Balm, 251
Honey Mask, 247
Honey Ointment, 287
Pet Bird Honey Treats, 324
Honeydew Sorbet, 234
Hops Anti-Anxiety Tea, 307
horehound leaves, 281
Hot Cross Buns, 114
hot drinks, 160–63
hot pepper. See cayenne pepper
hot water bath method, 72
housecleaning products. See cleaning products
household compounds, 354–58
household products, tips and

equipment for, 19–21
houseplant care, 382–85
Houseplant Food, 385
Hummingbird Nectar, Healthy, 327
Hummus, 150
hydrogen peroxide
cat care use, 323
oral hygiene use, 252
stain removal uses, 346

I

ice cream
alternative to, 229
Blueberry Ice Cream, 221
Butter Pecan Ice Cream, 227
Chocolate Chocolate Chip Ice Cream, 225
Coconut-Pineapple Ice Cream, 224
French Vanilla Ice Cream, 220
Honey Banana Ice Cream, 223
Ice Cream Cake, 227
lowering fat in, 222
Mint Chocolate Chip Ice Cream, 226
Peach Ice Cream, 222
Peppermint Ice Cream, 226
Rich Chocolate Ice Cream, 225
Rocky Road Ice Cream, 224
Strawberry Ice Cream, 223
ice cream makers, 220
iced tea recipes, 154
ices, 230
indigestion remedies, 276
infusions, herbal, 277
ingredient sources, 16, 20
insect bites, 284–85. See also itch relievers
insecticide recipes, 377–78, 381
insect repellents
Citronella Mosquito Candles, 365
clothing and scents as, 378
essential-oil based, 284
herbal, 381
insomnia remedies, 308–9
Interior Wall Cleaner, 336
Invigorating Oil for Fatigue, 309
Irish Soda Bread, 94
Italian Dressing, 40
Italian Herb Blend, 42
itch relievers, 285–88

J

jams, jellies, and marmalades
Apple Ginger Jelly, 80
Citrus Marmalade, 84
Dried-Apricot Jam, 76
Grape Jelly, 81
ingredients for, 76
jelling temperature, 81
Lemony Fig Jam, 77
Melon Ginger Jam, 78
Mint Jelly, 82
Peach Jam, 78
Pear Jam, 77
Seville Orange Marmalade, 83
Strawberry Jam, 79
Three-Berry Jam, 79
jelly bags, 82
jock itch remedy, 295
joint or muscle pain, 273, 301–3
juniper
Anti-Bruising Oil, 293
Invigorating Oil for Fatigue, 309
Muscle Soak, 302

K

Ketchup, 28
Ketchup Copper Polish, 340
kitchen cleaners, 342–45
kitchen equipment, 12–14
Kiwi Granita, 231
knives, 14

L

labels, on homemade products, 13, 18, 21
lady's mantle, 306
Laksa, Quick Shrimp, 190
Laksa Paste, 44
lamb, 177
Lasagna, 186
laundry products, 345–47, 368
lavender
Antibacterial Drawing Paste, 290
Antibacterial Oil, 290
Antifungal Foot Ointment, 295
Antifungal Solution, 296
Aromatic Moth-Repelling Sachets, 366
Athlete's Foot Powder, 295
in body oil, 259
Body Powder, 262
for burns, 293
for cold sores, 298
First-Aid Antiseptic, 291
Flea-Begone-Bandanna, 316
Flea Powder, 317
Fragrant Flea Treatment, 323
Headache Compresses, 305
Headache Massage Oil, 306
Headache Oil with Vitamin E, 307
Healing Oil Bath, 286
Healing Ointment, 292
Herbal Carpet Freshener, 336
for insomnia, 308, 309
for itch relief, 285, 287, 288
Soothing Footbath, 270
Summer Body Splash, 259
Laxative, 278
Lazy Person's Oven Cleaner, 343
leather cleaners, 339, 351
leftover foods, 13
Leg Massage Cream, 271
lemon balm
Calming Tea for Insomnia, 308
for cold sores, 297, 298
Lemon Balm Tea, 306
lemon essential oil
Bacteria-Fighting Citrus Mouthwash, 253
in body oil, 259
Summer Body Splash, 259
lemon extract, 260
lemongrass, 255, 259
lemons, lemon juice
Body Spray, 262
Cabinet Polish, 338
Candied Citrus Peels, 211
Citrus Disinfectant, 334
Citrus Marmalade, 84
Citrus Moisturizing Treatment, 258
Citrus Sorbet, 233
Cut-Lemon Brass and Copper Polish, 340
Facial Cleansing Mask, 246
for freezing fruit, 89
Highlight Rinse, 255
Lemonade Syrup, 156
Lemon Barley Water, 158
Lemon Frozen Yogurt, 228

Lemon Herb Marinade, 48
Lemon Lime Chutney, 75
Lemon Oil Furniture Polish, 338
Lemon Skin Toner, 245
Lemon Sorbet, 234
Lemon Squash, 157
Lemony Fig Jam, 77
as meat tenderizer, 47
Settler for Motion Sickness, 276
Soy and Sesame Marinade, 48
Tougher Toilet Bowl Cleaner, 349
Traditional Lemonade, 157
lemon verbena, 363
Lentil Soup, 191
licorice root, 276, 298
lime essential oil, 259
limes, lime juice
Citrus Cologne Splash, 260
Citrus Disinfectant, 334
Citrus Sorbet, 233
Lemon Lime Chutney, 75
Lime Sherbet, 232
Nontoxic Rust Remover, 349
Liniment, 303
linseed, 101
linseed oil, 20, 338
lip and mouth care, 251–54, 297–98
Liquid or Gel Soap, 264
Liver Paté, Chicken, 144
Liver Treats, Lucky (for dogs), 314
lobelia, 279
Lollipops, 205
Love Your Feet Cream, 270
luggage cleaner, 339

M

makeup removers, 242, 250
mangoes
freezing, 89
Mango and Passion Fruit Sauce, 58
Mango Chutney, 74
Mango Mousse, 217
manure
as free fertilizer, 373
Green Manure Soil Conditioner, 372
Houseplant Food, 385
marinades
antipasto, 143
goat cheese, 147
meat and seafood, 47–48
marmalades, 83–84
marshmallow root, 282
marshmallows
recipe for, 210
Rocky Road candy, 209
Rocky Road Ice Cream, 224
masks. See face care products
Massage Cream, 301
mayonnaise recipes, 29–30
Mayonnaise Scrub, Almond, 247
Meat Rub, Caribbean Spicy, 45
meat tenderizers, 47
melons
Honeydew Sorbet, 234
Melon Ginger Jam, 78
Melon Squares (for cats), 321
men's products, 272–73
menstrual cramp remedies, 304
meringues, 127
metal polishes, 340–41
Microwave Oven Cleaner, 343
Migraine Tea, 306
milk
Cinnamon Oatmeal Milk Bath, 266
Gentle Milk Bath, 266
Herbal Milk Bath for Sleeplessness, 309
Strawberries and Cream Bath Bags, 265
Strawberry Milk Sherbet, 233
Whitewash, 370
mineral deposit remover, 357
mineral oil, 317, 318
Minestrone, 191
mint
Anti-Bruising Oil, 293
Anti-Cramp Tea, 304
Antifungal Foot Ointment, 295
Chest Rub, 279
for congestion, 282
Decongestant Salve, 282
Deodorizing Minty Dog Wash, 316
Flea Powder, 317
Headache Massage Oil, 306
Herbal Inhalant, 283
Humidifier Booster, 283
Liniment, 303
Massage Cream, 301
Mint Chocolate Chip Ice Cream, 226
Mint Jelly, 82
Mints, 299
Mouthwash, 299
Muscle Soak, 302
Pastel Mint Patties, 207
Peppermint Ice Cream, 226
Poison Ivy Lotion, 285
Settler for Motion Sickness, 276
Spicy, Minty Mouthwash, 253
Spray for Fever, 284
Stomach-Calming Tea, 276
Toothpaste, 254, 299
Warm Herbal Body Treatment, 257
mirrors, for birds, 326
moisturizers, 243, 258
mold and mildew removers, 339
money savings, from homemade products, 10
Morning Sickness, Ginger Tea for, 304
mosquito repellents, 284, 365, 378
mothballs
Carpet Flea Remover, 367
Repellent for Four-Footed Pests, 375
Repellent for Houseplant Pests, 384
moth repellents, 364, 366
motion sickness remedies, 276–77
mousses, 216–17
mouth and lip care, 251–54, 297–98
mouthwash recipes
cold sore remedy, 298
for oral hygiene, 252–53, 299, 300
muesli, 26
muffins, 107–9, 325
mullein, 279, 283
Multigrain Bread, 100
multipurpose cleaners, 335, 347
muscle or joint pain, 273, 301–3
Muscle Relaxant for Cramps, 304
Muscle Rub, 273
mushrooms
freezing, 86
Mushroom Sauce, 57
Mushroom Wine Sauce, 54
Pasta with Mushroom Pesto, 184

mustard and mustard seed
antifungal footbath, 296
Dijon Mustard Sauce, 57
Mustard Marinade, 47
Mustard Powder Plaster, 280
Mustard recipe, 29
Mustard Seed Plaster, 279
Ringworm Paste, 290
myrrh, 295, 300

N

nail and hand care, 268–69, 357
nausea remedies, 276
Neck Moisturizer, Rich, 243
nettle, for hair care, 255
nibbles. See snacks and appetizers
Nontoxic Bathroom Cleaner, 348
Nontoxic Rust Remover, 349
Nontoxic Stain for Children's Wood Projects, 356
Nontoxic Toilet Bowl Cleaner, 349
normal skin, 243, 259
Nourishing Conditioner, 257
nuts and seeds. See also specific nuts
Banana Nut Bread, 96
Chocolate-Nut Frozen Bananas, 237
Fruit and Nut Cereal, 26
Premium Wild Bird Mix, 326
Spicy Nut Mix, 136
Wild Bird Food, 325

O

oats
Acne Facial Scrub, 288
Apricot Oat Bars, 141
Cinnamon Oatmeal Milk Bath, 266
Deep-Cleansing Facial, 247
Delectable Dog Biscuits, 313
Dry Cat Shampoo, 322
Fruit and Nut Cereal, 26
Granola, 27
Instant Dry Shampoo, 256
Muesli, 26
Oatmeal Bath for Hives, 287
Oatmeal Cookies, 128
Oatmeal Exfoliant, 249
Oatmeal Mix, 27
oil. See vegetable oil; specific types
Oil-Paint Stain, 355
oily skin, 243, 249, 259
ointments
Antifungal Foot Ointment, 295
Calendula Ointment, 292
Cold Sore Ointment, 297
Healing Ointment, 292
Honey Ointment, 287
tip for making, 295
olive oil. See also salad dressings
versus essential oils, 245
in furniture polish, 338
Globe Artichokes in Olive Oil, 147
herb-flavored, 35
Roasted Red Bell Peppers in Oil, 73
Warm Oil Hand Treatment, 269
olives, 95, 153
onions
Cough Suppressant, 280
French Onion Soup, 193
Pickled Onions, 70
Red Onion Relish, 71
oral hygiene products, 252–54, 299–301
orange essential oil, 262, 267
orange extract, in body splash, 260
oranges
Blood-Orange Champagne Granita, 230
Body Spray, 262
Candied Citrus Peels, 211
Citrus Disinfectant, 334
Citrus Marmalade, 84
Citrus Sorbet, 233
Orange Blossom, 157
Orange Cake, 119
Orange Ginger Marinade, 48
Orange Ice, 230
Seville Orange Marmalade, 83
ovens
cleaners for, 343–44
temperature calibration, 13

P

Pad Thai Noodles with Shrimp, 172
Paint and Tile Mold and Mildew Remover, 339
paints and stains
Finger Paints, 361
Nontoxic Stain for Children's Wood Projects, 356
Oil-Paint Stain, 355
Varnish-Based Stain, 356
Whitewash, 370
Pancake and Waffle Mix, 142
Pancakes, 61
Panna Cotta, 212
pantry staples. See specific foods or food categories
Paper Glue, 359
paraffin
Citronella Mosquito Candles, 365
Fire Starters, 369
Water Repellent for Exposed Wood, 370
parsley
Cheese and Parsley Bread, 93
for hair care, 255
Mints, 299
Salsa Verde, 32
passion fruit, 58, 229
pasta dishes
Fettuccine Alfredo, 181
Lasagna, 186
Pasta Puttanesca, 180
Pasta Salad, 197
Pasta with Classic Basil Pesto, 183
Pasta with Fresh Tomato Sauce, 180
Pasta with Mushroom Pesto, 184
Pasta with Seafood, 182
Pasta with Sun-Dried Tomato Pesto, 184
Penne All'amatriciana, 182
Penne with Four-Cheese Sauce, 181
Ravioli, 185
Spaghetti Bolognese, 179
Spaghetti with Speedy Tomato Sauce, 179
pasta recipes and tips, 62–63
pastry recipes, 123–25. See also pies and pastry
patchouli essential oil, 259
patch-tests, 18
pavlova, 127

peaches
Brandied Peaches, 217
freezing, 89
Peach Granita, 232
Peach Ice Cream, 222
Peach Jam, 78
Peachy Complexion Cream, 244
peanut butter
for dog care, 317
Finch and Canary Treat, 325
history of, 33
Peanut Butter Cookies, 129
Peanut Butter Cups, 209
recipe for, 33
Satay Sauce, 55
Wild Bird Food, 325
peanuts
Parrot Pops, 326
Peanut Brittle, 208
Rocky Road candy, 209
pears, 77, 218
peas, 87, 194
pecans
Butter Pecan Ice Cream, 227
Pecan Bread, 97
Pralines, 207
Rocky Road Ice Cream, 224
pectin, for jam, 76
Penne All'amatriciana, 182
Penne with Four-Cheese Sauce, 181
perspiration stains, 346
pest control products
garden, 374–81
household, 364–67
houseplant, 384
for people, 284
for pets, 316–17
pesto, 183–84
pet care
ant control for pet food bowls, 367
benefits of homemade, 15
birds, 324–27
cats, 319–23
dogs, 312–18
reptiles and fish, 329
rodents and rabbits, 327–29
pickles and relishes
Chili Jam, 67
Dill Pickles, 66
Pickled Cauliflower Florets, 69
Pickled Gherkins (cornichons), 67
Pickled Onions, 70
Pickled Spiced Plums, 71
Pickle Relish, 68
Red Onion Relish, 71
Sweet Pickles, 66
Tomato Relish, 69
pies and pastry
pastry recipes, 123–25
savory pies, 167, 176–78
sweet pies, 125–27
pineapple, 224
pine essential oil
Antifungal Foot Ointment, 295
Healing Oil Bath, 286
Muscle Soak, 302
Pine Floor Cleaner, 336
Pita Bread, 105
Pizza, 138
plantain leaves, for burns, 294
Play Bubbles, 360
Play Clay, Homemade, 361
Play Dough, Simple, 361
plums
freezing, 89
Pickled Spiced Plums, 71
Plum Sauce, 53
PMS Tea, 305
poinsettia care, 384
Poison Ivy Lotion, 285
pooper scoopers, 318
pork
Barbecued Spareribs, 168
Chili Con Carne, 166
Country Pork Sausages, 145
Ham, Pork, and Veal Terrine, 144
Pork Korma with Potatoes and Spinach, 171
Savory Meat Mix, 166
possum repellents, 374–75
potatoes
Oven-Baked French Fries, 137
Pork Korma with Potatoes and Spinach, 171
Potato Chips, 136
Potato Dinner Rolls, 110
Potato Salad, 196
for rust removal, 341
potpourri recipes, 363
pots and pans, 12, 14
Pottery Glue, 358
Potting Mix, General Purpose, 383
potting tables, 20–21
Pralines, 207
precautions
food products, 13
health and beauty product, 17–18
household and gardening product, 21
Pretzels, 137
psyllium husks, 278
puddings, 211–13
Puff Pastry, 124
pumpkin
Firm Stool Fix (for dogs), 318
freezing, 87
Sesame Pumpkin Bread, 95
punch, 158, 163

Q

Quesadillas, 149
Quiche Lorraine, 178
quick breads
Banana Nut Bread, 96
Beer Bread, 92
Carrot Bread, 97
Cheese and Parsley Bread, 93
Corn Bread, 93
Irish Soda Bread, 94
Olive and Sun-Dried Tomato Bread, 95
Pancakes, 142
Pecan Bread, 97
Savory Zucchini Bread, 92
Scones, 141
Sesame Pumpkin Bread, 95
Sweet Zucchini Bread, 98
Waffles, 142

R

rabbit food (pets), 328
rabbit repellents, 374
rags, recycled, 21
raisins, in breads, 104, 107
Ranch Dressing, 39
Ranch Dressing Mix, 38
raspberries
freezing, 89
Raspberry Sauce, 59, 127
Raspberry Sorbet, 234
Raspberry Vinaigrette, 36

Sparkling Fruit Bowl (punch), 158
Three-Berry Jam, 79
raspberry leaves, 277, 304
Ravioli, 185
ready meals. See take-out and ready-made foods
recycling, 21
Red Clay Stain Remover, 368
Red Curry Paste, 46
Red Wine Marinade, 47
relishes. See pickles and relishes
Repellent for Four-Footed Pests, 375
Repellent for Houseplant Pests, 384
reptile food (pets), 329
rewards, of homemade products, 10–11
rhubarb, 212, 380
rice
Basic Rice Pilaf, 175
Chinese Fried Rice, 174
Curry with Rice, 170
Low-Fat Chicken and Rice Dog Dinner, 312
Rice Pudding, 213
rice noodles, 172–73
Ringworm Paste, 290
Roasted Red Bell Peppers in Oil, 73
Rocky Road candy, 209
Rocky Road Ice Cream, 224
rodents, pet, 327–29
rolls, 110–15
Room Freshener Spray, 337
rose
Almond Rose Soap, 264
Essential Oil Itch Soother, 285
Lightly Scented Aftershave, 272
Relaxing Aromatic Bath, 309
Tired Eye Remedy, 242
rose geranium, 316, 317
rosemary
Anti-Bruising Oil, 293
for congestion, 282
Dandruff Treatment, 254
Energy Tea for Fatigue, 309
Flea Powder, 317
for hair care, 255
Insect Repellent, 381
Rosemary Shaving Soap, 272
rubbing alcohol
buying, 20
cleaning uses, 334, 335, 351
home remedy use, 303
mold and mildew removal, 339
pest control uses, 377, 380
rust removers
Nontoxic Rust Remover, 349
potatoes for, 341
Rust Remover, 369

S

sage, 255, 280
salad dressings
Balsamic Vinaigrette, 35
Blue Cheese Dressing, 39
Classic Vinaigrette, 34
French Dressing, 40
Garlic Vinaigrette, 35
Herb Dressing, 38
Herb Dressing Mix, 37
Herb Vinaigrette, 34
Italian Dressing, 40
Light Blue Cheese Dressing, 39
Ranch Dressing, 39
Ranch Dressing Mix, 38
Raspberry Vinaigrette, 36
Thai Salad Dressing, 38
Thousand Island Dressing, 40
Walnut Vinaigrette, 34
salads
Caesar Salad, 198
Classic Coleslaw, 195
Cobb Salad, 200
Creamy Chicken Salad, 198
Curried Chicken Salad, 199
Egg Salad, 197
Greek Salad, 195
Pasta Salad, 197
Potato Salad, 196
Salade Niçoise, 201
Shrimp Salad, 200
Thai Beef Salad, 196
Tuna Salad, 199
Turkey Salad, 199
Tuscan-Style Three-Bean Salad, 201
Salicylic Acid Corn Remover, 297
Saline Spray for Sinuses, 283
salmonella, 13, 30
salsas, 31, 32
salt
Almond Exfoliating Body Scrub, 261
Bath Cookies, 267
Electrolyte Drink, 277
Homemade Scrub Powder, 345
Red Clay Stain Remover, 368
Saline Spray for Sinuses, 283
Scouring Powder, 344
Soothing Footbath, 270
Strawberry Foot Scrub, 271
salves, 282, 287
sandalwood essential oil, 259
Sangria, 160
Sardine Balls (for cats), 320
Satay Sauce, 55
sauces
savory, 52–57, 167, 185, 186
sweet, 58–60, 127
Sausages, Country Pork, 145
scones, 141
scouring powders, 344–45, 347
seafood. See fish and seafood
Seafood Cocktail Sauce, 28
seasonings, 41–46
Seaweed Soil Conditioner, 372
seed-starting mixes, 382
sensitive skin, 243, 259
Septic Tank Activator, 350
Sesame Marinade, Soy and, 48
Sesame Pumpkin Bread, 95
Seville Orange Marmalade, 83
shampoo. See hair care products
shaving products
men's, 272–73
women's, 259
Shepherd's Pie, 177
sherbets, 232–33
shortbread, 131
shower caps, as dog bowl, 314
Showerhead Cleaner, 348
shrimp. See fish and seafood
Silver Shine, Quick and Easy, 341
Singapore Noodles, 173
sinus congestion remedy, 283
skin outbreaks, 288–91
Skin Rash Drying Paste, 286
skin toners, 244–45
skin types
body oils based on, 259
described, 243
sleeplessness remedies, 308–9

slippery elm, 281, 290
Slug and Snail Trap, 376
small appliances, 14
snacks and appetizers
Antipasto Platter, 143
Baba Ghanoush, 150
Beet Dip, 151
Chicken Liver Paté, 144
Chicken Nuggets, 139
Country Pork Sausages, 145
Curry Puffs, 149
Deviled Eggs, 146
Globe Artichokes in Olive Oil, 147
Guacamole, 151
Ham, Pork, and Veal Terrine, 144
Hummus, 150
Marinated Goat Cheese, 147
Oven-Baked French Fries, 137
Pizza, 138
Potato Chips, 136
Pretzels, 137
Quesadillas, 149
Spicy Nut mix, 136
Spinach-Feta Phyllo Triangles, 148
Tapenade, 153
Tzatziki, 153
soap
Almond Rose Soap, 264
Bug Blaster Soap Spray, 379
Cinnamon Soap, 265
Cleansing Soap, 292
Dishwashing Liquid, 342
Laundry Soap, 346
Liquid or Gel Soap, 264
Rosemary Shaving Soap, 272
Soap Repellent (for garden), 375
soap flakes, buying, 20
soil amendments, 371–73
soil mixes, for house plants, 382–83
soil testing, 20, 371
sorbets, 233–35
sore throat remedies, 281, 282
soup. See also cooking stocks
Beef Barley Soup, 187
Black Bean Soup, 188
Chicken Noodle Soup, 189
Cream of Tomato Soup, 190
French Onion Soup, 193
Gazpacho, 194
Gumbo, 192
Lentil Soup, 191
Minestrone, 191
New England Clam Chowder, 189
Quick Shrimp Laksa, 190
Split Pea Soup, 194
Vegetable Soup, 193
sour cream face mask, 248
Sourdough Bread, 106
southernwood, 366
Soy and Linseed Bread, 101
Soy and Sesame Marinade, 48
Spaghetti Bolognese, 179
Spaghetti with Speedy Tomato Sauce, 179
Spice Cake, 116
spikenard essential oil, 290
spinach, 148, 171
Split Pea Soup, 194
sprain and strain remedy, 303
spray bottles, recycled, 21
stainless steel polish, 341
stain removers, 346, 368
stains. See paints and stains
static electricity, 357
Steam Cough Relief, 280
Steam Treatment, 282
Steel Wool Soap Pads, 345
Sticky Buns, 115
stir-fried dishes, 169
stocks. See cooking stocks
Stomach-Calming Tea, 276
storage techniques
fresh pasta, 63
health and beauty products, 17, 260
household and gardening products, 21
leftover foods, 13
strawberries
Cheesecake with Strawberry Glaze, 120
Chocolate-Dipped, 219
freezing, 89
Rhubarb and Strawberry Compote, 212
Sparkling Fruit Bowl (punch), 158
Strawberry Foot Scrub, 271
Strawberry Frozen Yogurt, 228
Strawberry Ice Cream, 223
Strawberry Jam, 79
Strawberry Milk Sherbet, 233
Strawberry Pops, 236
Strawberry Sorbet, 235
Strawberry Yogurt Mask, 251
Three-Berry Jam, 79
Wine Poached Pears with Strawberries, 218
strawberry essential oil, 265
substitutions, in cooking
baking powder, 96
brown sugar, 167
buttermilk, 94
chocolate, 132
corn syrup, 210
cream, 178
tomato sauce, 180
sugar. See also candy
brown sugar substitute, 167
Cranberry Sugar Scrub, 261
Gargle Solution, 281
Healthy Hummingbird Nectar, 327
Hiccup Reliever, 277
for jam, 76
Septic Tank Activator, 350
Simple Sugar Scrub for Dry Skin, 261
Sugar Cookies, 131
for sweetening cold drinks, 155
Summer Body Splash, 259
Sunburn Cooler, 294
Sweet and Sour Sauce, 53
Sweet Pickles, 66
sweet potatoes, freezing, 87
sweet treats. See desserts and sweets
sweet woodruff, 308, 366

T

take-out and ready-made foods
deli-style dishes, 166–75
main-dish pies, 176–78
pasta dishes, 179–86
salads, 195–201
soups, 187–94
Tandoori Chicken, 175
tansy, 366
Tapenade, 153
Taramasalata, 152

Tartar Sauce, 31
tea, for sunburn, 294. See also cold drinks; hot drinks
tea tree oil
Antibacterial Drawing Paste, 290
Antibacterial Oil, 290
Antifungal Foot Ointment, 295
Antiseptic Lotion for Burns, 294
Cleansing Liquid for Acne, 289
for congestion, 282
First-Aid Antiseptic, 291
Healing Ointment, 292
for itch relief, 285, 288
Mouthwash for Cold Sores, 298
Natural Head Lice Treatment, 257
Oil Rub for Burned Skin, 293
Overnight Acne Cream, 289
Salve for Eczema or Dermatitis, 287
Toothpaste, 299
Teriyaki Marinade, 48
Thai Beef Salad, 196
Thai Green Chicken Curry, 171
Thai Salad Dressing, 38
Thick Hair Conditioner for Everyone, 256
Thousand Island Dressing, 40
Three-Berry Jam, 79
thyme
Antibacterial Oil, 290
Antifungal Solution, 296
Dandruff Treatment, 254
for hair care, 255
Insect Repellent, 381
tick removal, from pets, 323, 324
tile cleaners, 339, 348
Toffee Bars, 208
toilets
cleaners for, 349
Leaking Toilet Test, 358
tomatoes
Bloody Marys, 159
Cream of Tomato Soup, 190
Gazpacho, 194
Green Tomato Chutney, 75
Ketchup, 28
Olive and Sun-Dried Tomato Bread, 95
Oven-Dried Tomatoes, 73
Pasta Puttanesca, 180
Pasta with Fresh Tomato Sauce, 180
Pasta with Sun-Dried Tomato Pesto, 184
sauce substitution, 180
Spaghetti with Speedy Tomato Sauce, 179
Spicy Tomato Chutney, 74
Spicy Tomato Salsa, 31
stains from, 346
Tomato Herb Tarts, 167
Tomato Relish, 69
Tomato Sauce, 55, 185, 186
toothache remedies, 300–301
toothpaste
Deodorizing Minty Dog Wash, 316
recipes for, 254, 299
toxins
in commercial products, 19
essential oils as, 18
Tropical Pops, 237
Tuna Treats (for cats), 319
Turkey Salad, 199
Turtle and Reptile Treats, 329
tzatziki, 153

U

Upholstery Shampoo (for cars), 351

V

valerian root, 304
vanilla
Custard Sauce (créme anglaise), 59
French Vanilla Ice Cream, 220
homemade extract, 61
Vanilla Icing, 121
Varnish-Based Stain, 356
Veal Terrine, Ham, Pork, and, 144
vegetable oil
for dog care, 317
versus essential oil, 16, 245
Oil Spray Insecticide Concentrate, 381
vegetables
Antipasto Platter, 143
blanching, 85
bottling (canning), 68
freezing, 85–87
Stir-Fried Vegetables, 169
Vegetable Easter Egg Dyes, 360
Vegetable Soup, 193
Vegetable Stock, 51
vermouth, for flea control, 316
vinaigrettes, 34–36
vinegar. See also pickles and relishes; salad dressings
buying, 20
cleaning uses, 334, 335, 342, 343, 344, 348, 349
culinary uses, 47, 89
flavored, 37
health and beauty uses, 255, 288, 293
laundry uses, 345, 346, 347, 368
mold and mildew removal, 339
pest control uses, 317
rust removal, 369
unexpected uses, 357
Vinyl and Leather Interior Cleaner (for cars), 351
Vitamin E
Ear Mite Oil, 318
Headache Oil with Vitamin E, 307
tip for using, 248
vodka, 159, 316. See also wine and spirits

W

Waffle Mix, 61
Waffles, 142
wallpaper, cleaning, 335
Wallpaper Stripper, 354
walls
cleaners for, 335, 336
covering with fabric, 354
walnut leaves, for flea control, 317
Walnut Vinaigrette, 34
wart remedies, 291
washing soda
Automatic Dishwasher Detergent, 342
buying, 20
Quick and Easy Silver Shine, 341
water conservation, in garden, 372
weed control, 368, 369
White Goods Cleaner, 344
White Sauce, Basic, 56
Whitewash, 370
window cleaners, 334

Windshield Cleaner, 351
wine and spirits
Blood-Orange Champagne Granita, 230
Bloody Mary, 159
Brandied Peaches, 217
Cassis Sorbet, 233
Mushroom Wine Sauce, 54
Red Wine Marinade, 47
Sangria, 160
Wine Poached Pears with Strawberries, 218
wine stains, 346
witch hazel
Anti-Itch Wrap, 288
Compress for Bruises, 293
eye compresses, 243
Hemorrhoid Pads, 278
Lemon Skin Toner, 245
Refreshing Foot Spray, 271
women's problems, 304–7
wood ashes, 373, 376
wood protection products, 370. See also paints and stains
wrinkle treatments, 242, 249

Y

yarrow, 255
yeast and brewer's yeast
Facial Cleansing Mask, 246
for flea control, 317
Mask for Oily Skin, 249
Septic Tank Activator, 350
Slug and Snail Trap, 376
yeast breads
Brioche, 103
Challah, 102
Cinnamon-Raisin Swirl Bread, 104
ease of making, 99
Focaccia, 101
French Bread, 99
Multigrain Bread, 100
Pita Bread, 105
Sourdough Bread, 106
Soy and Linseed Bread, 101
Yeast Infection Cream, 305
yogurt
as meat tenderizer, 47
Strawberry Yogurt Mask, 251
Yeast Infection Cream, 305
yogurt, frozen, 228–29, 236
Youthful Skin Face Mask, 248

Z

zucchini breads, 92, 98

PHOTO CREDITS

iStock back cover tc, tr, br; 2cbr; 7c; 8tc, ctl, ctr, cbl, cbr, bc; 23; 49; 57; 96; 98; 105; 106; 110; 111; 114; 132; 205; 225; 229; 231; 235; 240c, l; 330.

Photolibrary 2tc, bl; 32c.

Shutterstock back cover tl, bl; 2tl, tr, ctl, ctc, ctr, cbl, cbc, bc, br; 3; 5; 7l, r; 8tr, ctc, cbc, bl, br; 9; 11; 12; 14; 15; 16tl; 16–17; 18; 19; 21; 22; 26; 29; 36; 44; 53; 55; 58; 62; 69; 73; 75; 79; 80; 84; 92; 103; 112; 116; 120; 123; 126; 136; 138; 143; 145; 146; 148; 151; 153; 154; 159; 163; 168; 170; 172; 174; 178–9; 183; 185; 186; 188; 191; 197; 199; 200; 208; 212; 214; 216; 219; 221; 238; 239; 240r; 241; 244; 248; 251; 255; 258; 262; 266; 270; 273; 274l, c, r; 275; 278; 283; 286; 291; 295; 296; 300; 302; 307; 308; 310l, c, r; 311; 315; 318; 322; 327; 329; 331; 332r; 333; 334–5; 339; 341; 342; 351; 352l, c, r; 353; 355; 359; 360; 363; 366; 371; 374; 375; 378; 380; 383; 384; 385.

DA2 Strategic Design front cover t

Rido/Shutterstock front cover bl

April Turner front cover bcl

Matka Wariatka front cover bcr

All other images are owned by Reader's Digest.